A Companion Guide to LAST'S ANATOMY

A Companion Guide to LAST'S ANATOMY

S. ALI MIRJALILI MD, PhD, PGDipSurgAnat, PGCertCPU

Senior lecturer, Anatomy and Medical Imaging Department, University of Auckland
Convenor of Science for Surgens Course, Department of Surgery, University of Auckland

QUENTIN FOGG BSc (HONS), PhD, FRCPS(GLasg)

Associate Professor in Clinical Anatomy, Department of Anatomy and Neuroscience, The University of Melbourne, Melbourne, Australia

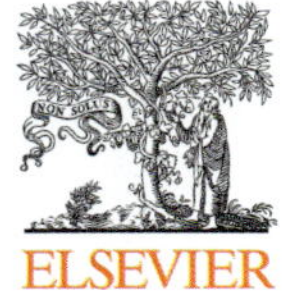

ELSEVIER

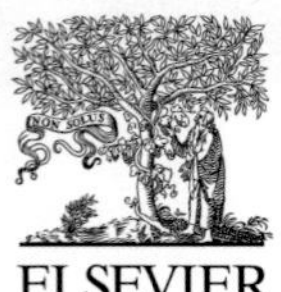

Elsevier Australia. ACN 001 002 357
(a division of Reed International Books Australia Pty Ltd)
Tower 1, 475 Victoria Avenue, Chatswood, NSW 2067

ISBN: 978-0-7295-4408-5

Notice

Practitioners and researchers must always rely on their own experience and knowledge in evaluating and using any information, methods, compounds or experiments described herein. Because of rapid advances in the medical sciences, in particular, independent verification of diagnoses and drug dosages should be made. To the fullest extent of the law, no responsibility is assumed by Elsevier, authors, editors or contributors for any injury and/or damage to persons or property as a matter of products liability, negligence or otherwise, or from any use or operation of any methods, products, instructions, or ideas contained in the material herein.

National Library of Australia Cataloguing-in-Publication Data

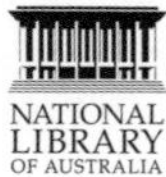

A catalogue record for this book is available from the National Library of Australia

Content Strategist: Larissa Norrie
Content Project Manager: Shivani Pal
Edited by Chris Wyard
Internal design: Standard
Index by SPi Global
Typeset by GW Tech
Printed in China

Last digit is the print number: 9 8 7 6 5 4 3 2 1

FOREWORD

A sound knowledge of the essentials of surgical anatomy and other clinically relevant anatomy, alongside a command of the essentials of clinical physiology and surgical pathology, are fundamental and indispensable requisites to good surgical training and assessment.

It is undeniable that, during the past two decades or more, the undergraduate medical curriculum worldwide has seen a steady decline in the emphasis placed on the study of anatomy. This is reflected both in the number of hours allocated to the study of anatomy and in the level of detail and intensity with which assessment of anatomical knowledge of students is undertaken in medical schools.

Regrettably, and perhaps consequentially, this development in the undergraduate medical environment has seen a concomitant and considerable diminution in the depth and breadth of anatomical knowledge that is currently imparted to surgical trainees and in the level to which their knowledge is assessed in postgraduate surgical examinations.

It is thus to the great credit of the Royal Australasian College of Surgeons (RACS) that the surgical curriculum and assessment designed and currently implemented by the RACS continues to place a considerable emphasis on the study of surgically relevant anatomy.

Against this background it is commendable that Dr S. Ali Mirjalili and Associate Professor Quentin Fogg have collaborated under the aegis of the RACS to present this *Companion Guide to Last's Anatomy: Regional and Applied*.

The two authors have blended their vast experience as teachers, trainers and published authors in the field of postgraduate surgical anatomy to bring out this most useful and richly illustrated study guide.

As the authors state clearly in their preface, their *Companion Guide* is not intended to supplant *Last's Anatomy*. Rather, it is meant to act as a complement to the parent textbook, by crystallising and reinforcing its anatomical principles and descriptions. Accordingly, the authors have been faithful to the regional approach to anatomy employed by Last, besides adhering scrupulously to the sequence of topics defined in *Last's Anatomy*.

The *Companion Guide* is set out in a clear, consistent and logical format. The prose is admirably concise, simple and easy to follow. The descriptions of topographical anatomy, organs, organ systems and blood supply are uniformly systematic, lucid and comprehensive. Numerous clinically significant facts and features not hitherto mentioned in *Last's Anatomy* have been introduced in the *Guide*, enhancing its appeal. 'The vein of Giacomini' in the section on the superficial veins of the lower limb is an example of one such novel entry! Another conspicuous feature of the *Guide* is that the text is supported throughout by a profusion of highly relevant, high-quality, colour illustrations comprising artwork as well as high-definition photographs of cadaver dissections. These illustrations, which are well integrated with the text, do much to facilitate comprehension and assimilation of the text.

I believe the *Guide* will serve as a concise and clinically oriented text of reference and will be ideal as a rapid review text for those preparing for a variety of examinations.

The *Companion Guide* should prove immensely useful to anyone preparing to take the Generic Surgical Science Examination (GSSE) whether as pre-vocational trainees or as surgical trainees in a dedicated surgical training programme. It should also be helpful as a quick and ready revision guide to anyone appearing for a specialty-specific surgical examination.

Finally, it is my very great pleasure to congratulate and compliment Drs Mirjalili and Fogg on putting their time and effort towards such a splendid and worthwhile enterprise and to the publisher Elsevier for their great part in delivering such a fine product.

Vishy Mahadevan MBBS PhD FDSRCSEng FRCS (Eng & Ed)
Emeritus Professor of Anatomy
Royal College of Surgeons of England;
Member of the Court of Examiners
Royal College of Surgeons of England;
Formerly: Barbers' Company Professor of Anatomy
and Professor of Surgical Anatomy
Royal College of Surgeons of England

PREFACE

Last's Anatomy: Regional and Applied has been a landmark surgical anatomy reference textbook since the 1950s and to this day remains one of the standard works for surgeons and surgeons in training. The book was first edited by Professor R. J. Last in 1954. The 9th edition, edited in the 1990s by Professor R. M. H. McMinn, is considered the standout surgical anatomy reference. Professor Last, an Australian, was a prominent and active surgeon and Professor McMinn, a Scotsman, was the consummate clinical anatomist; both had strong connections with the Royal College of Surgeons of England and were passionate and renowned educators.

Last's Anatomy: Regional and Applied (9th edition) remains the seminal surgical anatomy text in Australasia and was revised by one of the authors, Dr Ali Mirjalili, in 2019. Changes were minor but crucial in light of new anatomical research and modern minimally invasive surgery.

Dr Mirjalili has been teaching surgical anatomy for over a decade in Australasia and Professor Fogg has shared his 20 years of experience across Australia, North America and the UK. Learning surgical anatomy and achieving success in the Generic Surgical Sciences Examination (GSSE) (and equivalent exams globally) while juggling work on busy surgical units, is an unforgettable experience for any surgeon. We decided to write a companion guide to *Last's Anatomy* to help our postgraduate students and surgical trainees on this journey. This guide is by no means intended to replace this invaluable textbook, but to provide a concise companion for the time-poor reader. It is specifically designed to highlight key surgical anatomy and is supplemented by simple anatomical diagrams and photos of body donor dissections purposefully made for this edition. Illustrations are used to highlight particular anatomical relationships that are surgically important, or difficult to grasp. We hope that this companion will be the first stop when faced with an anatomical problem, and that it will encourage the reader to then dive deeper into the full versions of *Last's Anatomy*.

Beyond the GSSE, this resource will be invaluable for those undertaking study for specialty-specific anatomy examinations, or the anatomy component of Fellowship examinations, as well as being a familiar aid when needing some anatomical reassurance.

We would like to acknowledge Mr Sebastien Barfoot for his time proofreading and for his valuable comments. We would also like to thank Mr Robbie McPhee for digitally drawing all of the high-quality illustrations in the book. The cover images have been drawn (oil on paper) by Mr Parsoua Mahtash, a great realist painter, whom we also thank warmly.

S. Ali Mirjalili
Auckland, New Zealand

Quentin Fogg
Melbourne, Australia

CONTENTS

UPPER LIMB

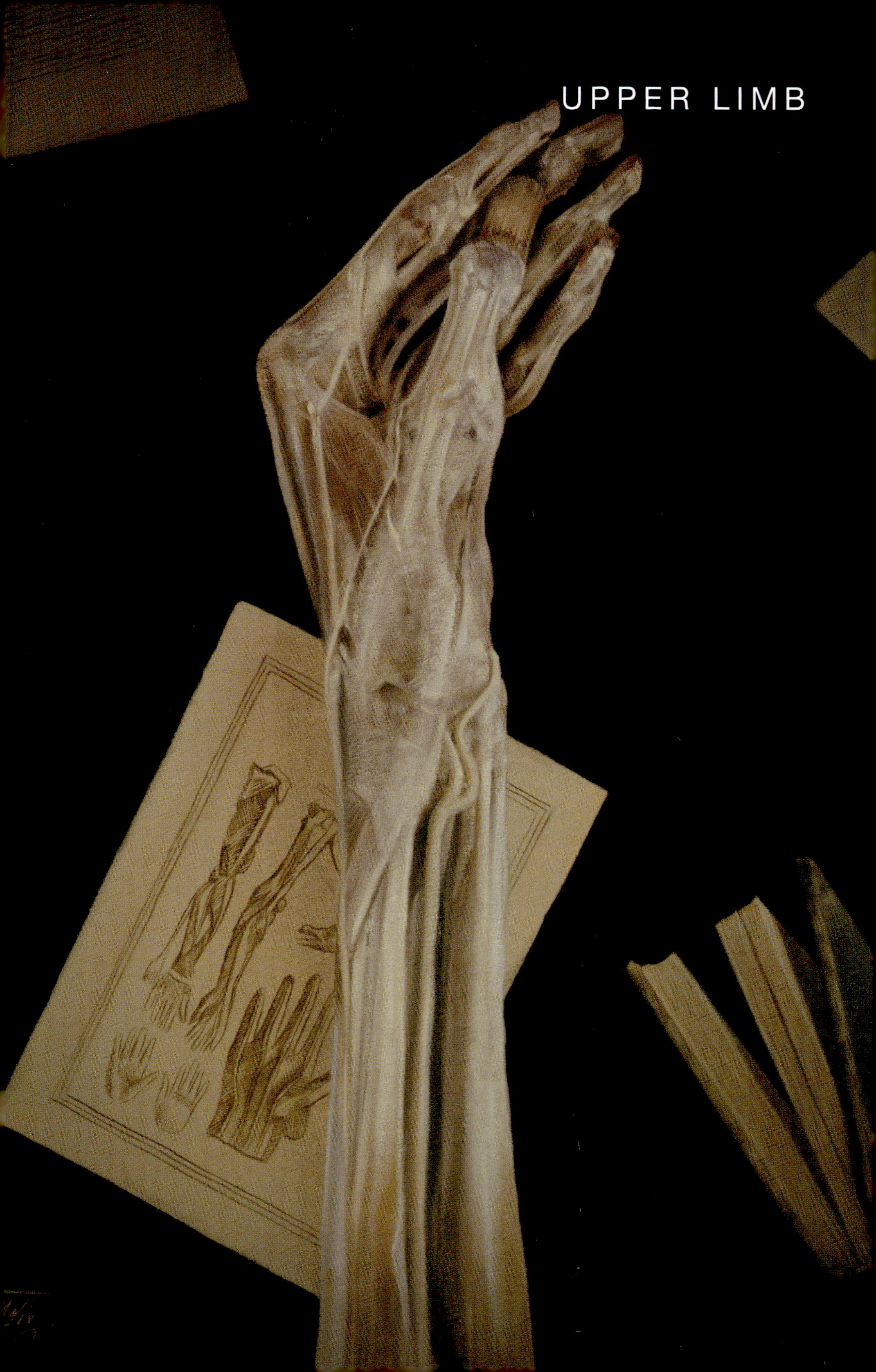

CHAPTER 1

Upper Limb

CHAPTER OUTLINE

Part 1 Pectoral Girdle

- Bones: the clavicle and scapula
- Joints: the sternoclavicular and acromioclavicular joints
- Remainder of attachment is purely muscular

BONES

Clavicle

The clavicle has an S-shaped contour which is convex at the medial aspect and concave at the lateral aspect. Its acromial end (lateral) is flat whereas the sternal (medial) end is more robust (quadrangular shape). It is the most commonly fractured bone in the body. The clavicle is most commonly fractured at the junction between the middle and lateral thirds. This is because (1) the strong coracoclavicular ligaments hold the lateral third in place and (2) the lateral third is flatter while the medial two-thirds are circular in cross-section, and therefore more resistant to fracture.

Scapula

The scapula (shoulder blade) is triangular. It has two surfaces (costal and dorsal), three borders (upper, medial and lateral) and three angles (superior, inferior and lateral). The spine is thick as it projects back from a horizontal attachment on the dorsal surface. Its posterior part slopes laterally towards the acromion. The acromion itself is rectangular, and articulates with the clavicle at the anterior end of its medial border. The glenoid cavity sits on the lateral border with two supraglenoid and infraglenoid tubercles lying above and below, respectively. The coracoid process originates from the glenoid process and curves forwards (Fig 1.1).

JOINTS

- The **sternoclavicular joint** (Fig 1.2A and B) is an atypical synovial joint with features of a ball and socket and separated into two cavities by a cartilaginous disc. The disc is attached

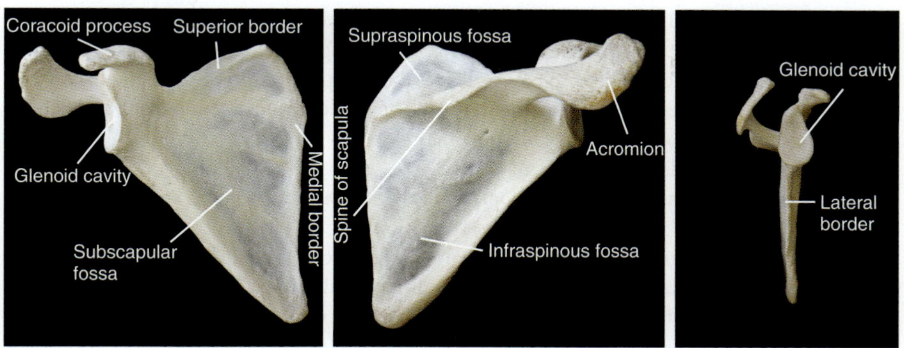

Fig. 1.1 Right scapula. Left: anterior view. Middle: posterior view. Right: lateral view.

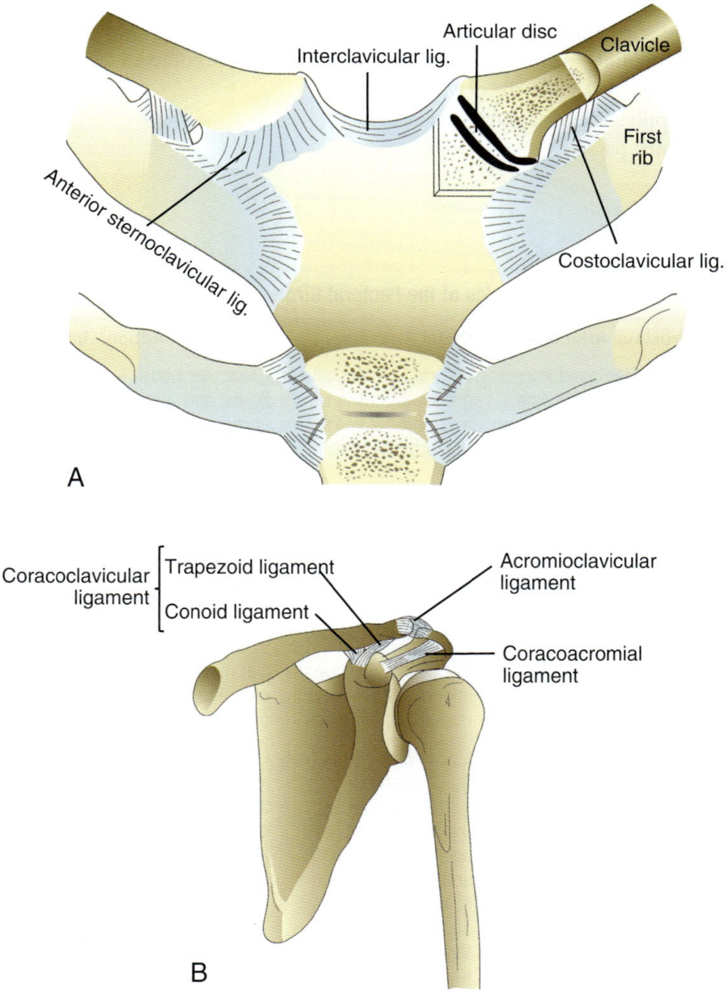

Fig. 1.2 **(A)** Anterior sternum and associated joints and ligaments (sternoclavicular joint). **(B)** Ligaments of the pectoral girdle, anterior view.

to the capsule as well as the medial end of the clavicle above and behind, and to the first costal cartilage below. Its articular surface is set at an angle of 45° to the transverse plane. The sternal end of the clavicle projects well above the upper margin of the manubrial facet. This is where the interclavicular ligament lies. The capsule is thickened in front and behind (anterior and posterior sternoclavicular ligaments).
  - Nerve supply: medial supraclavicular nerve
  - Movements: fulcrum is at the costoclavicular ligament and not the sternal end of the clavicle. About 40° rotation also occurs at this joint
  - Stability is maintained by ligaments – mainly by the costoclavicular ligament
- The **acromioclavicular joint** (see Fig 1.2B) is an atypical synovial joint between the overhanging lateral end of the clavicle and the underhanging medial border of the acromion. It is surrounded by a sleeve-like capsule.
- The **coracoclavicular ligament** (see Fig 1.2B) is extremely strong and provides the majority of the stability and much of the weight bearing support for the upper limb. The ligament has two parts:
  - **Trapezoid (lateral) –** from the trapezoid ridge of the coracoid to the trapezoid ridge on the under surface of the clavicle
  - **Conoid (medial) –** inverted cone from the knuckle of the coracoid to the conoid tubercle on the under surface of the clavicle
  - Nerve supply: lateral supraclavicular nerve
  - Movements: passive

MUSCLES

TABLE 1.1 ■ **Summary of the Muscles of the Pectoral Girdle**

	Proximal Attachment	Distal Attachment	Concentric Action	Innervation
Pectoralis major	Clavicular head from medial $^1/_2$ of clavicle, sternocostal head from lateral manubrium and sternum, six upper costal cartilages and external oblique aponeurosis	Lateral lip of bicipital groove of humerus and anterior lip of deltoid tuberosity	Clavicular head flexes and abducts arm, sternal head adducts and medially rotates arm	Medial pectoral nerve and lateral pectoral nerve (C5–8, T1)
Pectoralis minor	Anterior aspect of 3rd, 4th and 5th ribs	Medial and upper surface of coracoid process of scapula	Elevates ribs if scapula fixed	Medial pectoral nerve (C8–T1)
Subclavius	Costochondral junction of 1st rib	Subclavian groove on inferior surface of middle $^1/_3$ of clavicle	Depresses and steadies clavicle	Nerve to subclavius (C5, 6)
Trapezius	Medial third of superior nuchal line, ligamentum nuchae, spinous processes and supraspinous ligament to T12	Upper fibres to lateral $^1/_3$ of posterior border of clavicle, medial acromion and lateral spine of scapula, lower fibres to medial end of scapular spine as far as deltoid tubercle	Elevates and retracts scapula and rotates it during abduction of the arm	Spinal root of accessory nerve (CN XI)

TABLE 1.1 ■ **Summary of the Muscles of the Pectoral Girdle** (Continued)

	Proximal Attachment	Distal Attachment	Concentric Action	Innervation
Latissimus dorsi	All thoracic spines and supraspinous ligament from T7 down, lumbosacral spines via lumbar fascia, posterior third of iliac crest and lower four ribs	Floor of bicipital groove of humerus after spiralling around teres major	Extends, adducts and medially rotates arm and its costal attachment Helps with deep inspiration/ expiration	Thoracodorsal nerve (C6–8)
Rhomboid major	Spines of T2–5 and supraspinous ligament	Lower $^1/_2$ of posteromedial border of scapula	Retracts scapula and rotates to rest position	Dorsal scapular nerve (C5)
Rhomboid minor	Lower ligamentum nuchae, spines of C7/ T1	Small area of posteromedial border of scapula at level of the spine	Retracts scapula and rotates to rest position	Dorsal scapular nerve (C5)
Levator scapulae	Posterior tubercle of transverse processes of C1–4	Upper part of medial border of scapula	Raises medial border of scapula	Anterior rami of C3 and C4 (cervical plexus) and reinforced by dorsal scapular
Serratus anterior	Upper 8 ribs and anterior IC membranes from MC line	Inner medial border of scapula 1&2 digitations to upper angle, 3 & 4 costal margin and 5–8 inferior angle	Laterally rotates and protracts scapula	Long thoracic nerve (C5–7)

C = cervical, IC = intercostal, L = lumbar, MC = midclavicular, S = sacral, T = thoracic.

Part 2 Axilla (Fig 1.3)

- Space between the upper arm and side of the thorax, bounded in front and behind by the axillary folds and communicating superiorly with the posterior triangle of the neck
- Contains neurovascular structures and lymph nodes for the upper limb, side wall of the thorax and breast
  - Floor is the axillary fascia – extends from the serratus anterior fascia to the fascia of the arm
    - Suspended by the suspensory ligament
    - Attached in front and behind by axillary folds
  - Anterior wall is completed by the pectoralis major and minor, subclavius and clavipectoral fascia
  - Posterior wall extends lower and is formed by the subscapularis and teres major
  - Medial wall is formed by the upper parts of the serratus anterior (its limit defined as the level of the fourth rib)
  - Lateral boundary is the lips of the intertubercular groove of the humerus
  - Apex is formed by the clavicle, scapula and outer border of the first rib

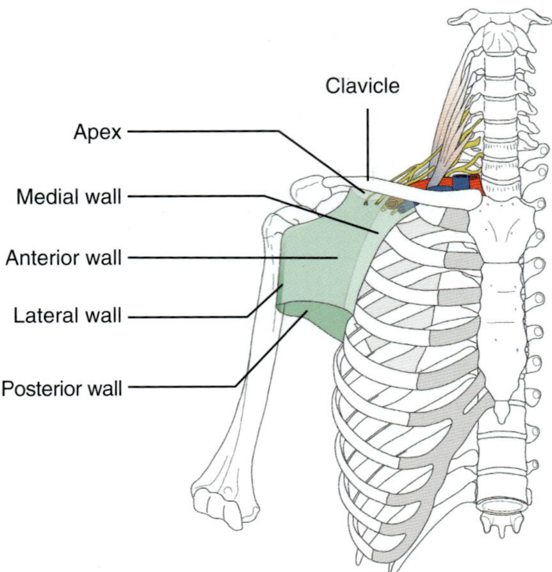

Fig. 1.3 Axilla and its relations.

SPACES (GATEWAYS) (Fig 1.4A and B)

- The quadrangular space lies between the subscapularis, teres major, humerus and long head of the triceps (anterior view) and the teres major, teres minor, humerus and long head of the triceps (posterior view) in the posterior wall of the axilla
  - Transmits the axillary nerve and the posterior circumflex humeral vessels, which lie inferior to the nerve
- The lower triangular space lies below teres major between the humerus and long head of the triceps
  - Transmits the radial nerve and profunda brachii vessels
- The upper triangular space lies medial to the long head of the triceps and above the teres major
  - Transmits the circumflex scapular artery

CONTENTS

- Transmits the neurovascular bundle from the neck to the upper limb
- Three cords of the brachial plexus are formed behind the clavicle and enter the axilla along the artery
- Cords embrace the **second part** of the axillary artery and veins
- The axillary artery is a continuation of the subclavian artery (at the lateral border of the first rib); it enters the axilla by passing over the first digitation of the serratus anterior muscle and is invested by axillary sheath fascia (from prevertebral)
  - The axillary artery becomes the brachial artery at the lower border of the teres major
  - It is divided into three parts by the pectoralis minor; the second part (behind the pectoralis minor) is embraced by three cords of the brachial plexus: lateral, medial and posterior (Fig 1.5A)
  - Branches (Fig 1.5B): **first part** has *one* branch, **second part** has *two* branches, **third part** has *three* branches
    - (first part) superior thoracic artery

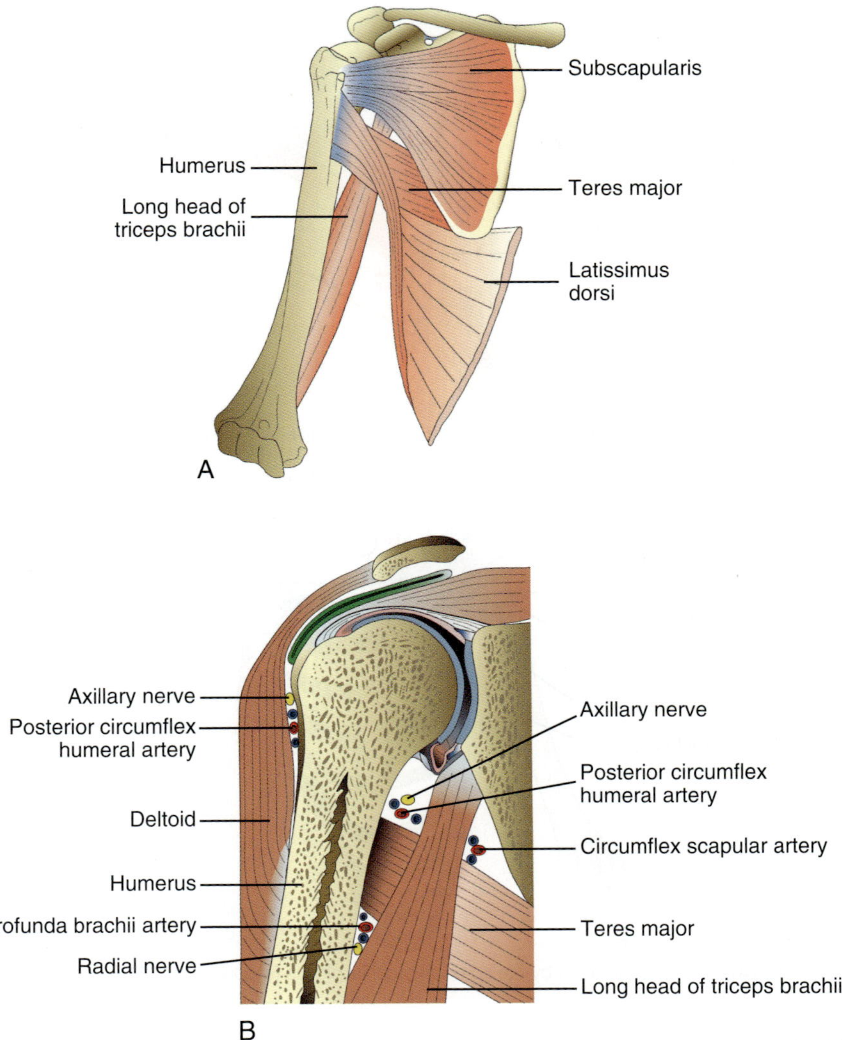

Fig. 1.4 (A) Muscular spaces (gateways) of the axilla. **(B)** Muscular spaces of the axilla and structures passing through (coronal view).

- (second part) thoracoacromial artery (has four branches: pectoral, deltoid, clavicular and acromial)
- (second part) lateral thoracic artery
- (third part) subscapular artery (largest branch and has two branches: circumflex scapular and thoracodorsal artery)
- (third part) anterior circumflex humeral artery
- (third part) posterior circumflex humeral artery

- Axillary vein is joined by the basilic vein at the posterior wall of the axilla
  - Beyond the first rib it continues as the subclavian vein
  - There is no axillary sheath around the vein

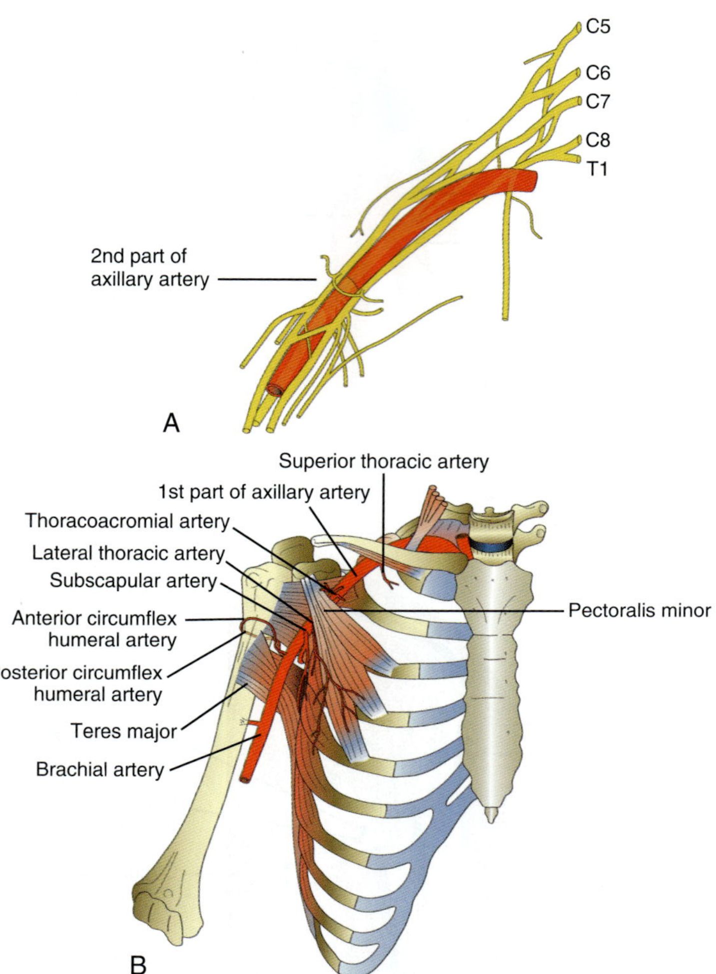

Fig. 1.5 **(A)** Axillary artery embraced by the cords of brachial plexus (second part). **(B)** Branches of the axillary artery.

BRACHIAL PLEXUS (Fig 1.6A and B)

TABLE 1.2 ■ **Summary of the Brachial Plexus**

Posterior Triangle		On 1st Rib (Behind the Clavicle)	2nd Part of Axillary (Posterior to Pectoralis Minor)	
Roots	**Trunks**	**Divisions**	**Cords**	**Terminal Branches**
C5, 6	Superior	Anterior branch of S & M	Lateral (C5–7)	Musculocutaneous & median
C7	Middle	Posterior branch of S, M & I	Posterior (C5–T1)	Radial & axillary
C8, T1	Inferior	Anterior branch of I	Medial (C8, T1)	Ulnar & median

A = anterior, C = cervical, I = inferior, M = middle, P = Posterior, S = superior, T = thoracic.

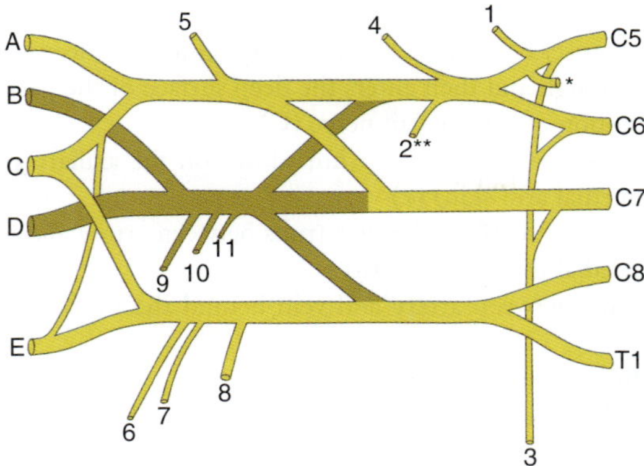

*Contribution to phrenic nerve (C3, 4, 5); ** Nerve to subclavius reported originating from the root or from the trunk.

A

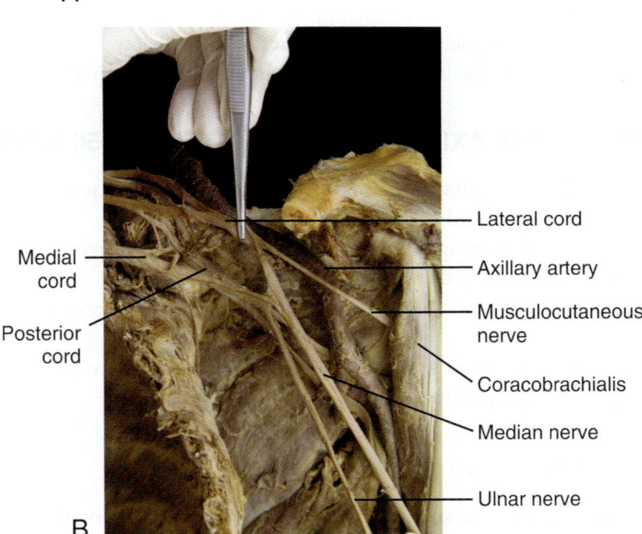

Fig. 1.6 Brachial plexus. **(A)** Schematic diagram. **(B)** Cadaveric dissection.

- **Branches from the roots** (supraclavicular part)
  - Dorsal scapular nerve C5 (passes behind the rhomboids) **(1** on Fig 1.6**)**
  - Nerve to subclavius (C5, C6) (passes in front of the subclavius) **(2)**
  - Long thoracic nerve C5, C6, C7 (passes behind the serratus anterior) **(3)**
- **Branches from the trunks**
  - Suprascapular nerve **(4)**
- **Branches from the lateral cord**
  - Lateral pectoral (innervates the pectoralis major together with the medial pectoral nerve) **(5)**
  - Musculocutaneous (perforates the coracobrachialis; innervates the coracobrachialis, biceps brachii, brachialis and ends as the lateral cutaneous nerve of the forearm) **(A)**
  - Lateral contribution of median nerve **(C)**

- **Branches from the medial cord**
  - Medial pectoral arises behind the axillary artery (enters the deep surface of the pectoralis minor, passes through and then enters the deep surface of the pectoralis major) **(6)**
  - Medial contribution of the median nerve **(C)**
  - Medial cutaneous nerve of the arm (runs down on the axillary vein and gives sensory supply to the medial arm skin) **(7)**
  - Medial cutaneous nerve of the forearm (runs between artery and vein and gives sensory supply to the medial forearm skin) **(8)**
  - Ulnar nerve (runs between artery and vein behind the medial cutaneous nerve of the forearm) **(E)**
- **Branches from the posterior cord**
  - Upper subscapular (small nerve to the subscapularis) **(9)**
  - Thoracodorsal (large nerve to the latissimus dorsi) **(10)**
  - Lower subscapular (supplying the lower part of the subscapular muscle and teres major) **(11)**
  - Axillary nerve (passes backwards through quadrangular space, behind the surgical neck of the humerus and innervates the deltoid and teres minor and gives sensory supply to a small patch on the lateral side of the upper arm) **(B)**
  - Radial nerve (largest branch and passes down through the lower triangular space into the radial groove between the lateral and medial heads of the triceps) **(D)**

LYMPH NODES IN THE AXILLA (APPROXIMATELY 35–50 NODES)

- Anterior or pectoral group lie along the medial wall of the axilla, receiving from the upper half of the anterior trunk and breast
- Posterior or subscapular group lie in the posteromedial wall, receiving from the upper half of the posterior trunk and axillary tail (Spence's tail)
- Lateral group lie along the medial side of the axillary vein, receiving from the above groups
- Central group lie in the fat of the axilla and collect from the above groups
- Apical group lie in the apex, receiving from all of the above

Part 3 Breast (Fig 1.7)

- Lies in the subcutaneous tissue (superficial fascia) of the anterior thoracic wall and the superficial fascia has two divisions: a superficial layer and a deep layer (posterior capsule)
- Base is from ribs two to six (from the midline to the midaxillary line)
- Overlies the pectoralis major, serratus anterior and a small part of the rectus sheath and the external oblique muscle
- Contains 15–20 lactiferous ducts, which converge on the nipple
- Posterior extension of the superficial fascia (behind the breast) condenses to form the posterior capsule
- Suspensory ligament (of Cooper) connects the dermis of the overlying skin to the posterior capsule
- Between the capsule and the pectoralis fascia is the submammary space

VASCULAR SUPPLY (Fig 1.8)

- Mainly the lateral thoracic artery
- The internal thoracic arteries, mainly through the second and third intercostal spaces, as well as the perforating branches of the intercostal arteries
- The pectoral branch of the thoracoacromial artery supplies the upper part

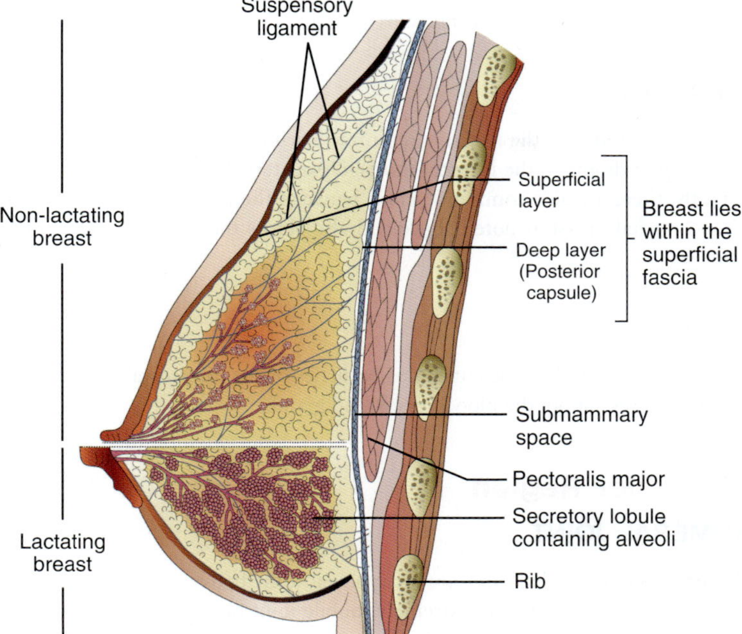

Fig. 1.7 Breast, sagittal section.

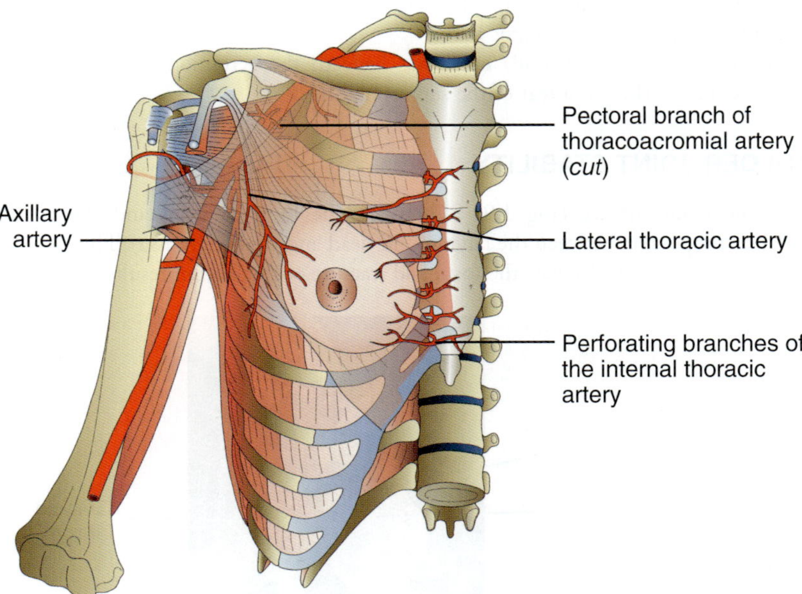

Fig. 1.8 Arterial supply of the breast (the breast is also supplied by the perforating branches of the intercostal arteries but is NOT shown in this diagram).

- Venous drainage is mainly by deep veins to the internal thoracic and axillary veins; some also drain to the posterior intercostal veins

LYMPH DRAINAGE

- The lateral part drains to the axillary and infraclavicular nodes
- The medial part drains to the internal thoracic/parasternal nodes
- Importantly, there are also communications between the lymph node groups draining the lateral and medial breast as noted above and also across the midline between the left and right breasts

NERVE SUPPLY

- The breast is innervated by the cutaneous branches of the intercostal nerves
- Sympathetic fibres supply the blood vessels and glands

Part 4 Shoulder Region

GLENOHUMERAL JOINT

The **glenohumeral joint** is a ball and socket synovial joint between the glenoid fossa of the scapula and the humeral head. It is an extremely mobile joint but inherently unstable and is the most commonly dislocated joint in the body. The most common dislocation is anterior dislocation, which typically occurs when the arm is abducted and externally rotated. The joint is least stable inferiorly when the shoulder is abducted.

Synovial membrane is attached around the glenoid labrum and lines the capsule and head/neck of the humerus. It herniates through the capsule to communicate with the subscapular bursa and sometimes with the infraspinatus bursa.

- The subacromial (subdeltoid) bursa lies beneath the acromion and normally does not connect unless there is a tear of the supraspinatus

SHOULDER JOINT STABILITY

- The **articular surface** (Fig 1.9) is between the humeral head and the glenoid fossa (4:1 disproportion between the large round head and the small fossa). The glenoid labrum (fibrocartilage ring) deepens the fossa and fracture of the labrum results in dislocation.

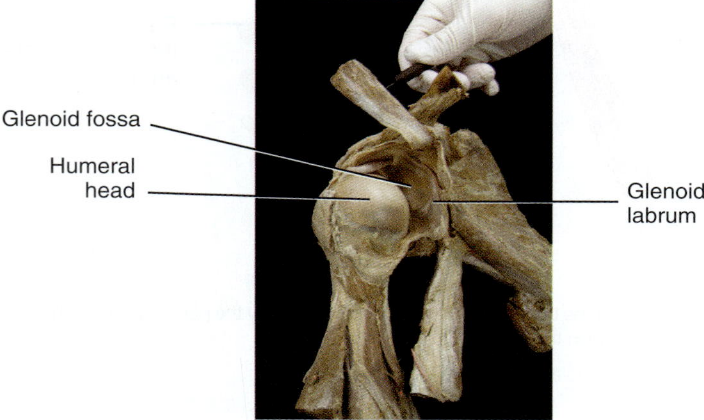

Fig. 1.9 Articular surfaces of the shoulder joint.

- **Glenohumeral ligaments** (Fig 1.10) (superior, middle and inferior) reinforce the capsule anteriorly. The coracohumeral ligaments are very strong. An upward displacement is prevented by the coracoacromial arch.
- The **joint capsule** is attached to the outer margins of the labrum and anatomical neck of the humerus *except* inferiorly, where it is attached to the surgical neck. The capsule is strong but lax inferomedially. At the upper end of the intertubercular groove, the capsule bridges the gap and forms the transverse humeral ligament.
- **Rotator cuff muscles** (Fig 1.11A and B) provide dynamic stability and include the supraspinatus, the infraspinatus, the teres minor and the subscapularis. Their tendons fuse with the lateral part of the joint capsule.
- **Long head of** the **biceps and** the **triceps** (see Fig 1.9): the long head of the biceps sinks 'through' the capsule and is intracapsular.
- **Negative intra-articular pressure**

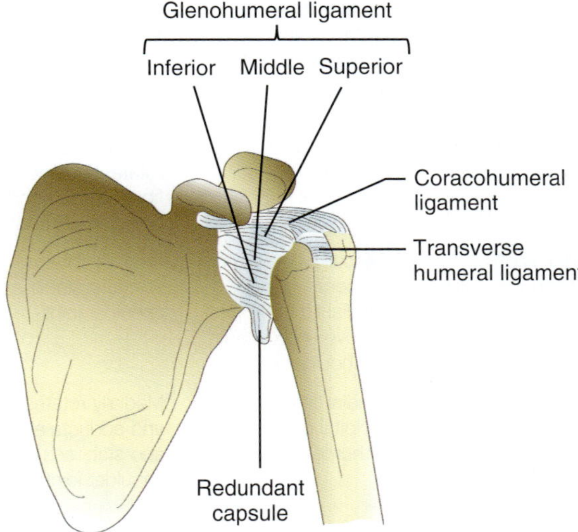

Fig. 1.10 Glenohumeral ligaments.

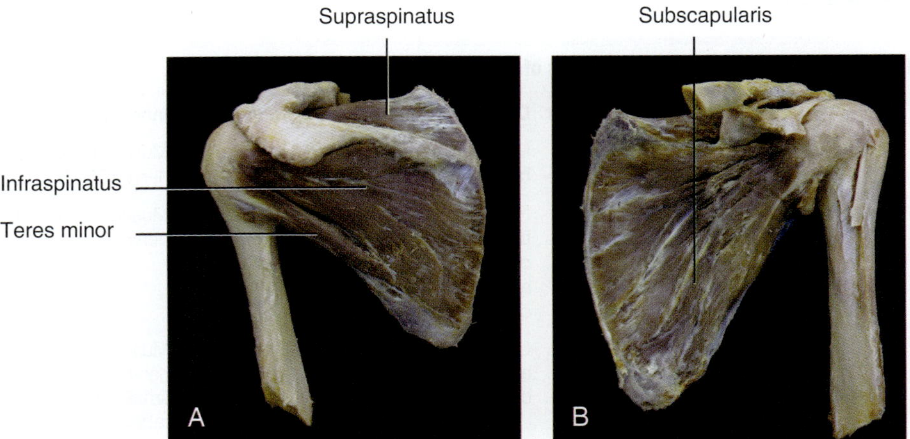

Fig. 1.11 Rotator cuff muscles. **(A)** Posterior view. **(B)** Anterior (costal) view.

MUSCLES OF THE SHOULDER REGION

TABLE 1.3 ■ **Summary of the Muscles of the Shoulder Region**

	Proximal Attachment	Distal Attachment	Concentric Action	Innervation
Supraspinatus	Medial $^{3}/_{4}$ of supraspinous fossa of scapula and upper surface of spine (bipenate)	Superior facet of greater tuberosity of humerus and capsule of shoulder joint	Abducts arm and stabilises shoulder joint	Suprascapular nerve (C5, 6)
Infraspinatus	Medial $^{3}/_{4}$ of infraspinatus fossa and fibrous intermuscular septa	Middle facet of greater tuberosity of humerus and capsule of shoulder joint	Laterally rotates arm and stabilises shoulder joint	Suprascapular nerve (C5, 6)
Teres minor	Middle $^{1}/_{3}$ of lateral border of scapula above teres major	Inferior facet of greater tuberosity of humerus and capsule of shoulder joint	Laterally rotates arm and stabilises shoulder joint	Axillary nerve (C5, 6)
Deltoid	Lateral $^{1}/_{3}$ of clavicle, acromion and spine of scapula	Middle of lateral surface of humerus (deltoid tuberosity)	Abducts arm, anterior fibres flex, medial fibres rotate, posterior fibres extend and lateral fibres rotate	Axillary nerve (C5, 6)
Subscapularis	Medial $^{2}/_{3}$ of subscapular fossa	Lesser tuberosity of humerus, upper medial lip of bicipital groove and capsule of shoulder joint	Medially rotates arm and stabilises shoulder joint	Upper and lower subscapular nerve (C5, 6)
Teres major	Lower 1/3 of lateral border of scapula below teres minor	Medial lip of the bicipital groove of humerus	Medially rotates and adducts arm and stabilises shoulder joint	Lower scapular nerve (C5, 6)

Part 5 Anterior Compartment of the Arm

MUSCLES

TABLE 1.4 ■ **Summary of the Muscles of the Anterior Compartment of the Arm**

	Proximal Attachment	Distal Attachment	Concentric Action	Innervation
Coracobrachialis	Coracoid process of scapula	Middle $^{1}/_{3}$ of medial border of humerus	Flexes and weakly adducts arm	Musculocutaneous nerve (C5–7)
Biceps brachii	**Long head** from supraglenoid tubercle of scapula **Short head** from coracoid process	Posterior border of bicipital tuberosity of radius & bicipital aponeurosis to deep fascia	Supinates forearm, flexes elbow and weakly flexes shoulder	Musculocutaneous nerve (C5, 6)
Brachialis	Anterior lower $^{1}/_{2}$ of humerus and medial and lateral intermuscular septa	Coronoid process and tuberosity of ulna	Flexes elbow	Musculocutaneous nerve (C5, 6), also small supply from radial nerve

The **neurovascular bundle** passes into the flexor compartment of the arm except:

- Posterior circumflex vessels and the axillary nerve are given off to the extensor compartment through the quadrangular space
- The radial nerve and the profunda brachii artery leave through the lower triangular space

BRACHIAL ARTERY

- A continuation of the axillary artery (at the lower border of the teres major and accompanied by venae comitantes) (see Fig 1.5B)
- The median nerve lies lateral then obliquely crosses in front of the artery to lie medially (Fig 1.12)
- The artery passes into the cubital fossa before dividing into radial and ulnar arteries
- The largest branch is the profunda brachii leaving through the lower triangular space
- Other major branches include the superior ulnar collateral (accompanies the ulnar nerve) and inferior ulnar collateral artery (consists of anterior and posterior branches) (Fig 1.13)

VEINS OF THE ARM (Fig 1.14)

- Axillary vein
- Venae comitantes accompany the brachial artery and all branches
- The basilic vein runs upwards (medially) and perforates deep fascia in the middle of the arm

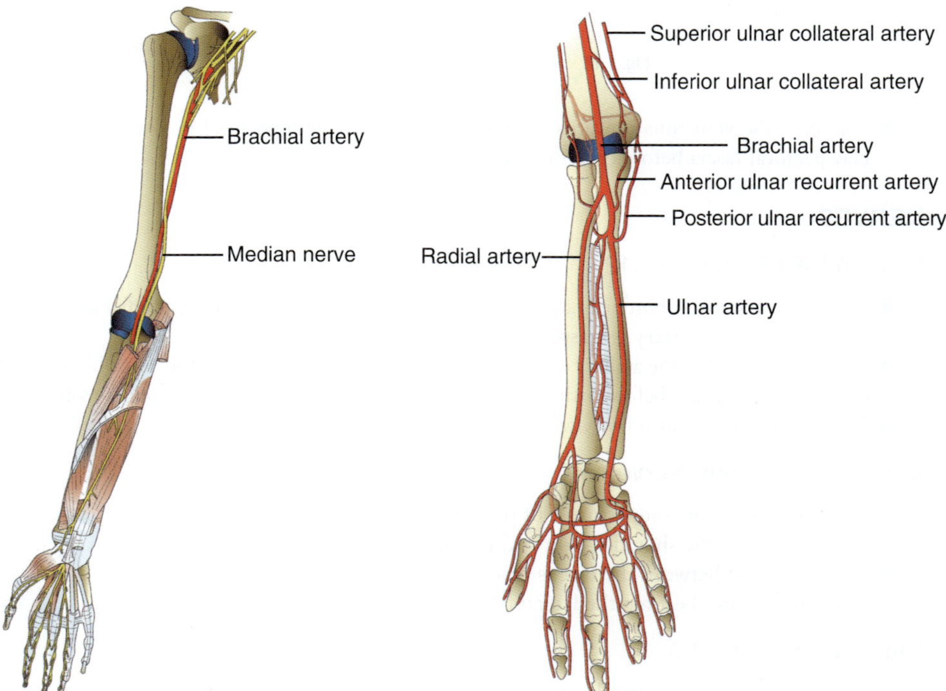

Fig. 1.12 Course of the median nerve.

Fig. 1.13 Arterial system of the elbow and forearm.

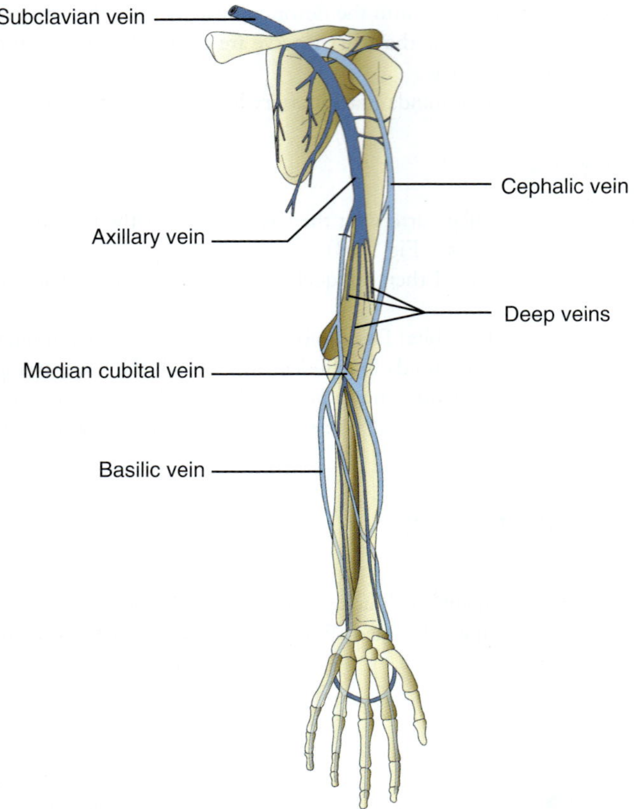

Fig. 1.14 Venous system of the upper limb.

- The cephalic vein runs upwards (laterally) then in the deltopectoral groove to pierce the clavipectoral fascia before entering the axillary vein

NERVES

Median Nerve (see Fig 1.12)

- Formed at the lower border of axilla by union of the contribution of the medial and lateral cords (the axillary artery is clasped between both cords)
- First it lies lateral to the axillary artery. Passing distally through the arm, the nerve lies in front of the brachial artery before sitting medial to the artery in the cubital fossa (elbow joint)
- No branches in the arm (*but does give sympathetic filaments and a twig to the elbow joint*)

Musculocutaneous Nerve

- Nerve of the flexor compartment of the arm
- Gives a twig to the shoulder joint and perforates the coracobrachialis and innervates it
- Proceeds to lie between the biceps brachii and brachialis supplying both muscles
- Remaining fibres become the lateral cutaneous nerve of the forearm

Ulnar Nerve (Fig 1.15)

- Lies posterior to the vessels and then inclines further back, piercing the medial intermuscular septum. Has no branches in the arm

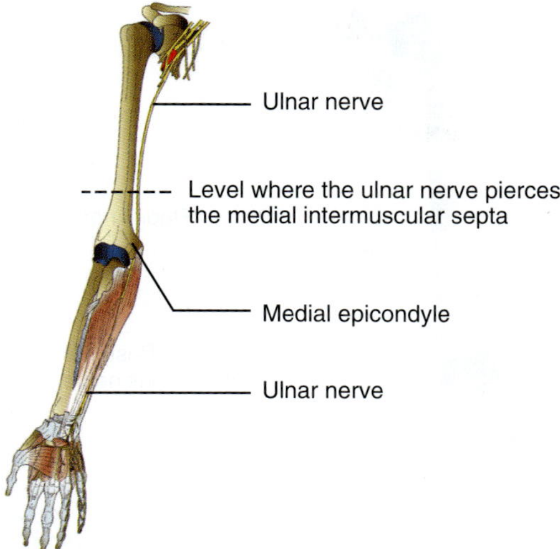

Fig. 1.15 Course of the ulnar nerve.

Medial Cutaneous Nerve of the Arm

- A small nerve, it lies anterior to the vessels and pierces the deep fascia of the upper arm, supplying skin on the front and medial sides of the upper part of the arm

Intercostobrachial nerve

- A lateral cutaneous branch of the second intercostal nerve, it supplies the axilla and skin on the medial side of the upper arm

LYMPHATICS

- An infraclavicular group of lymph nodes lie along the cephalic vein and a supratrochlear group lie in subcutaneous fat above the medial epicondyle

Part 6 Posterior Compartment of the Arm

MUSCLES

TABLE 1.5 ■ **Summary of the Muscles of the Posterior Compartment of the Arm**

Triceps brachii	Proximal Attachment	Distal Attachment	Concentric Action	Innervation
Long head	Infraglenoid tubercle of scapula	Posterior part of upper surface of olecranon process of ulna and posterior capsule of elbow joint	Extends elbow, stabilises shoulder and retracts capsule of elbow joint	Radial nerve (C6–8) (4 branches)
Lateral head	Upper 1/2 of posterior humerus			
Medial head	Lower 1/2 of posterior humerus			

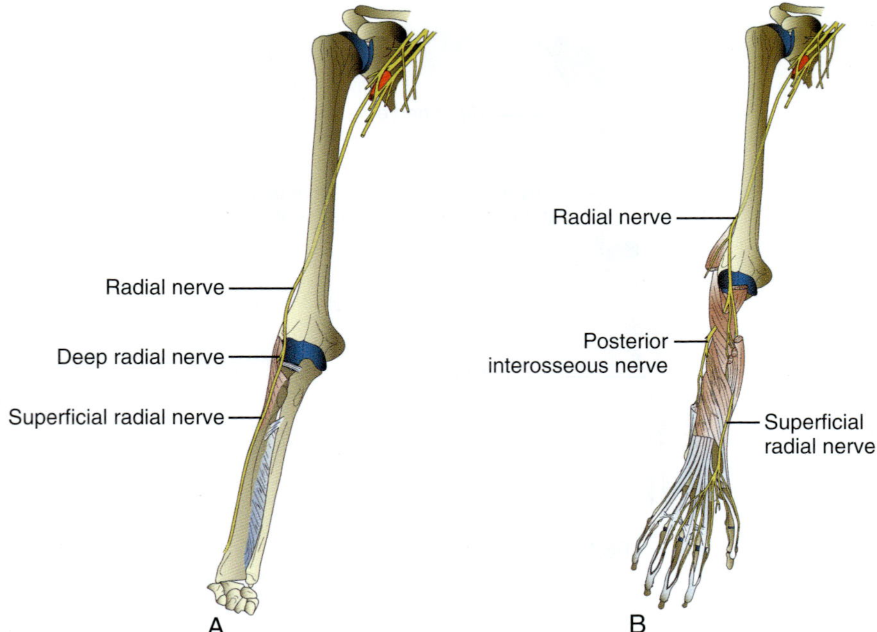

Fig. 1.16 Course of the radial nerve. **(A)** Anterior view. **(B)** Anterior view with a pronated forearm.

NERVES

Radial Nerve (Fig 1.16A and B)

- A continuation of the posterior cord (largest branch), it crosses beyond the posterior wall of the axilla then runs through the lower triangular space
- Accompanies the profunda brachii vessels and spirals obliquely downwards behind the humerus. At the lateral edge, the nerve comes into contact with the periosteum in the lower end of the spiral groove
- Then it pierces the lateral intermuscular septum to enter the anterior compartment before reaching the cubital fossa (under cover of the brachioradialis)
- Has four branches to the triceps
- Also gives origin to the lower lateral cutaneous nerve of the arm and the posterior cutaneous nerve of the forearm
- Crosses the elbow by passing anterior to the lateral epicondyle and splits into deep and superficial before the supinator. The deep radial passes through the two heads of the supinator to become the posterior interosseous nerve

Ulnar Nerve (see Fig 1.15)

- Passes through the lower part of the extensor compartment, then disappears by passing though the humeral and ulnar heads of the flexor carpi ulnaris into the forearm
- Lies in contact with the flexor carpi ulnaris along its course in the forearm

PROFUNDA BRACHII ARTERY

- Supply to the triceps brachii
- Passes through the lower triangular space then, at the lateral intermuscular septum, divides into anterior and posterior branches

ELBOW JOINT

- Humeroradial joint: a synovial hinge joint between the capitulum of the humerus and the radial head
  - The cylindrical head of radius is concave to fit the capitulum
- Humeroulnar joint: a synovial hinge joint between the trochlea of the humerus and the ulnar trochlear notch
  - The upper end of the ulna shows a deep trochlear notch
  - Engineering of the joint results in a carrying angle
- Communicates with the proximal radioulnar joint
- Capsule is attached to the humerus at the margins of the lower rounded ends of the articular surfaces (trochlea and capitulum)
  - Distally attached to the trochlear notch of the ulna and annular ligament – *not attached to radius*
  - The quadrate ligament prevents herniation
- The ulnar collateral (medial) ligament is triangular
  - Anterior band (strongest) – passes from the medial epicondyle of the humerus
  - Posterior band – from the medial border of the olecranon
  - Middle band – connects the anterior and posterior bands and houses the ulnar nerve
- Radial collateral (lateral) ligament is a single flattened band and extends from below the common extensor attachment and fuses with the annular ligament
- The annular ligament is attached to the radial notch of the ulna and slings around the head and neck of the radius
- Nerve supply is via the musculocutaneous, median, ulnar and radial nerves
- Movements: the only appreciable movement is flexion and extension (140°); the axis of the hinge lies obliquely
- Radioulnar joints
  - The **proximal joint** consists of annular ligament
  - The **distal joint** is closed distally by triangular fibrocartilage (the capsule is loose and pouches up to the pronator quadratus)

Part 7 Anterior Compartment of the Forearm

Flexor muscles of the forearm are arranged into groups of superficial and deep muscles.

SUPERFICIAL MUSCLES (FIVE MUSCLES)

TABLE 1.6 ■ **Summary of the Superficial Muscles of the Anterior Compartment of the Forearm**

	Proximal Attachment	Distal Attachment	Concentric Action	Innervation
Pronator teres	**Humeral head:** medial epicondyle, medial supracondylar ridge and medial intermuscular septum	Posterior to the most prominent part of lateral convexity of radius	Pronates forearm and flexes elbow	Median nerve (C6, 7)
	Ulnar head: medial border of coronoid process			
Flexor carpi radialis	Medial epicondyle	Bases of 2nd and 3rd MC via groove in trapezium	Flexes and abducts wrist	Median nerve (C6, 7)

Continued on following page

TABLE 1.6 ■ **Summary of the Superficial Muscles of the Anterior Compartment of the Forearm** (Continued)

	Proximal Attachment	Distal Attachment	Concentric Action	Innervation
Flexor digitorum superficialis	**Humeral head:** medial epicondyle of humerus and medial ligament of elbow **Ulnar head:** sublime tubercle & fibrous arch **Radial head:** whole length of anterior oblique line	Tendons split to insert onto sides of middle phalanges of medial 4 fingers	Flexes proximal IP joint and MCP/wrist	Median nerve (C7, 8, T1)
Palmaris longus	Medial epicondyle of humerus	Flexor retinaculum and palmar aponeurosis	Flexes wrist and tenses palmar aponeurosis	Median nerve (C7, 8)
Flexor carpi ulnaris	**Humeral head:** medial epicondyle of humerus **Ulnar head:** aponeurosis from medial olecranon and upper $^3/_4$ of ulna	Pisiform, hook of hamate, base of 5th MC via pisometacarpal and pisohamate ligaments	Flexes and adducts wrist and fixes pisiform during action of hypothenar muscles	**Ulnar nerve** (C7, 8, T1)

IP = interphalangeal, MC = metacarpal, MCP = metacarpophalangeal.

DEEP MUSCLES (THREE MUSCLES)

TABLE 1.7 ■ **Summary of the Deep Muscles of the Anterior Compartment of the Forearm**

	Proximal Attachment	Distal Attachment	Concentric Action	Innervation
Flexor digitorum profundus	Upper $^3/_4$ of anterior and medial surface of ulna as far around as subcutaneous border and narrow strip of interosseous membrane	Distal phalanges of medial 4 fingers	Flexes distal IP joints then 2° flexes IP and MCP joints and wrist	**Medial half** by ulnar nerve (C8, T1) **Lateral half** by median nerve (anterior interosseous) (C7, 8)
Flexor pollicis longus	Anterior surface of radius below anterior oblique line and adjacent interosseous membrane	Base of distal phalanges	Flexes distal IP joint	Median nerve (anterior interosseous) (C7, 8)
Pronator quadratus	Lower $^1/_4$ of anteromedial shaft of ulna	Lower $^1/_4$ of anterolateral shaft of radius and some interosseous membrane	Pronates forearm and maintains radius and ulna opposed	Median nerve (anterior interosseous) (C7, 8)

IP = interphalangeal, MC = metacarpal, MCP = metacarpophalangeal.

CUBITAL FOSSA (Fig 1.17A–C)

The cubital fossa is an important area of transition between the arm and the forearm. It is located anterior to the elbow joint and is a triangular depression.

- **Borders:** the brachioradialis muscle, the pronator teres and an imaginary horizontal line between the medial and lateral epicondyles

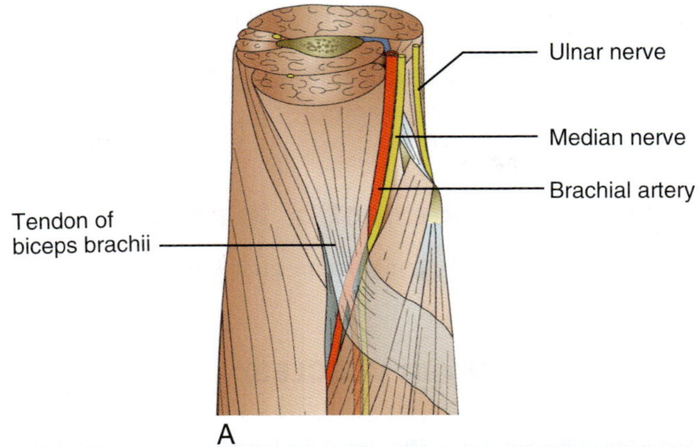

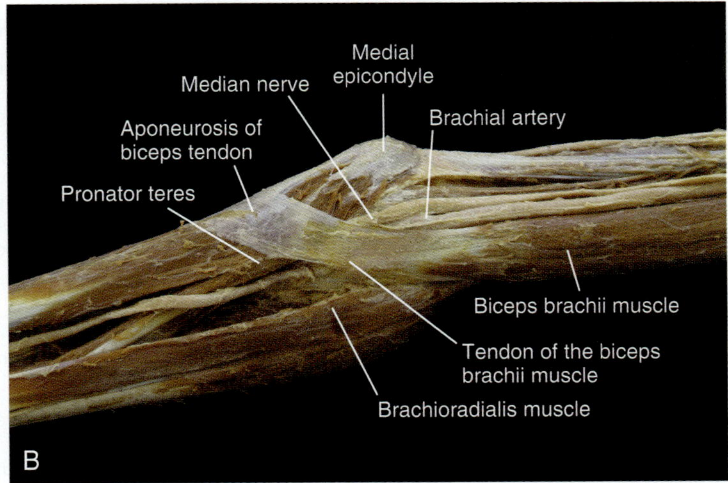

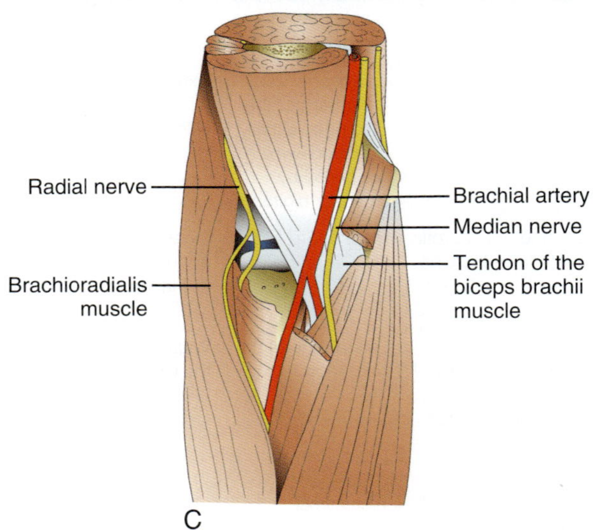

Fig. 1.17 Cubital fossa. **(A)** Superficial structures. **(B)** Cadaveric dissection. **(C)** Contents.

- **Roof:** superficial fascia, the lateral and medial cutaneous nerves of the forearm and the median cubital vein
- **Contents (lateral to medial):** the tendon of the biceps brachii muscle (with its aponeurosis), the brachial artery and the median nerve
- **Floor:** mainly the brachialis muscle

Part 8 Posterior Compartment of the Forearm

Extensor muscles of the forearm are arranged into groups of superficial muscles and deep muscles.

SUPERFICIAL MUSCLES (SEVEN MUSCLES)

TABLE 1.8 ■ **Summary of the Superficial Muscles of the Posterior Compartment of the Forearm**

	Proximal Attachment	Distal Attachment	Concentric Action	Innervation
Brachioradialis	Upper $^2/_3$ of lateral supracondylar ridge of humerus and lateral intermuscular septa	Base of styloid process of radius	Flexes arm at the elbow and brings the forearm into the midprone position	Radial nerve (before division into superficial and deep)
Extensor carpi radialis longus	Lower $^2/_3$ of lateral supracondylar ridge of humerus and lateral intermuscular septa	Posterior base of 2nd MC	Extends and adducts the hand at the wrist	Radial nerve (before division into superficial and deep)
Extensor carpi radialis brevis	CEA	Base of 3rd MC	Extends and adducts the hand at the wrist	Radial nerve (deep branch)
Extensor digitorum	CEA	Extensor expansion of all 4 fingers, 3 and 4 normally fuse with 5 only getting a slip	Extends all joints of fingers	Radial nerve (posterior interosseous nerve)
Extensor digiti minimi	CEA	Extensor expansion of the 5th finger, usually 2 tendons which are joined by extensor digitorum	Extends all joints of the little finger	Radial nerve (posterior interosseous nerve)
Extensor carpi ulnaris	CEA and aponeurotic sheath from the ulna	Base of 3rd MC	Extends and adducts the hand at the wrist	Radial nerve (posterior interosseous nerve)
Anconeus	Smooth surface at the lower extremity of posterior aspect of lateral epicondyle of humerus	Lateral side of the olecranon	Weak extensor of the elbow	Radial nerve (by a branch which runs through the medial head of triceps brachii)

CEA = common extensor attachment; MC = metacarpal

DEEP MUSCLES (FIVE MUSCLES)

TABLE 1.9 ■ **Summary of the Deep Muscles of the Posterior Compartment of the Forearm**

	Proximal Attachment	Distal Attachment	Concentric Action	Innervation
Supinator	**Deep part** from the supinator crest and fossa of the ulna **Superficial part** from the lateral epicondyle and lateral collateral ligament of the elbow and annular ligament	Neck and shaft of the radius	Supinate the forearm and acts alone only when the elbow is extended	Radial nerve (posterior interosseous nerve)
Abductor pollicis longus	Upper posterior surface of the ulna and middle 1/3 of the posterior surface of the radius and the interosseous membrane	Over tendons of radial extensors and brachioradialis to base of 1st MC and trapezium	Abducts and extends thumb at the CMC joint	Radial nerve (posterior interosseous nerve)
Extensor pollicis brevis	Lower 1/3 posterior shaft of radius and interosseous membrane	Over tendons of radial extensors and brachioradialis to base of the proximal phalanx of thumb	Extends MPC joint of the thumb	Radial nerve (posterior interosseous nerve)
Extensor pollicis longus	Middle 1/3 of posterior ulna and interosseous membrane	Base of distal phalanx of thumb	Extends IP and MCP joints of thumb	Radial nerve (posterior interosseous nerve)
Extensor indicis	Lower posterior shaft of the ulna and interosseous membrane	Extensor expansion of the index finger	Extends all joints of the index finger	Radial nerve (posterior interosseous nerve)

CMC = carpometacarpal, IP = interphalangeal, MC = metacarpal, MCP = metacarpophalangeal

COMMON EXTENSOR ATTACHMENT (CEA)

The CEA is a smooth area on the front of the lateral epicondyle and is for the attachment of the extensor carpi radialis brevis, the extensor digitorum, the extensor digiti minimi and the extensor carpi ulnaris. All four tendons are fused with each other and to the deep fascia.

EXTENSOR RETINACULUM

- A ribbon-like band (2.5 cm wide) lying obliquely across the extensor surface of the wrist joint
- Proximally attached to the radius above the styloid process and distally attached to the pisiform and triquetral bones

- Not attached to the ulna
- Maintains a constant tension throughout pronation/supination and holds down the extensor tendons
- From the extensor retinaculum, fibrous septa pass to the bones of the forearm with the extensor tunnel and divide into six compartments: the abductor pollicis longus, the extensor pollicis brevis, the extensor pollicis longus, the extensor digitorum and extensor indicis, the extensor minimi digiti, and the extensor carpi ulnaris

ANATOMICAL SNUFFBOX

The anatomical snuffbox is a concavity between the tendon of the extensor pollicis longus (ulnar side) and the tendon of the extensor pollicis brevis/abductor pollicis longus (radial side).

- The cutaneous branch of the radial nerve (superficial radial nerve) crosses over these tendons
- The radial artery lies deep to all three tendons
- Floor (proximal to distal): radial styloid, scaphoid, trapezium and base of the first metacarpal bone

BLOOD SUPPLY OF THE FOREARM

Arteries of the Forearm (see Fig 1.13)

- **Radial artery** – passes medially to the biceps tendon, across the supinator and over the tendon of the distal attachment of the pronator teres, the proximal attachment of the flexor digitorum superficialis, the proximal attachment of the flexor pollicis longus and the the distal attachment of the pronator quadratus
  - Passes deep to the tendons of the abductor pollicis longus/extensor pollicis brevis to cross snuffbox
  - In the upper part of the forearm it is overlapped by the brachioradialis
  - In the middle third of the forearm it has the superficial branch of the radial nerve lateral to it
  - Surface markings: along a line, slightly convex laterally, from medial to the biceps tendon (in the cubital fossa) to a point medial to the styloid process of the radius
- **Ulnar artery** – from the cubital fossa it passes deep to the pronator teres and the flexor digitorum superficialis near the median nerve, then lies over the flexor digitorum profundus
  - Surface markings: along a line, slightly convex medially, from medial to the biceps tendon (cubital fossa) to the radial side of the pisiform
- **Common interosseous artery** – a branch of the ulnar artery which divides into the anterior and the posterior interosseous arteries
  - The **anterior interosseous artery** lies deeply on the interosseous membrane between the flexor digitorum profundus and the flexor pollicis longus, and its perforating branches pierce the interosseous membrane to supply the deep extensor muscles
    - Nutrient vessels are given off to the radius and ulna
    - The artery passes through the interosseous membrane
  - The **posterior interosseous artery** passes between the bones in the forearm accompanying the posterior interosseous nerve and supplying the deep muscles of the extensor compartment. It fades out along its course and is supplemented by the anterior interosseous artery
- **Anastomosis around the elbow joint** is provided by the radial, ulnar and interosseous arteries which run upwards to anastomose with the descending articular branches of the profunda brachii and the ulnar collateral arteries
- **Anastomosis around the wrist joint** is provided by the anterior and posterior carpal branches from the radial and ulnar arteries to form the carpal arches

    - The anterior carpal arch – lies transversely across the wrist joint supplying the carpal bones and sends branches distally into the hand to anastomose with the deep palmar arch
    - The posterior carpal arch – lies transversally across the distal row of carpals, and sends dorsal metacarpal arteries distally into each metacarpal space

Veins of the Forearm (see Fig 1.14)

- Deep veins are plentiful and accompany arteries as venae comitantes
- Blood from the palm of the hand passes to the dorsum
    - From the radial side, it drains via the cephalic vein from the snuffbox
    - From the ulnar side, the basilic vein runs upwards and pierces the deep fascia halfway between the elbow and the axilla
- The median forearm vein drains subcutaneus tissue of the front of the wrist and forearm and divides into the median cephalic and median basilic veins

LYMPHATICS OF THE FOREARM

- Superficial lymphatics follow veins and deep ones follow arteries
    - Ulnar via basilic to supratrochlear nodes, and radial via cephalic to deltopectoral and infraclavicular nodes

NERVES OF THE FOREARM

Flexor Compartment

- Lateral cutaneous nerve of the forearm
    - A cutaneous continuation of the musculocutaneous nerve, which pierces the fascia above the elbow
- Medial cutaneous nerve of the forearm
    - Roughly symmetrical with the lateral cutaneous nerve
- Superficial branch of the radial nerve
    - Runs under the brachioradialis and is distributed to the radial two-thirds of the dorsum of the hand and the proximal parts of the dorsal surfaces of the thumb, index and middle fingers and half of the ring finger
- Median nerve
    - From the cubital fossa it runs between the two heads of the pronator teres and gives off a branch to the pronator teres
    - Then it runs between the flexor digitorum superficialis and the flexor digitorum profundus
    - Also supplies the flexor carpi radialis, the flexor digitorum superficialis and the palmaris longus
    - Gives off the anterior interosseous branch and innervates the flexor digitorum profundus (lateral half), the flexor pollicis longus, the pronator quadratus, the interosseous membrane and the periosteum
    - At the distal end of the forearm, it runs superficially between the tendon of the flexor carpi radialis and the palmaris longus before it continues through the carpal tunnel under the flexor retinaculum
    - Before the flexor retinaculum, it gives off a palmar branch (sensory) which crosses the wrist over the flexor retinaculum
    - It is cutaneous to the palmar aspect and nails of the flexor and nails of the three-and-a-half radial digits and a corresponding area of the palm (Fig 1.18)

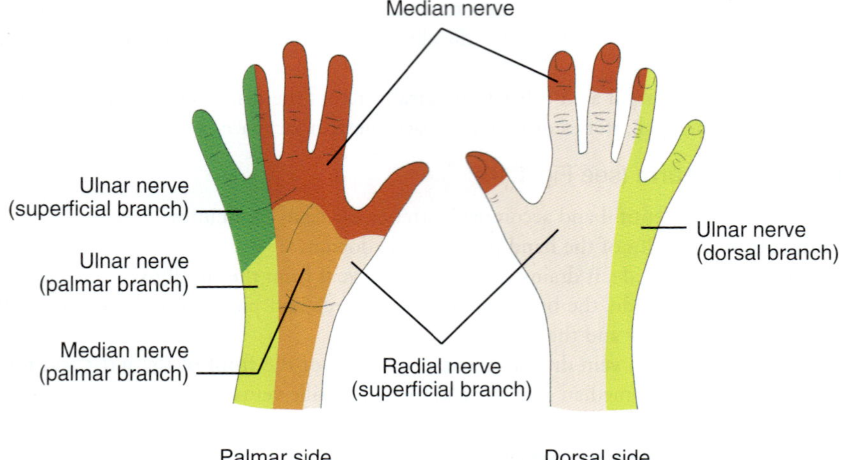

Fig. 1.18 Sensory distribution of the hand. Left: palmar view. Right: dorsal view.

- Ulnar nerve
  - Enters by passing between the two heads of the flexor carpi ulnaris
  - Lies between the flexor carpi ulnaris and the flexor digitorum profundus
  - Supplies the flexor digitorum profundus (medial half) and the flexor carpi ulnaris
  - Gives off a dorsal branch and innervates the dorsal side of the hand and ulnar one-and-a-half fingers
  - Gives off a palmar branch and passes over the flexor retinaculum and supplies skin over the hypothenar eminence and one-and-a-half fingers (palmar side) (see Fig 1.18)

Extensor Compartment

- Radial nerve
  - Splits into a deep branch and a superficial branch before supinator
  - The deep radial branch passes through the two heads of the supinator to become the posterior interosseous nerve
  - The superficial branch runs under the brachioradialis and then over the abductor pollicis longus, the extensor pollicis longus and the extensor pollicis brevis at the distal end of the forearm
  - Supplies all muscles of the extensor compartment: the brachioradialis, the extensor carpi radialis longus, the muscles arising from the common extensor attachment, the deep muscles of the extensor compartment and sensory supply to the interosseous membrane and the periosteum
  - It has no cutaneous branch in the forearm
  - Supplies the skin of the radial three-and-a-half digits (falling short of the nail beds) and a corresponding area of the dorsum (see Fig 1.18)
- Posterior interosseous nerve
  - Supplies the muscle arising from the common extensor attachment and deep muscles of the extensor compartment
  - Sensory supply to the interosseous membrane and the periosteum, with no cutaneous branch

Part 9 Wrist and Hand

DORSUM OF THE HAND

- Cutaneous innervation is by the radial nerve (three-and-a-half) and the ulnar nerve (one-and-a-half), with the distal phalanges supplied by the median and superficial ulnar (see Fig 1.18)
- Large veins forming the dorsal venous network (superficial to the extensor tendons) drain from the palm
- Wrist extensors (the extensor carpi radialis brevis and longus and the extensor carpi ulnaris) are inserted into the proximal part of the hand at the metacarpal bases
- More superficial are the extensor tendons of the fingers

WRIST JOINT

- Synovial joint formed proximally by the distal radius and articular disc (triangular fibrocartilage) and distally by the scaphoid, lunate and triquetral bones
- Triangular fibrocartilage holds the radius and ulnar together and separates the wrist (radiocarpal) from the radioulnar joint
- The capsule is thickened by the collateral ligaments and is much thicker in front than behind
- Two transverse rows of bones (four proximal and four distal):
  - Proximal row: scaphoid, lunate, triquetral and pisiform (lateral to medial)
  - Distal row: trapezium, trapezoid, capitate and hamate (lateral to medial)

PALM OF THE HAND

- Skin is characterised by the flexure creases which form by the palmaris brevis being attached directly to the dermis (panniculus carnosus)
- Cutaneous innervation is by superficial and palmar branches of the ulnar nerve, median nerve and radial nerve (see Fig 1.18)
- The palmar aponeurosis is the degenerated tendon of the palmaris longus; it fans out from the flexor retinaculum into four slips (one for each finger)
- Superficial fibres are inserted into the skin
- The main part divides and inserts into the deep transverse ligament of the palm
- Its function is mechanical and gives attachment to the skin to aid in gripping
- The flexor retinaculum is a strong band attached to the scaphoid tubercle and trapezium ridge (laterally/radial side), and the pisiform and hook of the hamate (medially, ulnar side)
  - Muscles of thenar and hypothenar eminences arise from the retinaculum and several structures pass across it
  - Both the tendon of the palmaris longus and the palmar aponeuroses are fused to the retinaculum
  - The ulnar nerve lies on the retinaculum (alongside the pisiform) with the ulnar artery on its radial side. The ulnar nerve divides into superficial and deep branches after passing the retinaculum

Thenar Eminence

Three short muscles originating from the flexor retinaculum:

- Abductor pollicis brevis arises from the flexor retinaculum and scaphoid tubercle and is inserted into the radial side of the proximal phalanx and extensor policis longus
- Flexor pollicis brevis arises from the flexor retinaculum and trapezium and is inserted into the radial sesamoid of the thumb and proximal phalanx

- Opponens pollicis lies deep to the above, arises from the flexor retinaculum and trapezium and is inserted into the radial border of the metacarpal bone of the thumb
- All three muscles are supplied by the recurrent branch (muscular branch) of the median nerve which comes off the median nerve after it passes through the carpal tunnel

Hypothenar Eminence

- Abductor digiti minimi: arises from the pisiform and flexor retinaculum and is inserted into the ulnar side of the proximal phalanx and into the extensor expansion
- Flexor digiti minimi brevis: arises from the flexor retinaculum and is inserted into the base of the proximal phalanx
- Opponens digiti minimi: arises from the flexor retinaculum and hamate hook and is inserted into the ulnar side of the fifth metacarpal bone
- All three muscles are supplied by the deep branch of the ulnar nerve

Digital Nerves

- Lie immediately deep to the superficial palmar arch
- Divide into the proper palmar digital nerves (arteries lie dorsal to the nerve) and are destined to supply fingertip pads and nail beds
- Superficial branch of the ulnar nerve divides into medial (medial side of the little finger) and lateral (lateral side of the little finger and medial side of the ring finger)
- Median nerve enters beneath the flexor retinaculum
    - Medial branch: divides into two and supplies palmar skin, the cleft and adjacent sides of the ring and middle fingers and the cleft and adjacent sides of the middle and index fingers. The latter branch supplies the second lumbrical muscle
    - Lateral branch: supplies the palmar skin, the radial side of the index finger, and the whole of the thumb. The branch to the index finger supplies the first lumbrical muscle
    - Muscular branch (recurrent): curls upwards around the distal border of the flexor retinaculum to supply the thenar muscles

Carpal Tunnel (Fig 1.19)

- A bony gutter with passage of the superficial and profundus tendons, the flexor pollicis longus and the median nerve
- All eight tendons (superficial and profundus tendons) share a common synovial sheath which is reflected inwards (i.e. opening towards the radial side)

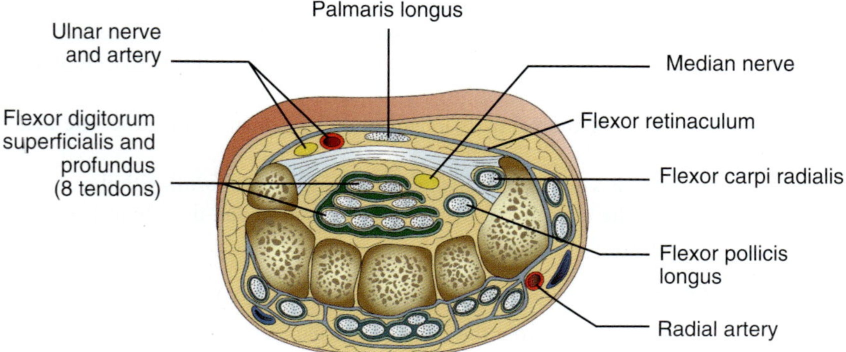

Fig. 1.19 Carpal tunnel and its contents, transverse section.

Carpal Tunnel Syndrome

- Main symptom is compression of the median nerve and results in wasting of the thenar muscles and anaesthesia over the radial three-and-a-half digits. There is no anaesthesia over the thenar eminence as this is usually supplied by the palmar branch, which passes superficially to the flexor retinaculum.

Adductor Pollicis

- Lies deeply in the palm in contact with metacarpal bones and interossei
  - **Transverse head:** arises from the whole length of the palmar border of the third metacarpal bone and inserts into the base of the proximal phalanx and the tendon of the extensor pollicis longus
  - **Oblique head:** arises from the second and third metacarpals and adjacent carpal bones and the fibres of this head run edge to edge with the transverse head and converge with it on the ulnar sesamoid
- Supplied by the deep branch of the ulnar nerve

RADIAL ARTERY IN THE HAND

- Slopes across the anatomical snuffbox over the trapezium and passes into the hand between the two heads of the first dorsal interosseous. Between the first dorsal interosseous and the adductor pollicis, the artery divides into two large branches
- Gives off the arteria radialis indicis and the princeps pollicis artery before passing between the two heads of the adductor pollicis to form the deep palmar arch (Fig 1.20)
- Deep palmar arch: an arterial arcade formed by the radial artery and anastomosing with the deep branch of the ulnar artery

Superficial Palmar Arch (Often Not a Complete Arch)

- An arterial arcade lying superficially (just deep to the palmar aponeurosis) as a direct continuation of the ulnar artery
- Gives off the palmar digital artery (little finger), and three common palmar digital arteries
- All are directed towards the nail beds

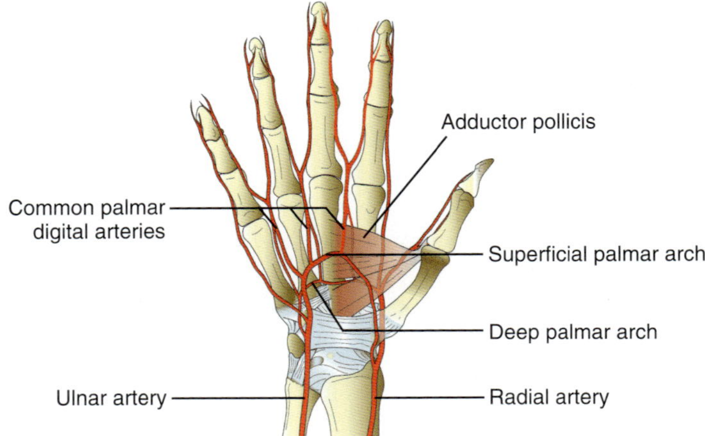

Fig. 1.20 Arterial supply of the hand.

ULNAR NERVE IN THE HAND (See Fig 1.15)

- Enters the hand beneath the flexor carpi ulnaris tendon, then runs on the flexor retinaculum, where it divides into superficial and deep branches after passing the retinaculum
  - Superficial branch: supplies the palmaris brevis, then continues on as digital nerves to one-and-a-half fingers. The small palmar branch supplies the skin over the hypothenar muscles
  - Deep branch: supplies the three hypothenar muscles, two lumbricals (ulnar side), all interossei and the adductor pollicis

INTEROSSEI MUSCLES

- **Palmar interossei** are smaller and arise from their own metacarpal bone
- **Dorsal interossei** are larger and arise from the adjacent sides of the metacarpal bones of the space in which they lie. There is no distal attachment to the first and fifth proximal phalanges and there is one on each side of the third proximal phalanx
- Action: **palmar interossei** adduct towards the middle finger (PAD) and the **dorsal interossei** abduct (DAB).
- All are supplied by the deep branch of the ulnar nerve

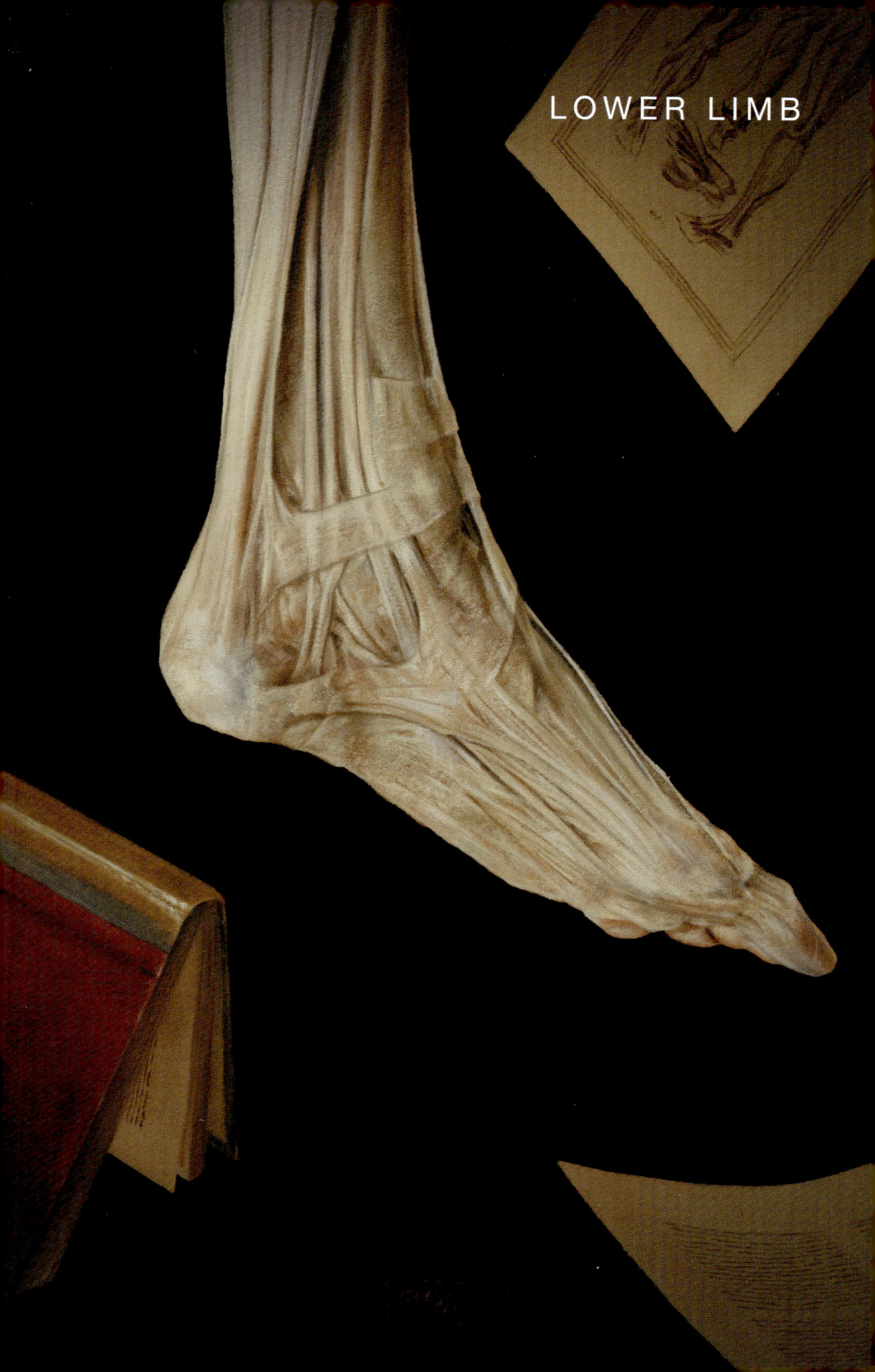

LOWER LIMB

CHAPTER 2

Lower Limb

CHAPTER OUTLINE

Part 1 Anterior Compartment of the Thigh

SKIN AND SUBCUTANEOUS TISSUE

Contains cutaneous nerves, lymphatic vessels and nodes, the small and great saphenous veins together with their tributaries and superficial branches of the femoral artery.

Superficial Nerves (Fig 2.1)

Cutaneous nerves are derived from the first three lumbar nerves.

- Ilioinguinal nerve: a collateral branch of the iliohypogastric nerve (L1), it passes through the anterior abdominal wall in the neurovascular plane (supplying lower parts of the conjoint tendon). It then emerges on the front of the spermatic cord at the superficial inguinal ring. It also supplies: the root of the penis, the anterior third of the scrotum and a small area of the thigh
- Femoral branch of the genitofemoral nerve (L1, 2): it lies on the psoas and passes with the external iliac artery and the femoral artery into the femoral sheath, then pierces it anteriorly to supply the skin over the femoral triangle
- Medial femoral cutaneous nerve: a branch of the anterior division of the femoral nerve, it supplies the medial side of the thigh with terminal twigs to the patellar plexus
- Intermediate femoral cutaneous nerve: a branch of the femoral nerve, it passes vertically downwards beneath the fascia lata to supply the front of the thigh down to the knee
- Lateral femoral cutaneous nerve: a branch of the lumbar plexus, it passes beneath and then within the iliac fascia and then beneath (or through) the inguinal ligament just medial to anterior superior iliac spine (ASIS). It divides into anterior and posterior branches which separately pierce the fascia lata below the lateral end of the inguinal ligament
  - Anterior branch (L3): supplies the anterolateral surface of the thigh
  - Posterior branch (L2): supplies the posterolateral aspect of the thigh

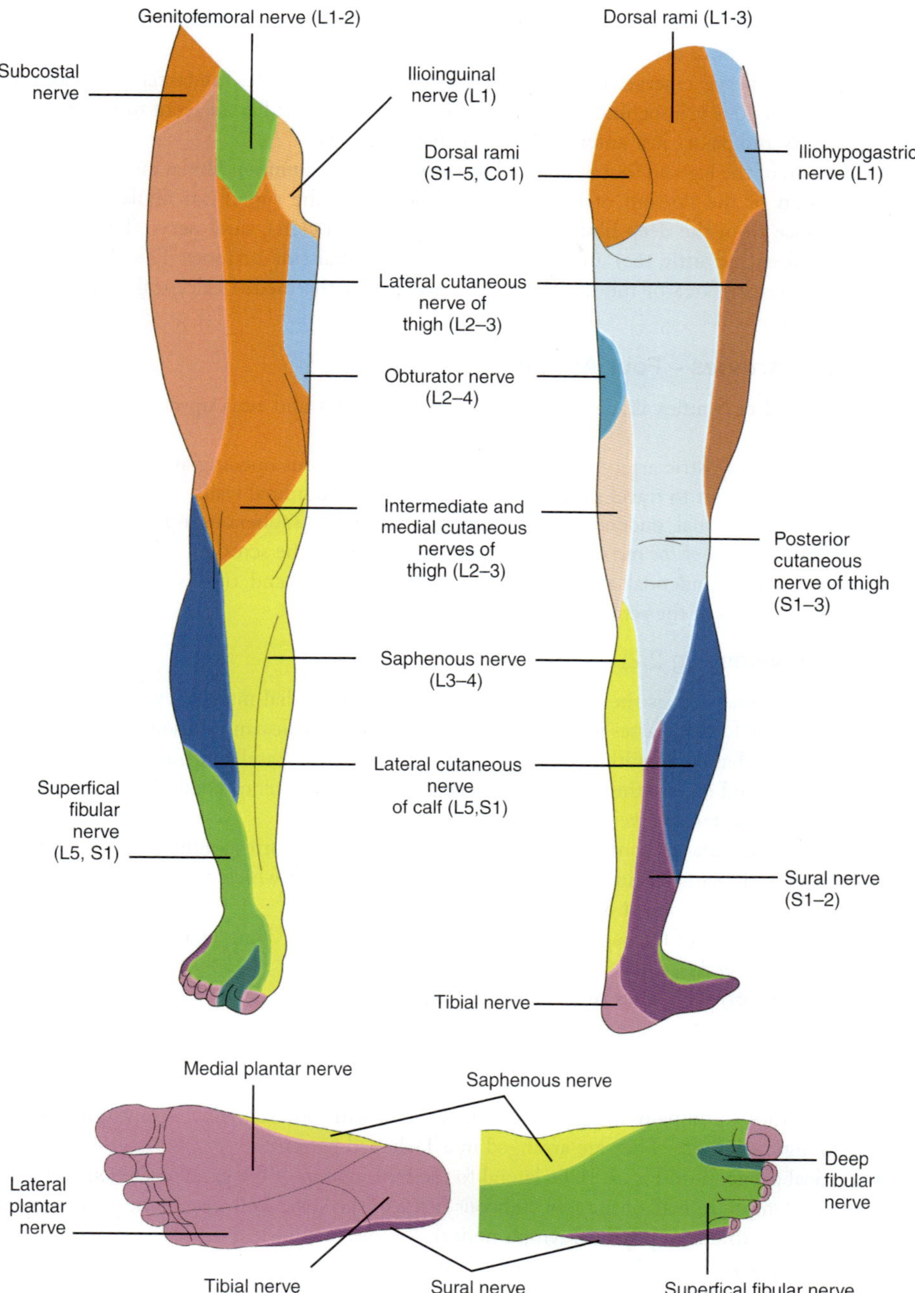

Fig. 2.1 Sensory distribution of the lower limb.

- Obturator nerve (L2–4): sends cutaneous branches to supply the medial aspect of the thigh
- Most of the posterior skin of the thigh is supplied by the posterior cutaneous nerve of the thigh (S1–3), which extends part way down the back of the calf where the sural nerve takes over

- Patellar plexus: a fine network of communicating branches that is formed from twigs of many of the above nerves
- Saphenous nerve: emerges from the adductor canal and perforates the fascia lata to join the great saphenous vein behind the medial aspect of the knee. It lies adjacent to the vein as it descends and passes just anterior to the medial malleolus
- The skin of the leg and foot is supplied by the saphenous, common fibular and tibial nerves. The skin of the dorsum of the foot is innervated by the superficial fibular nerve with assistance from the deep fibular nerve (first interdigital cleft), sural nerve (lateral margin of the foot and little toe) and saphenous nerve (medial side of foot). The skin over the weight-bearing area of the heel is mostly supplied by the medial calcaneal branch of the tibial nerve

Superficial Arteries – Four Arteries

- Superficial circumflex iliac artery: pierces the fascia lata and runs upwards to supply the ASIS
- Superficial epigastric artery: emerges through the saphenous opening and then crosses the inguinal ligament to travel superiorly up the anterior abdominal wall
- Superficial external pudendal artery: emerges from the saphenous opening and passes medially *in front of the spermatic cord* to supply the skin of the scrotum
- Deep external pudendal artery: emerges further medially and travels *behind the cord* to supply the skin of the scrotum

Superficial Veins (Fig 2.2)

The great saphenous vein is the upward continuation of the medial marginal vein of the dorsal venous arch of the foot. It passes just anterior to the medial malleolus and runs up the medial side of the leg. It lies a hand's breadth behind the medial border of the patella. It travels up the medial side of the thigh and pierces the cribriform fascia covering the saphenous opening in the femoral triangle to enter the femoral vein on its anteromedial aspect.

- Numerous tributaries converge on the upper end, generally corresponding with the arteries
- The great saphenous vein contains up to 20 valves, most of which are below the knee but there is a constant one at the saphenofemoral junction
- Surface anatomy of the saphenofemoral junction is about 2–3 cm lateral to and just below the pubic tubercle

The small (short) saphenous vein originates from the lateral side of the foot behind the lateral malleolus and ascends the calf posteriorly in the midline.

Lymph Nodes and Vessels (Fig 2.3)

Large lymphatics accompany the great saphenous vein, with other channels converging on the superficial inguinal nodes. They are arranged in a T-shaped pattern:

- Vertical group (1 on Fig. 2.3): lie lateral to the termination of the great saphenous vein and receive lymph from all of the subcutaneous tissue of the lower limb except the posterolateral calf (which drains to popliteal lymph nodes)
- Lateral group (2): lie laterally below the inguinal ligament and receive lymph from the buttock, ipsilateral flank and back below the umbilicus
- Medial group (3): lie medially below the inguinal ligament and receive lymph from the anterior abdominal wall below the umbilicus and perineum including the distal segment of the anal canal and vagina and the external genitalia (*but NOT the testicle*)
- Efferents: converge towards the saphenous opening to drain into the deep inguinal nodes (medial to the femoral vein)

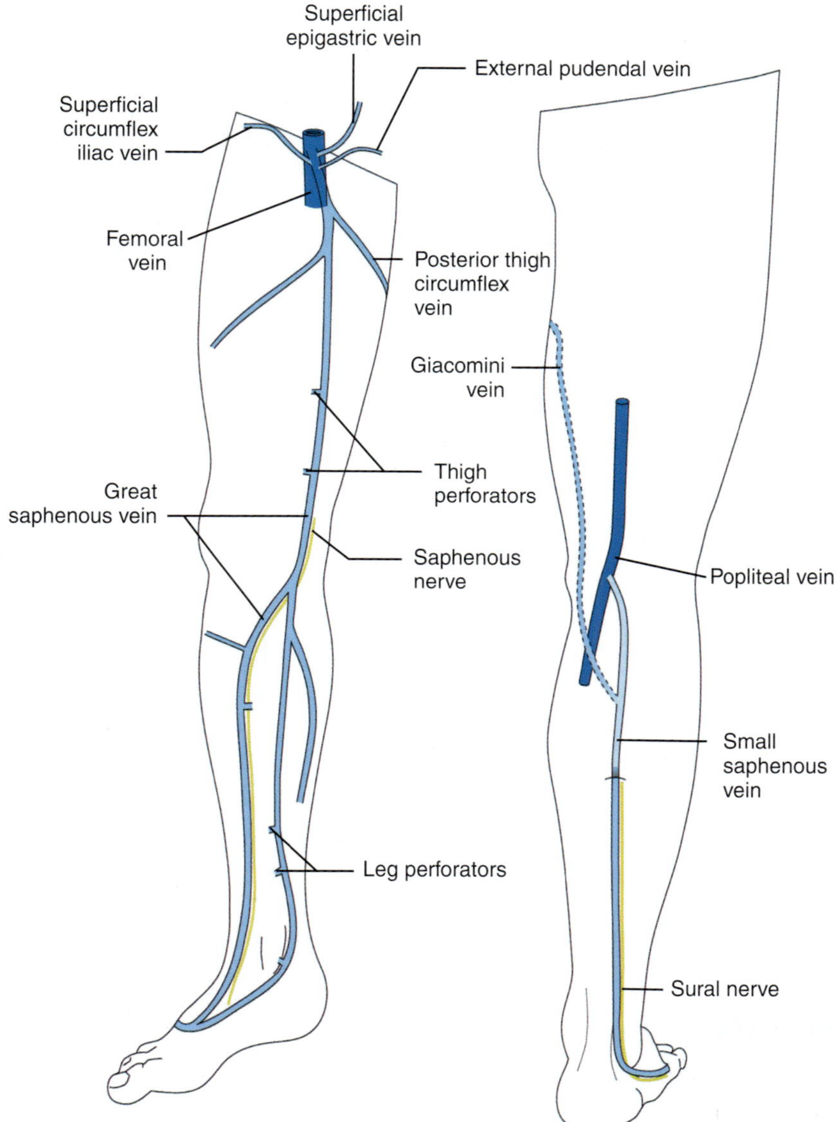

Fig. 2.2 Superficial veins of the lower limb. Left: Anterior view. Right: Posterior view.

- The deep inguinal nodes include one or two lymph nodes inside the femoral canal. They receive lymph from three sources: superficial inguinal nodes, deep lymphatics accompanying the lower limb arteries, and, *importantly*, lymphatics from the glans penis and clitoris

Superficial Fascia

Scarpa's fascia extends below the inguinal ligament and fixes to the fascia lata.

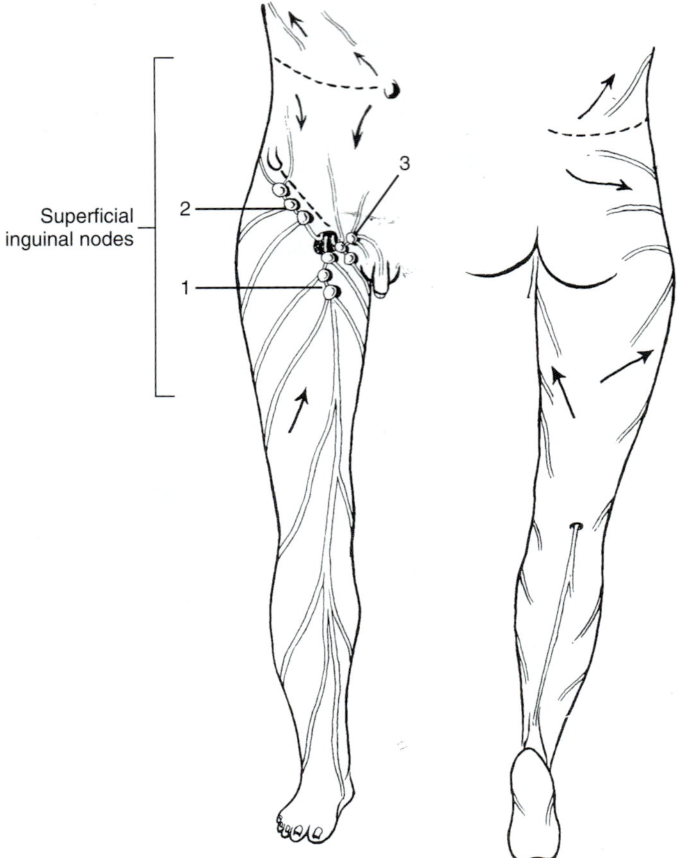

Fig. 2.3 Superficial lymphatics of the lower limb (superficial inguinal lymph nodes).

FASCIA LATA (Fig 2.4)

This is a thickening of the fascia extending vertically downwards to be inserted on exposed bony points around the knee joint. It is attached along a line from the pubic tubercle, the inferior border of the inguinal ligament, the anterior superior iliac spine and the outer lip of the iliac crest as far back as the posterior gluteal line, where it turns inferiorly along the sacrum and sacrotuberous ligament to reach the ischial tuberosity. From here, it turns superiorly to attach to the ischiopubic ramus and body of the pubic bone. The fascia splits twice into two layers to enclose the tensor fascia latae laterally and the gluteus maximus posteriorly.

- The arrangment of the fascia lata on its anteromedial part creates a small defect in the fascia which is covered by a layer of loose connective tissue called the cribrifom fascia, and is perforated by the great saphenous vein and lymphatics. This defect is called the saphenous opening
- Innervation: superior gluteal nerve

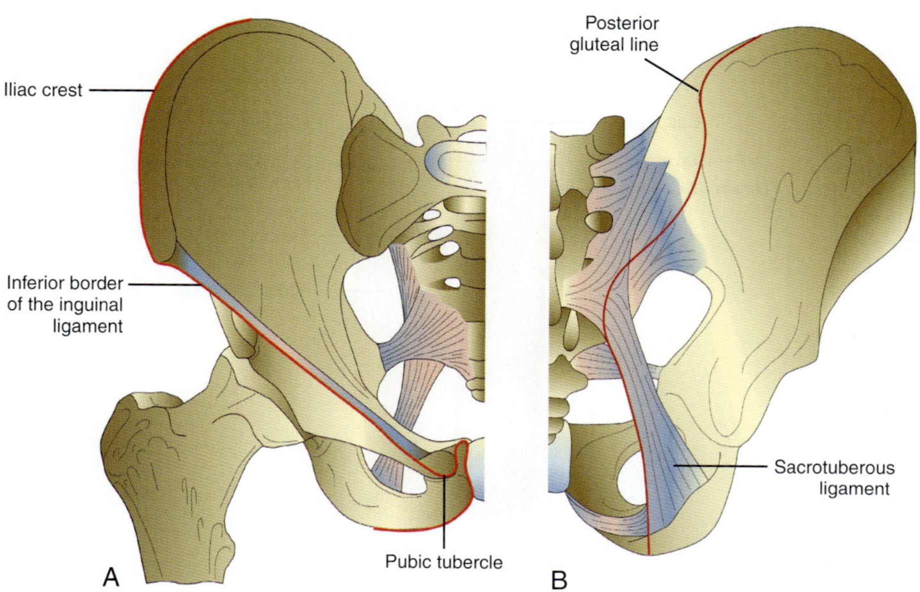

Fig. 2.4 Origin of the fascia lata. **(A)** Anterior view. **(B)** Posterior view.

Tensor Fascia Lata

This is a thin triangular sheet of muscle enclosed by the fascia lata. It originates from the iliac crest between the anterior superior iliac spine and the tubercle and inserts distally into the fascia lata of the iliotibial tract. The muscle is innervated by the superior gluteal nerve (L4, 5, S1).

Iliotibial Tract (Iliotibial Band)

This is a longitudinal thickening of the fascia lata, which extends along the lateral aspect of the thigh between the tubercle of the iliac crest and a facet on the anterolateral surface of the lateral tibial condyle. The tract encloses the tensor fascia lata and the major part of the gluteus maximus is inserted into it posteriorly. In the lower thigh, the lateral intermuscular septum connects the iliotibial tract to the linea aspera of the femur.

FEMORAL TRIANGLE (Fig 2.5)

Boundaries

- Lies between the inguinal ligament (base), the medial border of the sartorius (lateral border) and the medial border of the adductor longus (medial border) creating a gutter-shaped floor
- The roof is formed by the fascia lata, subcutaneous tissue and skin
- From lateral to medial, the floor is formed by the iliacus, psoas, pectineus, adductor brevis (small portion) and the adductor longus

Contents

- The femoral nerve, femoral artery, femoral vein and femoral canal containing lymphatics (from lateral to medial)

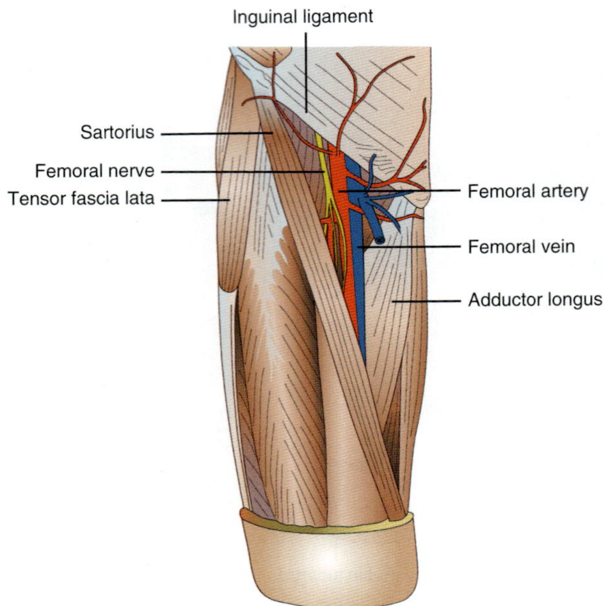

Fig. 2.5 Boundaries and contents of the femoral triangle.

TABLE 2.1 ■ **Muscles Forming the Borders and Floor of the Femoral Triangle**

Muscle	Proximal Attachment	Distal Attachment	Concentric Action	Innervation
Sartorius	Anterior superior iliac spine	Just medial to tibial tuberosity in front of gracilis and semitendinosus	Flexes, abducts and laterally rotates the thigh at the hip	Femoral nerve (L2–4)
			Flexes and medially rotates the leg at the knee	
Iliacus	Iliac fossa	Lesser trochanter and adjacent distal area of femur	Flexes the hip	Femoral nerve (L2, 3)
Psoas major	T12–L5 intervertebral discs and adjacent margins of vertebral bodies and transverse process of L1–5	Lesser trochanter and adjacent distal area of femur	Flexes the hip	Anterior primary rami of L1–3 (mainly L2)
Pectineus	Pectineal line of pubis	Upper end of femur below lesser trochanter	Flexes and adducts the thigh	Femoral nerve (L2, 3) ± Obturator nerve (L2, 3)
Adductor longus	Body of pubis	Lower $^2/_3$ of linea aspera	Adducts the hip	Obturator nerve (L2–4)
Adductor brevis	Inferior ramus and body of pubis	Upper $^1/_3$ of linea aspera	Adducts the hip	Obturator nerve (L2–4)

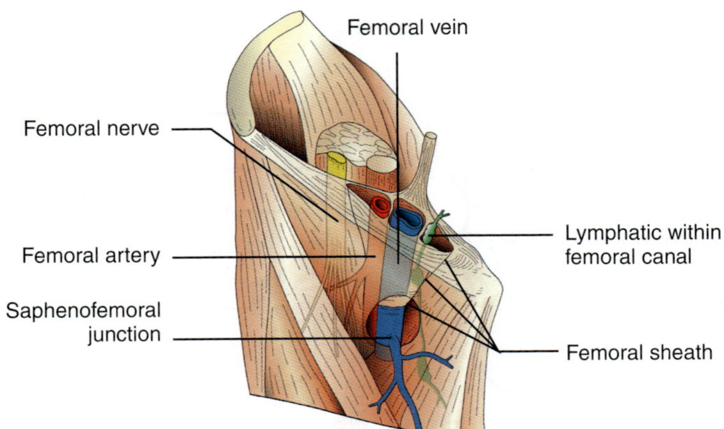

Fig. 2.6 Femoral sheath and its relations.

Femoral Sheath (Fig 2.6)

This is a funnel-shaped prolongation of two fasciae surrounding the femoral vessels passing beneath the inguinal ligament.

- It is formed by the transversalis fascia anteriorly and the iliacus fascia posteriorly. These both fuse with adventitia of the femoral artery and vein about an inch below the inguinal ligament. The sheath's presence allows for freedom of movement
- The sheath has three compartment: lateral (contains the femoral artery), intermediate (contains the femoral vein) and medial (the femoral **space** or **canal** contains fat, lymphatics and lymph nodes)
- The femoral branch of the genitofemoral nerve also lies within the sheath adjacent to the femoral artery, but pierces the sheath just distal to the inguinal ligament to supply the skin of the upper anterior part of the femoral triangle
- The femoral ring (entrance to the femoral canal) has four boundaries:
  - *Anteriorly* by the inguinal ligament
  - *Medially* by the crescentic lateral edge of the lacunar ligament
  - *Posteriorly* by the pectineal ligament
  - *Laterally* by the femoral vein

FEMORAL ARTERY (Fig 2.7)

- Enters midway between the anterior superior iliac spine and the pubic symphysis (surface marking)
- Courses downwards to enter the adductor canal at the apex of the femoral triangle and disappears below the sartorius
- Has four small branches below the inguinal ligament (in the femoral triangle) and then gives off the large profunda femoris artery
- Branches arising below the inguinal ligament are: the superficial epigastric artery, superficial circumflex iliac artery, superficial external pudendal artery and deep external pudendal artery

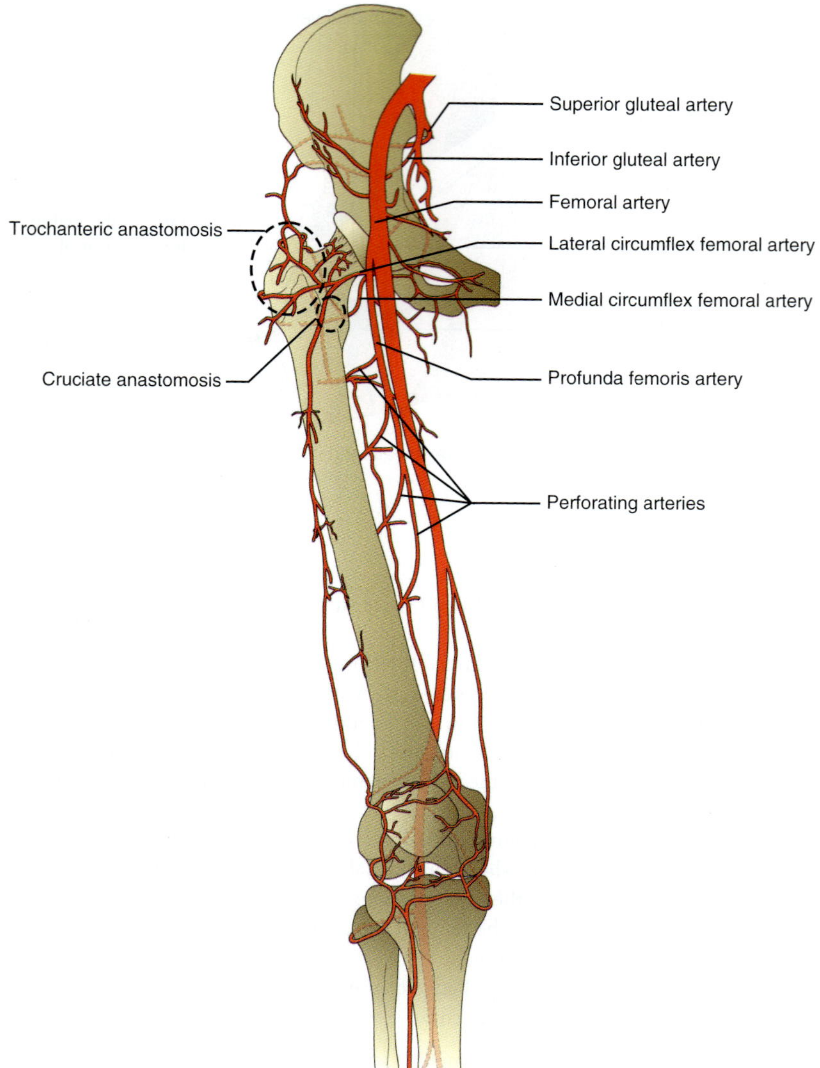

Fig. 2.7 Branches of the femoral artery.

- Profunda femoris – a vessel of the thigh muscles, arises about 4 cm below the inguinal ligament just beyond the termination of the femoral sheath and has a number of branches:
  - **Lateral circumflex femoral artery:** arises from the lateral side of the profunda femoris artery. It passes laterally *between the superficial and deep branches of the femoral nerve*
    - Ascending branch: runs up under under the sartorius and tensor fascia lata along the vastus lateralis and may contribute to the trochanteric anastomosis before ending in the arterial anastomosis around the anterior superior iliac spine
    - Transverse branch: crosses the vastus lateralis to contribute to the cruciate anastomosis
    - Descending branch: descends between the vastus lateralis and the vastus medialis and ends at about the level of the distal femur
  - **Medial circumflex femoral artery:** arises from the medial side of the profunda artery and passes backwards, ending by dividing on the quadratus femoris into an ascending (to the

trochanteric anastomosis) and a transverse branch (to the cruciate anastomosis). This branch is the dominant supply to the hip joint

- **Perforating arteries** (4 in number): pass through adductor magnus backwards and upwards, and supply the adductor muscles and hamstrings

- Both the *medial and lateral circumflex femoral* arteries contribute to two arterial anastomostic networks around the hip. The most important is the trochanteric anastomosis, which lies near the trochanteric fossa of the femur, creating an extracapsular arterial ring around the femoral neck. There is also a cruciate anastomosis lying posteriorly at the level of the lesser trochanter near the lower edge of the femoral attachment of the quadratus femoris.

Femoral Vein

- The continuation of the popliteal vein as it passes up through the adductor hiatus
- Receives a tributary corresponding to the profunda femoris artery
- The great saphenous vein joins its anteromedial side at the saphenofemoral junction. The femoral vein is differentiated from the great saphenous vein by not having tributaries at this point

Femoral Nerve

- A nerve of the extensor/anterior compartment, formed from the anterior rami L2–4
- Enters the thigh lateral to the femoral sheath and within a few centimetres divides into superficial (or anterior) and deep (or posterior) groups, which are often separated by the *lateral circumflex femoral artery*
- Superficial group:
  - Cutaneous (two): intermediate and medial femoral cutaneous nerves
  - Muscular (two): sartorius and pectineus
- Deep group:
  - Cutaneous: saphenous nerve to the medial side of the leg and foot
  - Muscular: quadratus femoris
    - Supplies the hip joint
    - Nerve to the rectus femoris (ususally two branches) and
    - Nerve to the vastus medialis (large branch), others to the vastus lateralis and intermedius
    - Nerve to the articularis genus

Quadriceps Femoris

TABLE 2.2 ■ **Summary of the Quadriceps Femoris Muscle**

Muscle	Proximal Attachment	Distal Attachment	Concentric Action	Innervation
Rectus femoris	Straight head from anterior inferior iliac spine; reflected head from ilium just above acetabulum	Quadriceps tendon and patella and continues as patellar ligament	Extends the leg at the knee and flexes the thigh at the hip	Femoral nerve (L2–4)
Vastus lateralis	Lateral margins of femur (intertrochanteric line, greater trochanter, gluteal tuberosity, linea aspera and lateral supracondylar line) and lateral intermuscular septum		Extends knee	
Vastus intermedius	Upper $^{2}/_{3}$ of anterior and lateral shaft of femur		Extends knee	
Vastus medialis	Medial margins of femur (intertrochanteric line, pectineal line, linea aspera, and medial supracondylar line) and medial intermuscular septum		Extends knee	

Adductor Canal (Fig 2.8)

The adductor canal (subsartorial or Hunter's canal) is an intermuscular gutter on the medial aspect of the thigh extending from the apex of the femoral triangle to the adductor hiatus, which is an opening in the tendon of the adductor magnus adjacent to the femur just above the knee. The canal is triangular in cross-section and is bounded:

- Posteriorly by the adductor longus above and the adductor magnus below
- Anterolaterally by the vastus medialis
- Anteromedially (the roof of the canal) by a strong layer of fascia under the sartorius

The adductor canal contains the:

- Femoral artery lying between the saphenous nerve and the femoral vein at all levels in the thigh. Its descending genicular branch is given off just above the hiatus
- Nerve to the vastus medialis
- Saphenous nerve, which communicates with cutaneous branches of the obturator nerve and the medial cutaneous nerve of the thigh in the canal

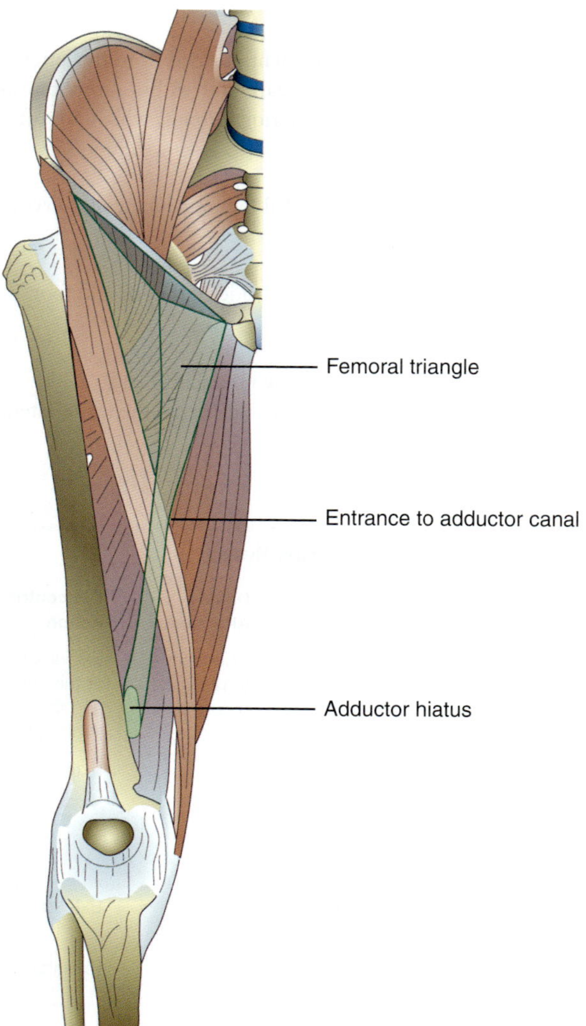

Fig. 2.8 Adductor canal and its relations.

Part 2 Medial Compartment of the Thigh

The medial (or adductor) compartment of the thigh is separated from the anterior (or extensor) compartment by the medial intermuscular septum passing from the linea aspera of the femur over the anterior surface of the pectineus, the adductor longus and the lower part of the adductor magnus to the fascia lata. There is no intermuscular septum between the medial compartment and the posterior (or flexor) compartment containing the hamstring muscles.

ADDUCTOR MUSCLES

TABLE 2.3 ■ **Summary of the Adductor Muscles**

Muscle	Proximal Attachment	Distal Attachment	Concentric Action	Innervation
Gracilis	Outer surface of the ischiopubic ramus	Medial surface of proximal tibia	Adducts hip Flexes knee and medially rotates the flexed knee	Obturator nerve (L2–4)
Adductor longus	Body of pubis	Lower $^2/_3$ of linea aspera	Adducts the hip	
Adductor brevis	Inferior ramus and body of pubis	Upper $^1/_3$ of linea aspera	Adducts the hip	
Adductor magnus	Adductor portion: ischiopubic ramus	Posterior surface of proximal femur, linea aspera and upper part of medial supracondylar line	Adducts hip	
	Hamstring portion: ischial tuberosity	Adductor tubercle and lower part of medial supracondylar line	Extends hip	Sciatic nerve: tibial part

OBTURATOR ARTERY

The obturator artery emerges from the obturator foramen along with the obturator vein and nerve. It then divides into medial and lateral branches, which encircle the outer aspect of the obturator membrane deep to the obturator externus, and anastomoses with the medial circumflex femoral artery (cruciate anastomosis).

- From the lateral branch arises a small acetabular branch to the hip joint through the acetabular notch into the ligament of the head of femur.

OBTURATOR NERVE

The obturator nerve (L2–4) is formed in the lumbar plexus within the psoas major. It runs downwards on the medial side of the psoas and exits the pelvis through the obturator foramen. It splits into two divisions; the anterior division descends in front of adductor brevis and the posterior division behind:

- Anterior division: passes in front of the obturator externus above and the adductor brevis below and runs downwards behind the pectineus and adductor longus. It sends a branch to the hip joint, communicates with cutaneous branches of the femoral nerve in the adductor canal and supplies skin on the medial aspect of the thigh (subsartorial plexus)
  - Supplies the adductor longus, brevis and gracilis

- Posterior division: passes through the obturator externus and then runs downwards *behind* the adductor brevis and on the adductor magnus. It enters the popliteal fossa via the adductor hiatus and sends a twig to the kee joint, which accompanies the middle genicular artery
  - Supplies the adductor magnus muscle and obturator externus

Part 3 Gluteal Region and Hip Joint

The gluteal (buttock) region lies on the posterior aspect of the pelvis and extends from the iliac crest above to the gluteal fold below, and from a line joining the greater trochanter and anterior superior iliac spine laterally to the midline. The region provides a conduit for various muscles, vessels and nerves passing between the pelvis and the lower limb. The gluteal region has two groups of muscles classified rather loosely as superficial and deep (see table below).

GREATER AND LESSER SCIATIC FORAMINA (Fig 2.9)

The sacrotuberous and sacrospinous ligaments convert the greater and lesser sciatic notches of the pelvis into greater and lesser sciatic foramina, respectively.

The Greater Sciatic Foramen Boundaries

- Superiorly and anteriorly by the greater sciatic notch of the hip bone, posteriorly by the sacrotuberous ligament, and inferiorly by the sacrospinous ligament and ischial spine

The Lesser Sciatic Foramen Boundaries

- Anteriorly by the lesser sciatic notch of the hip bone, posteriorly by the sacrotuberous ligament, and superiorly by the ischial spine and sacrospinous ligament
- The lesser sciatic foramen transmits four structures: the tendon of the obturator internus, the nerve to the obturator internus, the pudendal nerve and the internal pudendal vessels

Numerous neurovascular structures emerge from the pelvis above or below the piriformis through the greater sciatic notch. The piriformis ('pear-shaped') is a key landmark in the gluteal region. It originates in the pelvis from the anterior surface of the sacrum and exits through the greater sciatic foramen, which it largely fills.

Emerging from the pelvis through the greater sciatic foramen above the upper border of piriformis are the:

- Superior gluteal nerve (L4, 5, S1), which runs laterally between the gluteus medius and the gluteus minimus and ends in the tensor fascia lata
- Superior gluteal artery, which gives off a superficial branch that supplies the gluteus maximus and the overlying skin, and a deep branch, which follows the same course as the nerve before dividing into an upper branch that reaches the ASIS and a deep branch that joins the trochanteric anastomosis

Emerging from the pelvis through the greater sciatic foramen below the lower border of piriformis are the:

- Inferior gluteal nerve (L5, S1, 2), which pierces the deep surface of the gluteus maximus
- Inferior gluteal artery, which runs with the nerve to supply the piriformis and gluteus maximus and gives off branches to the trochanteric and cruciate anastomoses
- Sciatic nerve (L4, 5, S1–3), which exits the pelvis through the greater sciatic foramen below the piriformis, lateral to the inferior gluteal and pudendal nerves and vessels. It runs over the posterior surface of the acetabulum (with the nerve to the quadratus femoris on its deep surface) and descends vertically over the obturator internus, gemelli and quadratus femoris to enter the posterior compartment of the thigh on the posterior surface of the adductor magnus

TABLE 2.4 ■ **Summary of the Gluteal Muscles**

Muscle		Proximal Attachment	Distal Attachment	Innervation	Concentric Action
Superficial	Gluteus maximus	Gluteal surface of ilium behind posterior gluteal line; fascia over erector spinae; dorsal sacrum and lateral coccyx; sacrotuberous ligament; fascia over gluteus medius	Iliotibial tract (superficial fibres) and gluteal tuberosity of proximal femur (deep fibres)	Inferior gluteal nerve (L5, S1, 2)	• Powerful thigh extensor (climbing stairs, running, raising trunk from bent forward position) • Lateral hip rotation • Extends knee (via iliotibial tract) • Assists with hip abduction
	Gluteus medius	Gluteal surface of ilium between iliac crest above and anterior and posterior gluteal lines below; overlying fascia	Lateral surface of greater trochanter	Superior gluteal nerve (L4, 5, S1)	• Abduct thigh • Prevent pelvic tilt when contralateral foot is lifted off ground in walking & running • Medial rotation of hip
	Gluteus minimus	Gluteal surface of ilium between anterior and inferior gluteal lines	Anterosuperior surface of greater trochanter and hip joint capsule		
Deep	Piriformis	Pelvic surface of S2–4 sacral segments between anterior sacral foramina	Apex of greater trochanter	Anterior rami of S1, 2	• Lateral rotation of hip • Abduction of hip when sitting
	Obturator internus	Deep surface of obturator membrane on pelvic side wall	Tendons fuse and insert into medial aspect of greater trochanter	Nerve to obturator internus (L5, S1, 2)	• Lateral rotation of extended hip (abducts flexed hip)
	Gemellus superior	Ischial spine			
	Gemellus inferior	schial tuberosity		Nerve to quadratus femoris (L4, 5, S1)	
	Quadratus femoris		Quadrate tubercle on intertrochanteric crest		• Lateral rotation of hip
	Obturator externus	Outer surface of obturator membrane and adjacent bone	Trochanteric fossa of femur	Obturator nerve (L2–4)	• Lateral rotation of extended hip (abducts flexed hip)

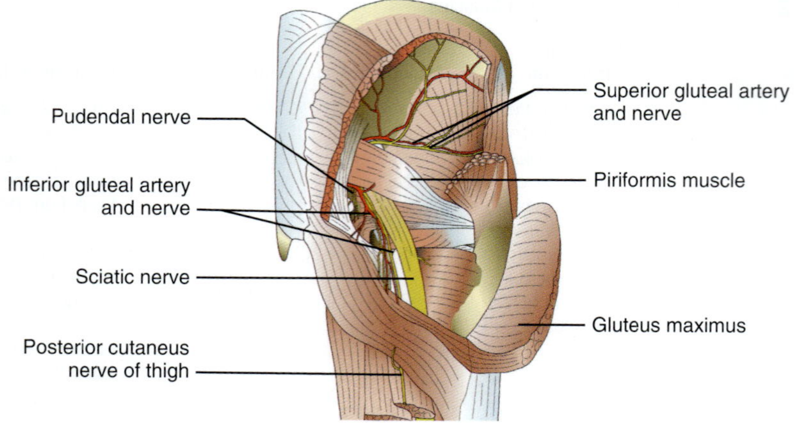

Fig. 2.9 Structures emerging through the greater and lesser sciatic foramina.

and deep to the biceps femoris. The posterior femoral cutaneous nerve and inferior gluteal artery lie on its medial side. The point of division of the sciatic nerve into its tibial and common fibular components is near the apex of the popliteal fossa, but a high division is not uncommon

- Posterior cutaneous nerve of thigh (S2, 3) (the posterior femoral cutaneous nerve), which runs medial to the sciatic nerve deep to the gluteus maximus. It travels down the back of the thigh deep to the fascia lata but superficial to the hamstring muscles before piercing the deep fascia behind the knee. Thereafter, it runs with the small saphenous vein about half way down the calf. It supplies the skin of the gluteal region, the posterior perineal region and the posterior aspect of the thigh and leg
- Pudendal nerve (S2–4), which makes only a brief appearance in the gluteal region. After emerging from the greater sciatic foramen below the piriformis, it turns around the sacrospinous ligament just medial to the ischial spine over the sacrospinous ligament to enter the perineum via the lesser sciatic foramen
- Internal pudendal artery, which follows a similar course on the lateral side of the pudendal nerve, crossing the tip of the ischial spine to enter the perineum (it is the dominant blood supply of the perineum and external genitalia)
- A nerve to the obturator internus (L5, S1, 2)
- A nerve to the quadratus femoris (L4, 5, S1)

HIP JOINT

The hip joint is a synovial joint of ball and socket type. The centre of the joint lies slightly below and lateral to the middle of the inguinal ligament.

Articular Surfaces

- Articulation occurs between the almost spherical femoral head and the cup-shaped acetabulum
- The femoral head forms roughly two-thirds of a sphere and is covered by hyaline cartilage except at the pit (fovea) where the ligament of the head of the femur (ligamentum teres) is attached

- The hemispherical acetabulum contains a C-shaped area of hyaline cartilage. Its concavity is deepened by the acetabular labrum, which covers slightly more than a hemisphere of the femoral head and spans the acetabular notch inferiorly, attaching to the outer edge of the transverse acetabular ligament
- The ligament of the head of the femur attaches to the transverse acetabular ligament

Capsule

The fibrous capsule is loose but strong and surrounds the head and neck of the femur.

- The capsule is medially attached to the circumference of the acetabular margin and the transverse acetabular ligament. Laterally the capsule surrounds the head and neck of the femur and extends to the intertrochanteric line on the femur anteriorly and two-thirds of the way along the femoral neck posteriorly
- The capsule is thicker anterosuperiorly and relatively thin posteroinferiorly, reflecting the distribution of biomechanical stress
- Some capsular fibres are reflected back along the neck of the femur as far as the articular margin of the femoral head; these retinacular fibres contain small arteries mostly from the trochanteric anastomosis that supply the head and neck of the femur
- The capsule has an inner collar of circular fibres (zona orbicularis), which clasp the femoral neck, and outer longitudinally oriented fibres

The synovial membrane is attached to the acetabular labrum and the transverse acetabular ligament and lines the internal surface of the joint capsule. It is reflected back up the neck of the femur, overlying the retinacular fibres, as far as the articular margin of the femoral head. The acetabular fat pad and ligament of the head of the femur are enclosed within a sleeve of synovial membrane that attaches to the margins of the acetabular fossa and fovea on the head of the femur.

Ligaments (Fig 2.10)

In addition to the two intrinsic ligaments of the hip joint, the ligament of the head of the femur and the transverse acetabular ligament, the fibrous capsule is reinforced by three extrinsic ligaments, each of which arises from a separate component of the hip bone and blends with the joint

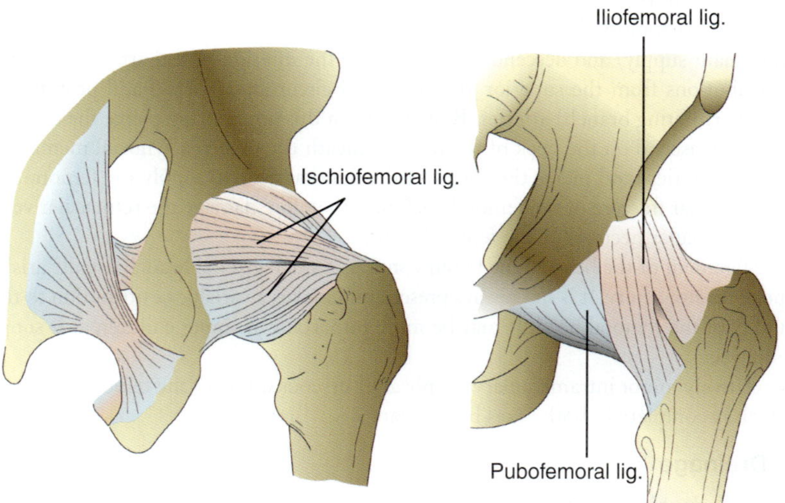

Fig. 2.10 Ligaments of the hip joint. Left: Posterior view. Right: Anterior view.

capsule; the iliofemoral ligament lies anterosuperiorly, the pubofemoral ligament lies inferiorly and the ischiofemoral ligament lies posteriorly.

- All three ligaments spiral around the femoral neck and become increasingly taut with hip extension
- The iliofemoral ligament limits external rotation, the pubofemoral ligament limits abduction, and the ischiofemoral ligament limits internal rotation
- The hip joint capsule is least taut when the hip is partially flexed, abducted and externally rotated and so this is the most comfortable position for a patient with a painful hip joint effusion

Relations

- Anteriorly (from medial to lateral): the pectineus and the overlying femoral vein, the tendon of the psoas major and the overlying femoral artery, the iliacus with the femoral nerve in the groove between it and the tendon of the psoas major, and the straight head of the rectus femoris together with the deep layer of the iliotibial tract fascia
- Superiorly (from medial to lateral): the reflected head of the rectus femoris and gluteus minimus
- Inferiorly: the obturator externus
- Posteriorly (from superior to inferior): the piriformis, the tendon of the obturator internus with the gemelli separating the joint from the sciatic nerve, the tendon of the obturator externus and an ascending branch of the medial circumflex femoral artery separating the joint from the quadratus femoris and sciatic nerve

Bursae

The joint may communicate with the subtendinous iliopsoas bursa via a small gap between the iliofemoral and the pubofemoral ligaments.

Blood Supply (Fig 2.11A and B)

The hip joint receives an arterial supply from several sources:

1. The head and intracapsular part of the neck of the femur is supplied from the trochanteric anastomosis, an extracapsular arterial ring encircling the neck of the femur just distal to the attachment of the fibrous capsule of the joint. It lies in the region of the trochanteric fossa. It is an anastomosis between the deep branch of the medial circumflex femoral artery (dominant supply) and descending branches of the inferior gluteal artery, with or without contributions from the superior gluteal, lateral circumflex femoral and profunda femoris (first perforating branch) arteries. Branches from this arterial ring pierce the capsule of the hip joint, ascend on the neck of the femur beneath the reflected synovial membrane (retinacular arteries) and pierce the cortex of the femoral neck to supply the femoral head. An intracapsular fracture of the femoral neck may therefore damage the retinacular vessels and cause avascular necrosis of the femoral head
2. The ligament of the head of the femur contains a small arterial branch usually arising from the obturator artery. It is not always present and makes a variable contribution to the blood supply of the femoral head. It may be more important in young children as it supplies the epiphysis
3. A relatively minor intramedullary supply after osseous union of the femoral head and neck, which is complete in both sexes by 18 years

Lymph Drainage

Drainage from the hip is to the inguinal and internal iliac lymph nodes.

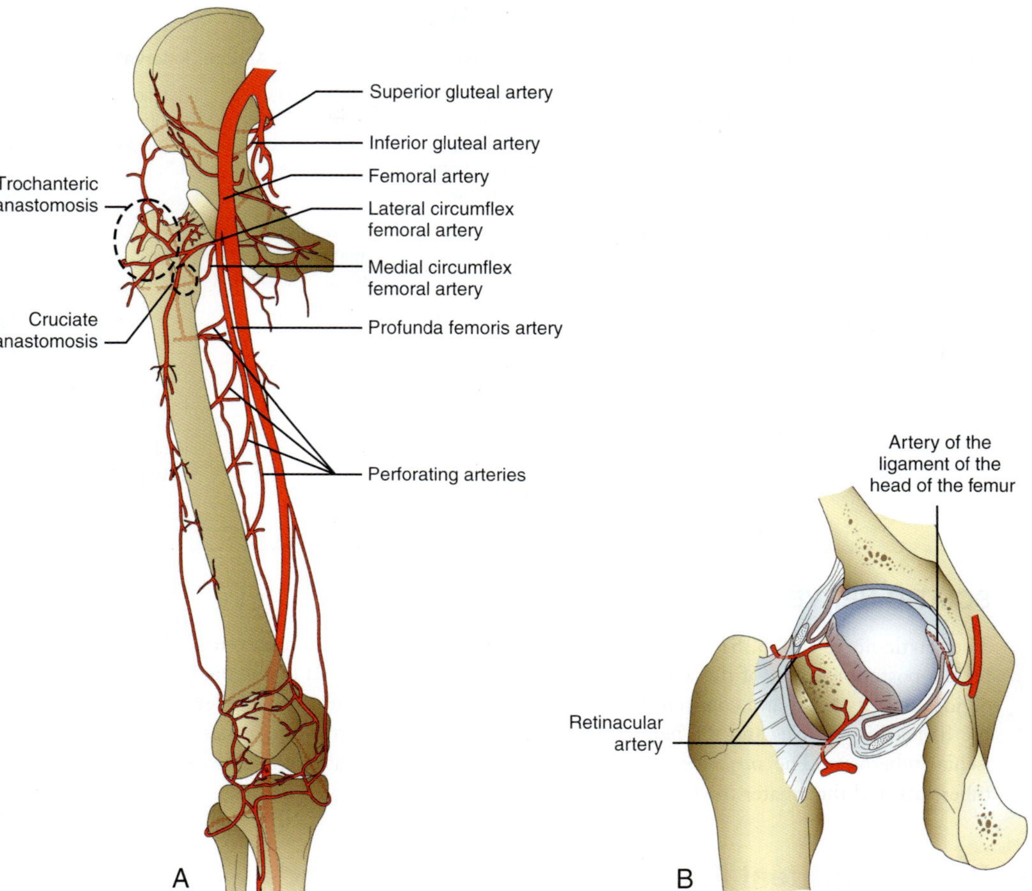

Fig. 2.11 **(A)** Femoral artery and blood supply of the hip (cruciate and trochanteric anastomosis). **(B)** Blood supply of the hip joint (artery of the head of the femur and retinacular arteries).

Nerve Supply

The anterior capsule of the hip joint is innervated by the femoral and obturator nerves and the posterior capsule by the sciatic nerve, superior gluteal nerve and nerve to the quadratus femoris.

Part 4 Posterior Compartment of the Thigh

The hamstring muscles (semimembranosus, semitendinosus and long head of the biceps femoris) arise from the ischial tuberosity, cross both the hip and knee joints, and the are supplied by the tibial component of the sciatic nerve (L5, S1, 2).

The short head of the biceps femoris arises from the femur and is not a true hamstring muscle; it is supplied by the common fibular component of the sciatic nerve. The hamstring muscles flex the knee but they also extend the hip joint, as in straightening the trunk after bending forwards at the hips.

TABLE 2.5 ■ **Summary of the Muscles of the Posterior Compartment of the Thigh**

Muscle	Proximal Attachment	Distal Attachment	Concentric Action	Innervation
Semimembranosus	Ischial tuberosity (superolateral facet)	Posterolateral surface of medial tibial condyle, fascia over popliteus and oblique popliteal ligament	Flexes and medially rotates knee; extends hip	Sciatic nerve: tibial component (L5, S1, 2)
Semitendinosus	Ischial tuberosity (medial facet)	Medial surface of proximal tibia	Flexes and medially rotates knee; extends hip	
Biceps femoris	Long head: ischial tuberosity (medial facet)	Head of fibula (around lateral collateral ligament of knee)	Flexes and laterally rotates knee Long head extends hip	
	Short head: lateral lip of linea aspera			Sciatic nerve: common fibular component (L5, S1, 2)

SCIATIC NERVE

The sciatic nerve (L4, 5, S1–3) runs vertically through the posterior compartment of the thigh on the posterior aspect of the adductor magnus deep to the long head of the biceps femoris. It divides into its tibial and common fibular (peroneal) components at a variable level. It supplies the hamstring muscles and the hamstring component of the adductor magnus arising from the ischial tuberosity. The *surface marking* of the nerve is from the midpoint between the ischial tuberosity and the greater trochanter to the apex of the popliteal fossa.

Part 5 Popliteal Fossa, Knee Joint and Leg

POPLITEAL FOSSA (Fig 2.12)

This is a diamond-shaped depression behind the flexed knee.

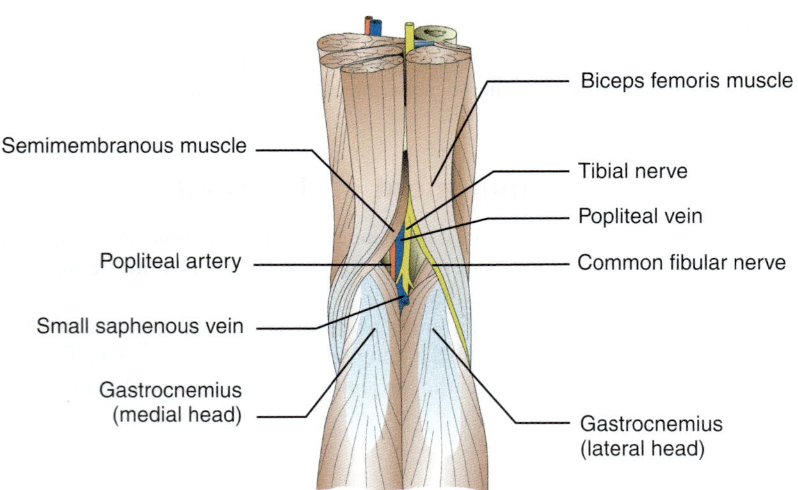

Fig. 2.12 Popliteal fossa and its contents.

Boundaries

- Medial border: superiorly, the semimembranosus and the overlying semitendinosus; inferiorly, the medial head of the gastrocnemius
- Lateral border: superiorly, the biceps femoris; inferiorly, the lateral head of the gastrocnemius with the underlying plantaris muscle
- Floor (from superior to inferior): the posterior surface of the distal femur, the capsule of the knee joint reinforced by the oblique popliteal ligament, and the posterior aspect of the proximal tibia covered by the popliteus and its fascia
- Roof: the popliteal fascia, which merges with the fascia lata proximally and the fascia cruris distally

Contents

- **Common peroneal nerve**
  - Slopes downwards medial to the biceps femoris and passes superficial to the lateral head of the gastrocnemius before spiralling around the neck of the fibula (where it can be rolled against the bone). It then passes deep to the fibularis longus and divides into its two terminal branches: the deep and superficial fibular (peroneal) nerves
  - Gives numerous branches:
    - Sural communicating nerve
    - Lateral cutaneous nerve of the calf
    - Genicular branches
- **Tibial nerve**
  - Runs vertically down in the middle of the fossa and then passes deeply between the heads of the gastrocnemius
  - Gives motor branches to all muscles that arise in the popliteal fossa
  - Has only one cutaneous nerve – the sural nerve – which pierces the deep fascia (replacing the posterior cutaneous nerve of the thigh) and passes down in the subcutaneous fat
  - Genicular nerves
- **Popliteal vessels and lymphatics**
  - The popliteal artery is the deepest of the structures. The muscular branches are given to the muscles in the popliteal fossa (end-artery type) and genicular branches (upper/superior medial and lateral, and lower/inferior medial and lateral) (Fig 2.13A). The middle genicular artery pierces the oblique popliteal ligament and the posterior capsule of the knee joint to supply the cruciate ligaments (Fig 2.13B).
  - The popliteal vein lies between the nerve and the artery and receives the termination of the small saphenous vein
  - Popliteal lymph nodes are distributed around the popliteal vessels and drain to the deep inguinal lymph nodes

There are two additional structures in the subcutaneous tissue of the popliteal fossa: the **posterior cutaneous nerve of the thigh** and the **small saphenous vein**.

- **Popliteus**
  - Originates from the popliteal surface of the tibia and inserts onto a pit just below the epicondyle on the lateral surface of the lateral condyle of the femur
  - Lies within the joint capsule
  - Supplied by the tibial nerve
  - Functions: with the knee fully extended and the foot planted (i.e. the tibia is fixed), the popliteus rotates the femur laterally on the tibia, thereby '*unlocking*' the knee at the beginning of flexion

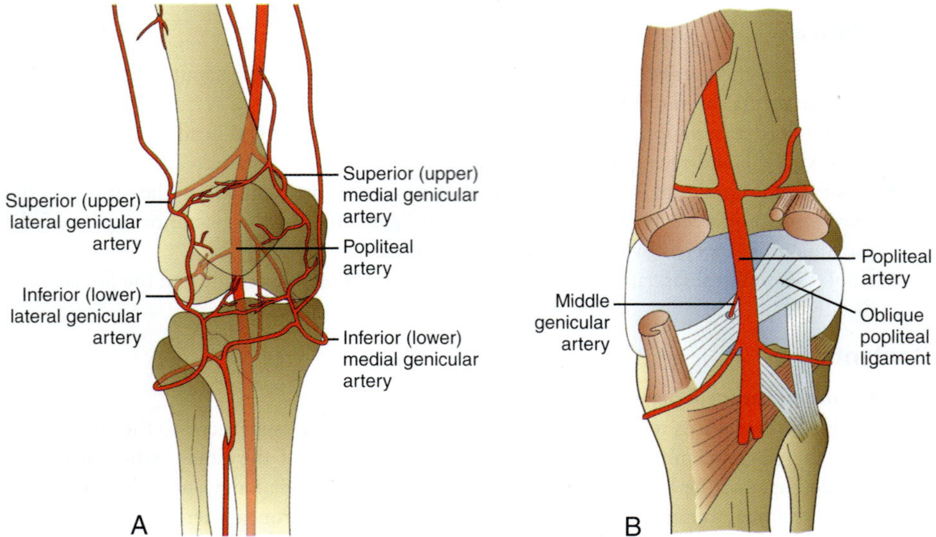

Fig. 2.13 **(A)** Arterial system of the knee. **(B)** Arterial system of the knee, posterior view.

KNEE JOINT

The knee joint is the largest synovial joint in the body and is adapted for weight-bearing and locomotion. It can be regarded as a complex hinge joint with tibiofemoral and patellofemoral components.

Articular Surfaces

- The distal femur has two large condyles separated posteriorly by a deep intercondylar fossa and fused anteriorly at the patellar surface (trochlear groove)
- The tibial plateau has two shallow concave facets; the medial facet is confined to the plateau but the lateral facet slopes slightly backwards over the posterior margin of the lateral tibial condyle
- The articular surface of the patella consists of a broad lateral and a narrow medial facet divided by a shallow vertical ridge

Capsule (Fig 2.14)

The fibrous capsule encloses the articular cavity and the intercondylar region. It is thicker anteriorly and posteriorly, where it is reinforced by tendinous expansions from surrounding muscles. The capsule is attached to the articular margins of the femur, patella and tibia.

- It is deficient at two main sites: anteriorly, where the knee joint communicates with the suprapatellar bursa, and posterolaterally, where the capsule extends down over the tendon of popliteus to the head of the fibula as the arcuate popliteal ligament

Synovial membrane lines most of the fibrous capsule, but diverges from it at several sites:

- Where it is reflected around the cruciate ligaments, which are therefore intracapsular but extrasynovial
- Where it extends approximately a hand's breadth above the patella between the quadriceps tendon and the distal femur as the suprapatella bursa
- Around the tendon of the popliteus

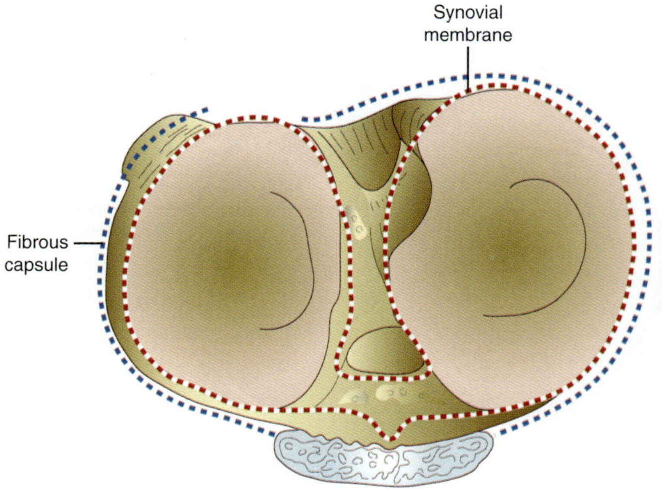

Fig. 2.14 Attachments of the capsule and synovial membrane of the knee joint.

- Deep to the patellar tendon, where it is invaginated by the extrasynovial infrapatellar fat pad, creating a midline infrapatellar synovial fold or 'plica' that sweeps up to attach to the femoral intercondylar fossa
  - The synovial membrane is also attached to the superior and inferior peripheral margins of each meniscus. The healthy knee normally contains only a few millilitres of synovial fluid

Ligaments (Fig 2.15A and B)

Consist of extracapsular and intracapsular ligaments, which play a major role in the stability of the knee.

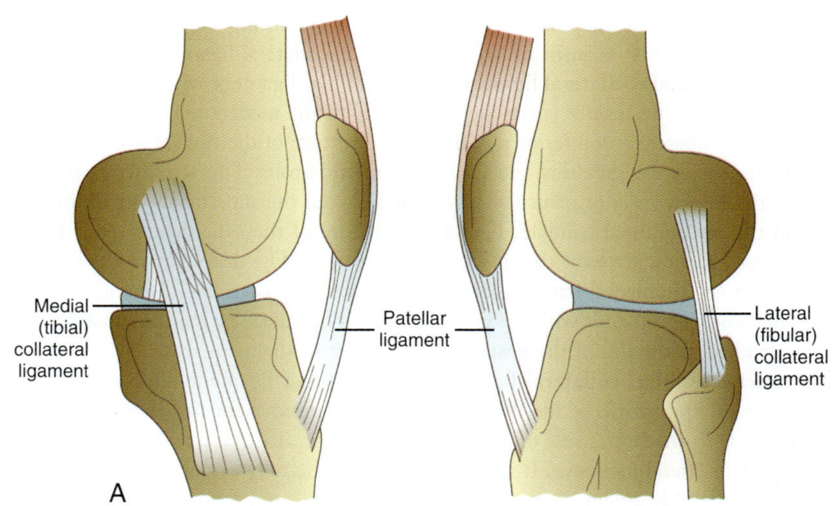

Fig. 2.15 **(A)** Ligaments of the knee.

Continued on following page

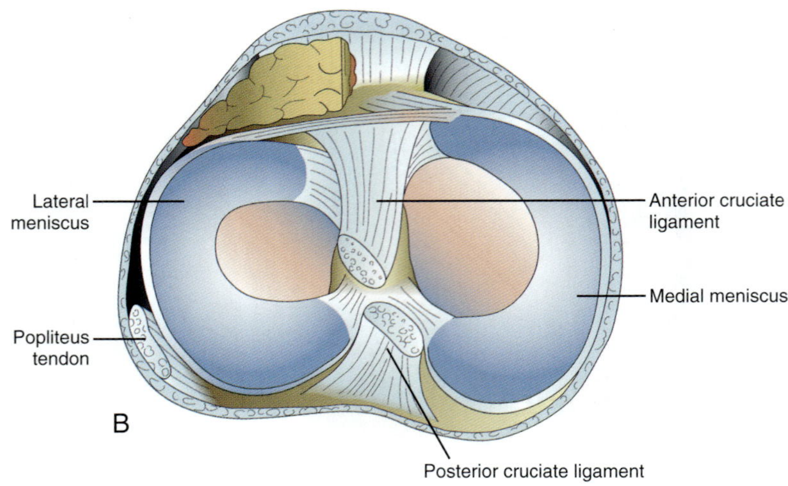

Fig. 2.15, cont'd (B) Menisci and their relations.

Extracapsular Ligaments.

1. Patellar ligament – extends from the patella to the tibial tuberosity and represents the continuation of the quadriceps femoris tendon. It is inserted into a smooth oblique area on the tibial tuberosity
2. Patellar retinacula – pass posteriorly from the medial and lateral margins of the patella and patellar ligament; they are a multilayered sheet of fibrous tissue. These are the medial and lateral patellar retinacula, which are continuous with the lower margins of the vastus medialis and lateralis muscles. They blend with the underlying joint capsule and collateral ligaments and insert into their respective tibial condyles inferiorly. The upper part of the medial patellar retinaculum has a discrete thickening, the medial patellofemoral ligament, which passes from the superomedial border of the patella to the anterior aspect of the medial epicondyle of the femur; it is a key factor in stabilising the patella
3. Collateral ligaments – consist of lateral and medial collateral ligaments:

   The **medial (tibial) collateral ligament** is a broad, flat ligament with superficial and deep components. The former is attached superiorly to the medial epicondyle just below the adductor tubercle and inferiorly to the medial surface of the tibia above and behind the attachment of the sartorius, gracilis and semitendinosus. The semimembranosus bursa and the medial inferior genicular vessels lie between the superficial part of the ligament and the medial tibial condyle. The oblique nature of the superficial part of the medial collateral ligament means that it is taut in extension. The deep part of the ligament extends from the medial femoral condyle above to the posterolateral margin of the tibial plateau below; it blends with the underlying joint capsule. The medial collateral ligament is attached to the rim of the posterior horn of the medial meniscus

   The **lateral (fibular) collateral ligament** is a cord-like ligament attached superiorly to the lateral epicondyle of the femur just above the groove for the popliteus tendon and inferiorly to the lateral side of the head of the fibula. It is not attached to the knee joint capsule or lateral meniscus. It is also most taut in the fully extended knee

   - The collateral ligaments protect the knee from valgus and varus stresses
4. **Oblique popliteal ligament** – a tendinous expansion from the distal attachment of the semimembranosus that passes superolaterally to blend with the capsule of the knee joint

and the tendon of the lateral head of the gastrocnemius at the lateral femoral condyle. It is perforated by the middle genicular vessels and the articular branch of the obturator nerve. This ligament reinforces the posterior capsule of the knee joint and is a major restraint against hyperextension

5. **Arcuate popliteal ligament** – passes superiorly from the head of the fibula and fuses with the posterior aspect of the joint capsule and the underlying tendon of the popliteus
6. **Popliteofibular ligament** – passes superiorly from the head of the fibula to the tendon of popliteus just below the joint line and is an important posterolateral stabiliser. In addition, a fabellofibular ligament may be identified passing superiorly from the head of the fibula to a cartilaginous or bony sesamoid bone (fabella) in the lateral head of gastrocnemius

Intracapsular Ligaments. The two strong cruciate ligaments lie in the intercondylar region of the knee inside the capsule of the joint (but outside the synovial membrane) and connect the tibia to the femur. They are named from their tibial origins.

1. The **anterior cruciate ligament (ACL)** is attached to the anterior part of the intercondylar area of the tibia and ascends posteriorly in the intercondylar fossa to attach to the lateral femoral condyle
2. The **posterior cruciate ligament (PCL)** is attached to the posterior part of the intercondylar area of the tibia and a small adjacent area on the posterior surface of the tibia. It ascends anteriorly in the intercondylar fossa to the medial femoral condyle
   - Each cruciate ligament is about 4 cm long, just over 1 cm wide and composed of two discrete bundles of collagen fibres
   - The cruciate ligaments are critical to anteroposterior stability of the knee, especially the weight-bearing flexed knee
   - The ACL prevents anterior displacement of the tibia on the femur, while the PCL prevents posterior displacement of the tibia
   - The ACL limits backward displacement of the lateral femoral condyle in full extension of the knee, resulting in medial rotation of the femur and 'locking' of the knee joint.
   - The ACL prevents hyperextension of the knee and provide rotational stability, while the PCL prevents hyperflexion

Menisci (see Fig 2.15B)

The medial and lateral menisci are crescentic, intracapsular, fibrocartilaginous structures covering approximately two-thirds of the tibial articular surface. Their upper surfaces are concave to optimise congruency with the femoral condyles. They are wedge-shaped in cross-section and only their outer margins are vascularised. Their thin avascular central regions are nourished by synovial fluid. The meniscal horns are richly innervated, while the remainder of the meniscus is relatively insensitive. The menisci are attached to the tibial plateau via meniscal horns and are also loosely attached at their outer margins to the periphery of the tibial condyles (via so-called coronary ligaments). The anterior horns of both menisci are interconnected anteriorly by a transverse ligament.

1. The lateral meniscus is C-shaped with a relatively uniform breadth. Its posterior horn gains two additional attachments: to the tendon of popliteus, which is attached to its periphery and separates it from the lateral collateral ligament, and to the medial femoral condyle by anterior and/or posterior meniscofemoral ligaments that pass in front of and behind the PCL, respectively. These attachments cause the lateral meniscus to be more mobile than the medial meniscus
2. The medial meniscus is comma-shaped with a broader posterior horn; the attachments of its horns to the tibial plateau embrace those of the smaller lateral meniscus. Posteriorly, its periphery is attached to the knee joint capsule and medial collateral ligament,

rendering it much less mobile than the lateral meniscus and therefore much more prone to injury

- Functions: improve congruency between the tibial and the femoral articular surfaces, act as shock absorbers, spread load-bearing over a wider surface area, and provide proprioceptive information

Bursae (Fig 2.16)

- There are numerous bursae around the knee joint
- The largest is the **suprapatellar bursa**; a small muscle, the articularis genus, is attached to the apex of this synovial pouch and pulls it proximally away from the joint in extension
- A bursa lies beneath each head of the gastrocnemius; the one beneath the medial head often communicates with the knee joint and sometimes with the semimembranosus bursa between the medial head of gastrocnemius and the semimembranosus tendon
- Other bursae around the knee include: the prepatellar bursa, subcutaneous and deep infrapatellar bursae, a bursa deep to the tendon of popliteus, the pes anserine bursa deep to the distal tendons of the sartorius, gracilis and semitendinosus, and several bursae related to the medial collateral ligament

Blood Supply (Fig 2.17)

- There is a rich arterial anastomosis around the knee that supplies the capsule and joint structures
- The network receives contributions from (i) the genicular branches of the popliteal artery, (ii) the descending genicular branch of the femoral artery and (iii) a recurrent branch from the anterior tibial artery
- The middle genicular artery supplies the cruciate ligaments

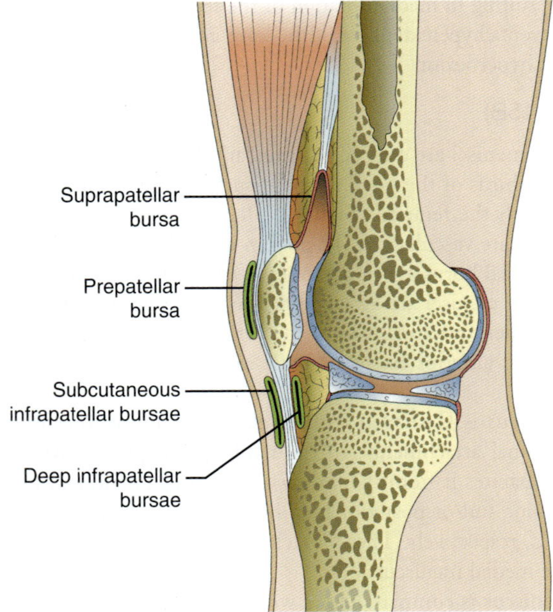

Fig. 2.16 Bursae of the knee, sagittal section.

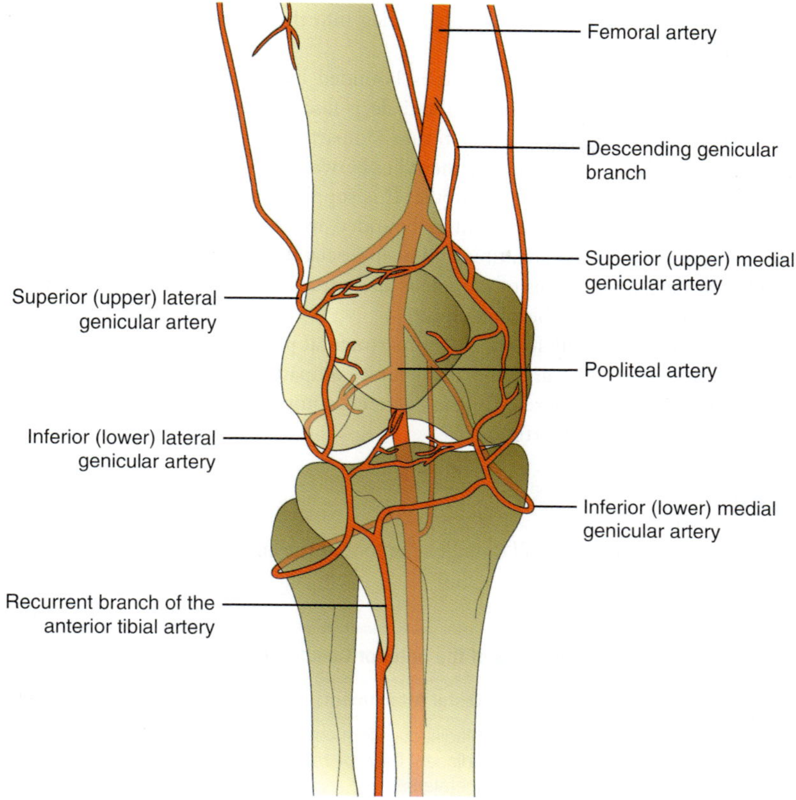

Fig. 2.17 Blood supply of the knee.

Lymph drainage

- Popliteal lymph nodes

Nerve supply

- The joint capsule and ligaments are supplied by articular branches of nerves supplying the muscles acting on the joint (Hilton's law)
- Innervated by the femoral, sciatic (tibial and common fibular nerves) and obturator nerves

Part 6 Anterior Compartment of the Leg

LEG

The leg is the anatomical region between the knee and ankle joints containing the tibia and fibula united by an interosseous membrane. The leg is invested in a stocking of deep fascia (fascia cruris) that encloses the leg muscles, but does not cover the palpable subcutaneous surface of the tibia, fusing instead with the periosteum along the medial and lateral borders of the bone. The tibialis anterior and the extensor digitorum longus gain attachment to its deep surface. Inferiorly, the deep fascia of the leg blends with the periosteum of the malleoli and is continuous with both the extensor and the flexor retinacula. Two intermuscular septa (anterior and posterior) extend from the deep fascia to the fibula and divide the leg into three osteofascial compartments, each supplied by their own nerve:

- The anterior (extensor) compartment is bounded by the tibia, interosseous membrane, fibula, anterior intermuscular septum and deep fascia. It is the least expansile. The deep fibular nerve innervates the muscles in this compartment
- The lateral (fibular/evertor) compartment lies between the anterior and posterior intermuscular septa and the deep fascia and fibula. It is supplied by the superficial fibular nerve
- The posterior (flexor) compartment is bounded by the posterior intermuscular septum, fibula, interosseous membrane, tibia and deep fascia; it has superficial and deep parts separated by the deep aponeurosis of the soleus and a transverse layer of fascia. The nerve of the posterior compartment is the tibial nerve
- The arterial supply loosely follows a compartmental pattern with the anterior tibial artery supplying muscles in the anterior and lateral compartments, the popliteal and posterior tibial arteries supplying muscles in the posterior compartment, and the fibular artery contributing to all three compartments

MUSCLES

The muscles in this compartment all dorsiflex the foot at the ankle; this action is important when walking.

TABLE 2.6 ■ **Summary of the Muscles of the Anterior Compartment of the Leg**

Muscle	Proximal Attachment	Distal Attachment	Concentric Action	Innervation
Tibialis anterior	Upper 1/2 of the lateral shaft of tibia and interosseous membrane and overlying deep fascia	Medial cuneiform and adjacent base of 1st metatarsal	Dorsiflexion of ankle and inversion of the foot	Deep fibular nerve (L4, 5)
Extensor hallucis longus	Middle 1/2 of anterior shaft of fibula and interosseous membrane	Dorsal aspect of base of distal phalanx of great toe	Extension of great toe and dorsiflexion of ankle	Deep fibular nerve (L5)
Extensor digitorum longus	Lateral condyle of tibia, proximal anterior surface of fibula, interosseous membrane and overlying deep fascia	Extensor hoods over proximal phalanges with slips to base of middle and distal phalanges of lateral 4 digits	Extension of lateral 4 toes and dorsiflexion of ankle	Deep fibular nerve (L5, S1)
Fibularis (peroneus) tertius	Lower 1/3 of anterior surface of fibula and interosseous membrane	Dorsum of base of 5th metatarsal	Dorsiflexion of ankle and eversion of foot	Deep fibular nerve (L5, S1)

ANTERIOR TIBIAL ARTERY (Fig 2.18)

- Major artery to the anterior compartment
- From the popliteal bifurcation it passes forwards into the anterior compartment of the leg through an opening in the interosseous membrane just medial to the neck of the fibula and it then descends on the interosseous membrane

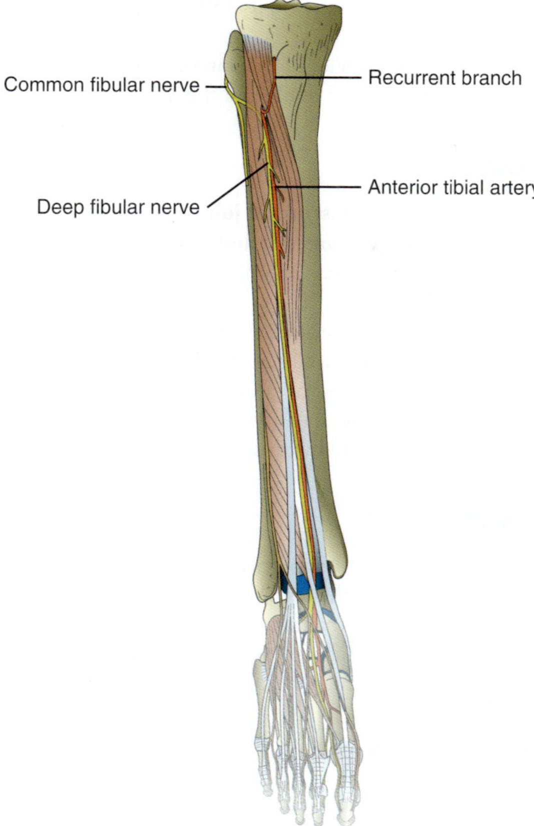

Fig. 2.18 Anterior tibial artery and deep fibular nerve.

- Contributes to the arterial anastomosis around the knee by a recurrent branch
- Crosses the ankle joint midway between the malleoli, where it becomes the dorsalis pedis artery; here it is palpable between the tendons of the tibialis anterior and the extensor hallucis longus
- Contributes to an arterial anastomosis around the ankle by malleolar branches
- The anterior compartment is also supplied by a perforating branch from the fibular artery that passes anteriorly through the inferior aperture in the interosseus membrane to anastomose with a branch of the anterior tibial artery

DEEP FIBULAR NERVE (see Fig 2.18)

- Originates in the lateral compartment deep to the fibularis longus as one of the two divisions of the common fibular nerve (L4, 5, S1, 2)
- Continues its course around the fibular neck piercing the anterior intermuscular septum and runs obliquely forwards deep to the extensor digitorum longus to the front of the interosseous membrane, where it lies with the anterior tibial artery between the extensor digitorum longus and the tibialis anterior

- Descends with the artery and lies lateral to it at the ankle, where it divides into its terminal branches
- In the leg, it supplies the four muscles of the anterior compartment and conveys sensation from the periosteum of the tibia and fibula and the ankle joint

TIBIOFIBULAR JOINT

- Superior tibiofibular joint: a plane **synovial joint** between the lateral tibial condyle and the fibular head. It is reinforced by anterior and posterior ligaments and the tendon of the biceps femoris. The joint sometimes communicates with a posterior bursa deep to the popliteus tendon.
- Inferior tibiofibular joint: usually considered to be a **fibrous joint** (syndesmosis) between the medial convex surface of the distal end of the fibula and the concave fibular notch of the tibia. The joint is reinforced by anterior, posterior and interosseous tibiofibular ligaments and plays a key role in the stability of the ankle joint. The fibula is capable of only a small amount of rotation associated with ankle movements.

INTEROSSEOUS MEMBRANE

This connects the interosseous borders of the tibia and fibula and separates the anterior and posterior osteofascial compartments of the leg. Most of its fibres run obliquely down from the tibia to the fibula, resisting downward traction on the latter. The membrane has two notable apertures: for the anterior tibial artery above and the perforating branch of the fibular artery below; both arteries run forwards into the anterior compartment.

Part 7 Dorsum of the Foot

The following structures are present on the dorsum of the foot: the long tendons of the extensor digitorum longus and the extensor hallucis longus, the extensor digitorum brevis, and the neurovascular structures, comprising the dorsalis pedis artery and the deep and superficial fibular nerves.

- All of these structures except the superficial fibular nerve run under the extensor retinacula
- The dorsalis pedis artery is the continuation of the anterior tibial artery after it crosses the ankle joint midway between the malleoli
- The deep fibular nerve lies lateral to the anterior tibial/dorsalis pedis artery at the ankle joint and runs forwards on the dorsum of the foot deep to the tendons to supply the skin of the first interdigital cleft

Part 8 Lateral Compartment of the Leg

The two muscles in this compartment evert the foot at the ankle. The fibularis longus helps to maintain the lateral longitudinal and transverse arches of the foot. Both tendons pass behind the lateral malleolus under the superior fibular retinaculum. They run forwards on the lateral surface of the calcaneus under the inferior fibular retinaculum, where they are separated by the fibular trochlea (the fibularis brevis above and the fibularis longus below). The fibularis longus runs in a groove on the undersurface of the cuboid bone, which is converted into a tunnel by the long plantar ligament, and crosses the sole of the foot obliquely to its attachment site. Both tendons share a common synovial sheath as far as the fibular trochlea; thereafter, each tendon has a separate sheath.

TABLE 2.7 ■ **Summary of the Muscles of the Lateral Compartment of the Leg**

Muscle	Proximal Attachment	Distal Attachment	Concentric Action	Innervation
Fibularis longus	Head and upper $^2/_3$ of lateral side of fibula	Base of first metatarsal and adjacent medial cuneiform	Eversion of foot and weak plantarflexion of ankle Fibularis longus helps to maintain lateral longitudinal and transverse arches of the foot	Superficial fibular nerve (L5, S1)
Fibularis brevis	Lower $^2/_3$ of lateral side of fibula	Tuberosity on lateral side of base of fifth metatarsal		

FIBULAR ARTERY

- The lateral compartment muscles are supplied by perforating branches from the fibular artery, running in the posterior compartment of the leg, and by branches of the anterior tibial artery
- The fibular artery usually arises from the posterior tibial artery about 2 cm below its origin and descends between the tibialis posterior and the flexor hallucis longus
- Gives off muscular and fasciocutaneous branches and a nutrient artery to the fibula
- At the level of the ankle joint, gives off a perforating branch that passes anteriorly through the inferior aperture in the interosseus membrane to reinforce the arterial supply to the anterior compartment of the leg and foot
- Terminates as calcaneal branches

SUPERFICIAL FIBULAR NERVE (Fig 2.19)

- One of the two divisions of the common fibular nerve (L4, 5, S1, 2)
- Descends deep to the fibularis longus and innervates the muscles of the lateral compartment of the leg along with the overlying skin

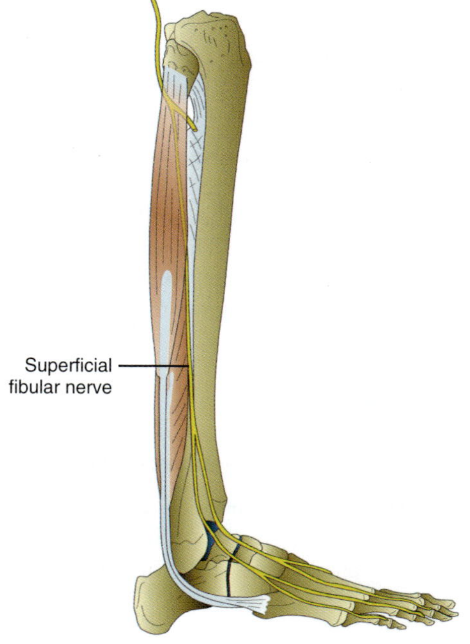

Fig. 2.19 Superficial fibular nerve and its relations.

- Pierces the deep fascia in the lower leg and enters the foot, dividing into medial and lateral branches that supply the skin over the dorsum of the foot

Part 9 Posterior Compartment of the Leg

The posterior compartment (the calf) has superficial and deep muscles separated by the deep aponeurosis of the soleus and a transverse layer of fascia. The superficial gastrocnemius and the soleus muscles act as powerful plantar flexors of the ankle. The two heads of the gastrocnemius converge as a broad aponeurosis on the anterior surface of the muscle. The aponeurosis gradually narrows and incorporates the soleus tendon on its deep surface forming the subcutaneous calcaneal, or Achilles tendon. The tendon has a mean length of 15 cm and its fibres are spiralled to assist with elastic recoil. Distally, it is attached to a transverse area on the middle third of the posterior surface of the calcaneus, with a bursa and fat pad located between the tendon and the bone and another bursa between the tendon and the skin. The soleus is a large, powerful, multipennate, flattened muscle with proximal attachments to the tibia and fibula. The neurovascular bundle descends on the deep surface of the muscle. Of the two muscles, the gastrocnemius is stated to be the more propulsive, as in running or jumping, whereas the soleus is more postural as in maintaining standing balance.

SUPERFICIAL MUSCLES OF THE LEG

TABLE 2.8 ■ **Summary of the Superficial Muscles of the Posterior Compartment of the Leg**

Muscle	Proximal Attachment	Distal Attachment	Concentric Action	Innervation
Gastrocnemius	**Lateral head:** lateral surface of lateral femoral condyle **Medial head:** posterior surface of medial femoral condyle	Posterior surface of calcaneus via Achilles tendon	Plantarflexion of ankle Flexion of knee	Tibial nerve (S1, 2)
Soleus	Head and upper 1/4 of fibula, soleal line and middle 1/3 of medial border of tibia, and fibrous arch between tibia and fibula		Plantarflexion of ankle	

The deep muscles consist of the popliteus (described in Part 5), the tibialis posterior, the flexor hallucis longus and the flexor digitorum longus. The tendons of the latter three muscles pass under the flexor retinaculum to enter the sole of the foot, where the tendon of the flexor hallucis longus crosses deep to the tendon of the flexor digitorum longus.

DEEP MUSCLES OF THE LEG

TABLE 2.9 ■ **Summary of the Deep Muscles of the Posterior Compartment of the Leg**

Muscle	Proximal Attachment	Distal Attachment	Concentric Action	Innervation
Flexor digitorum longus	Medial part of posterior surface of tibia below soleal line	Base of distal phalanges of lateral 4 digits	Flexion of lateral 4 toes Plantarflexion of ankle	Tibial nerve (S1, 2)

TABLE 2.9 ■ **Summary of the Deep Muscles of the Posterior Compartment of the Leg** (Continued)

Flexor hallucis longus	Distal posterior surface of fibula and adjacent interosseous membrane	Base of distal phalanx of great toe	Flexion of great toe (important for 'toe-off' in the gait cycle) Plantarflexion of ankle Supports medial longitudinal arch of foot	Tibial nerve (S1, 2)
Tibialis posterior	Posterior surface of tibia below soleal line, interosseous membrane and adjacent fibula	Tuberosity of navicular, medial cuneiform, and bases of metatarsals 2–4	Inversion of foot Plantarflexion of ankle Supports medial longitudinal arch of foot	Tibial nerve (L4, 5)

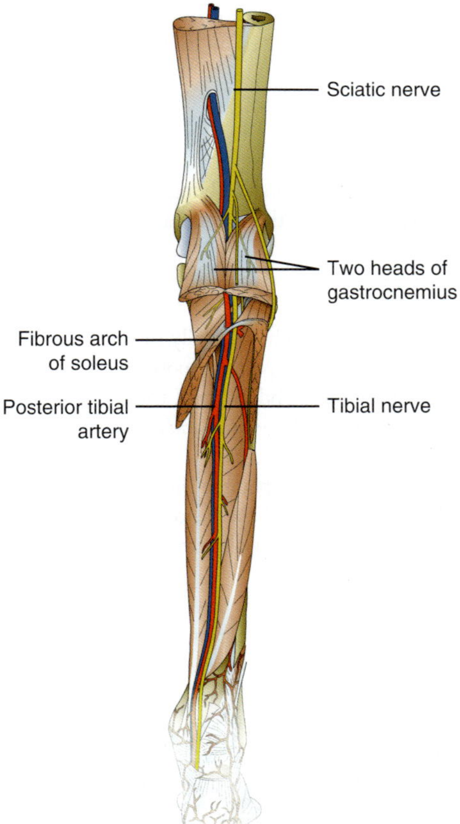

Fig. 2.20 Posterior tibial artery and tibial nerve.

POSTERIOR TIBIAL ARTERY (Fig 2.20)

- Passes under the fibrous arch of the soleus and descends in a neurovascular plane between the superficial and the deep muscles of the posterior compartment
- Gives off a nutrient artery to the tibia, muscular branches to posterior compartment muscles, and branches to the Achilles tendon and the overlying skin of the calf

- Its largest branch is the fibular (peroneal) artery, which often arises about 2 cm beyond the origin of the posterior tibial artery
- At the ankle, the posterior tibial artery is palpable midway between the medial malleolus and the calcaneal tendon
- Passes under the flexor retinaculum and divides into medial and lateral plantar arteries

TIBIAL NERVE (see Fig 2.20)

- Leaves the popliteal fossa between the two heads of the gastrocnemius
- Travels with the posterior tibial artery down the calf deep to the soleus
- Gives off articular branches to the knee and ankle, a cutaneous branch (the sural nerve) and branches to the muscles in the posterior compartment; the branches to gastrocnemius, soleus and popliteus originate high in the leg between the two heads of gastrocnemius
- Lies just under the deep fascia in the distal third of the calf and passes behind the medial malleolus, passing under the flexor retinaculum, where it gives off the cutaneous medial calcaneal nerve and terminates by dividing into the medial and lateral plantar nerves

Part 10 Sole of the Foot

The sole of the foot is covered by thick skin overlying specialised subcutaneous tissue containing multiple skin ligaments. Deep to this are the plantar aponeurosis and four muscle layers.

MUSCLES

- The four muscle layers are shown schematically in Fig 2.21 and are summarised below:
  - **Layer 1:** immediately deep to the plantar aponeurosis, consisting of three short muscles (the flexor digitorum brevis and abductors of the big and little toes)
    A neurovascular plane containing the medial and lateral plantar vessels and nerves lies between the first and second layers
  - **Layer 2:** consists of the quadratus plantae muscle, the tendon of the flexor hallucis longus, the four lumbrical muscles and the flexor digitorum longus tendons
  - **Layer 3:** consists of three short muscles, the flexor digiti minimi brevis, the adductor hallucis and the flexor hallucis brevis
  - **Layer 4:** consists of the four dorsal and three plantar interossei together with the tendons of the fibularis longus and tibialis posterior

ARTERIES

- The posterior tibial artery divides into medial and lateral plantar branches, which run between the first and second layers of the sole of the foot

NERVES

- The medial and lateral plantar nerves (S1–3) originate from the tibial nerve. The medial plantar nerve is larger and is the major sensory nerve of the sole of the foot, including the plantar aspect of the medial three-and-a-half toes. It also supplies 4 intrinsic muscles: the abductor hallucis, the flexor digitorum brevis, the flexor hallucis brevis and the first lumbrical. All of the other intrinsic muscles of the foot are innervated by the lateral plantar nerve, which also provides sensation to the lateral aspect of the anterior sole and plantar surface of the lateral one-and-a-half toes

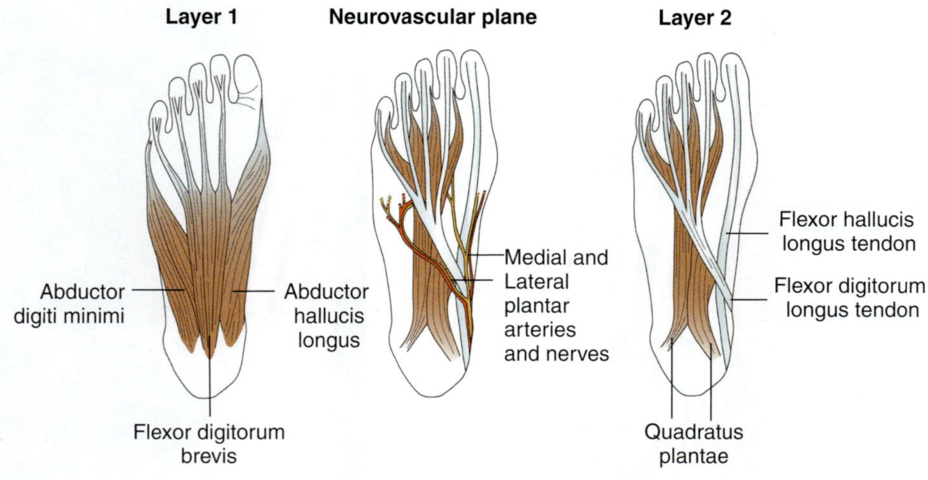

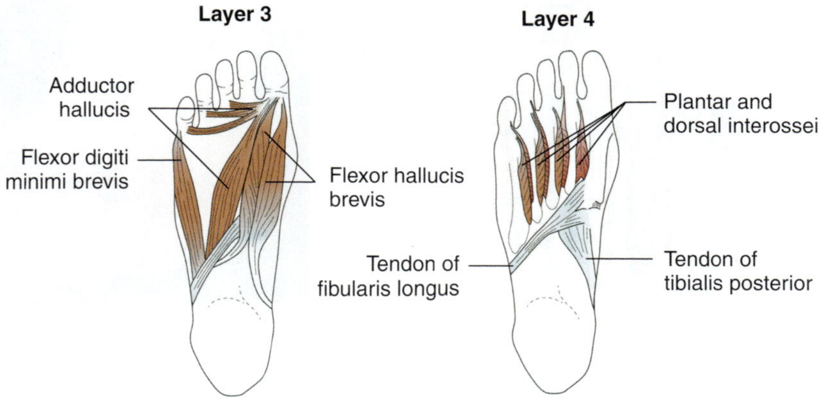

Fig. 2.21 Muscles layers of the foot.

Part 11 Ankle and Foot Joints

ANKLE RETINACULA

These are localised thickenings of deep fascia at the ankle to prevent bowstringing of the tendons.

Extensor Retinacula

There are two extensor retinacula: superior and inferior.

- The **superior extensor retinaculum** is attached to the anterior borders of the tibia and fibula above the ankle. It binds the tendons of the anterior compartment of the leg. *The superficial fibular nerve crosses the retinaculum superficially while the anterior tibial vessels and deep fibular nerve pass deep to the retinaculum* (Fig 2.22)
- The **inferior extensor retinaculum** is Y-shaped. It is attached laterally to the upper surface of the calcaneus and diverges medially as two limbs, one of which is attached to the medial malleolus and the other to the medial side of the plantar aponeurosis

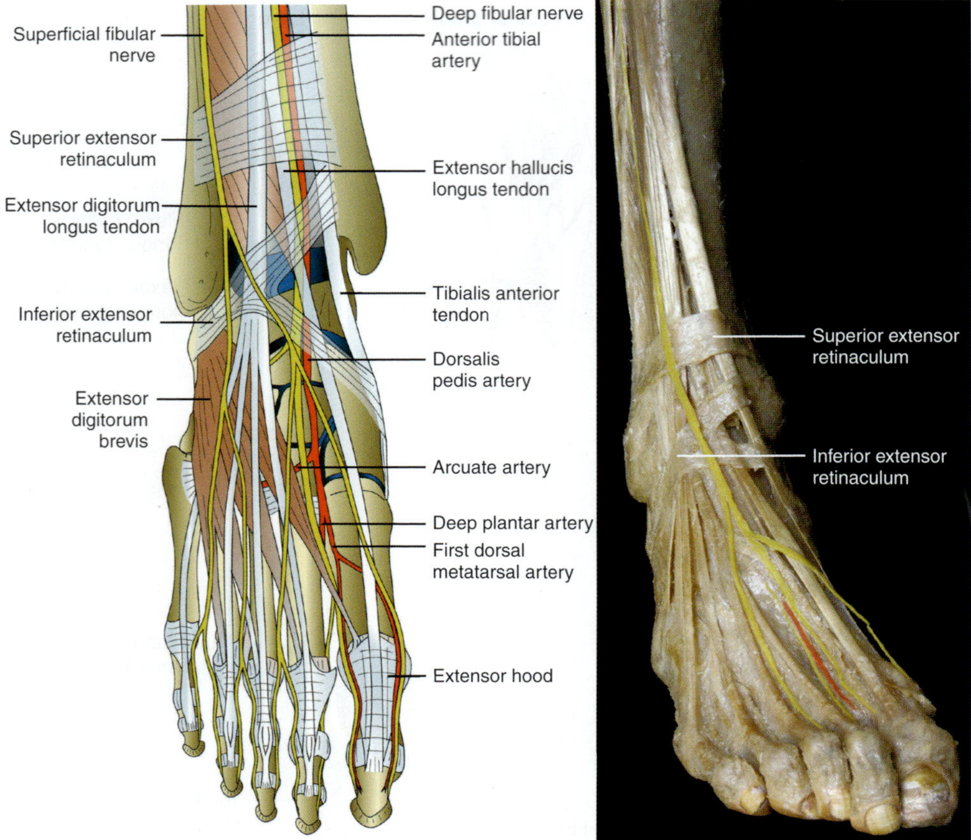

Fig. 2.22 Extensor retinacula and their relations.

Flexor Retinaculum

The flexor retinaculum extends posteroinferiorly from the medial malleolus to the medial side of the calcaneus. Inferiorly, it merges with the plantar aponeurosis. The retinaculum covers a gutter between the tibia and the calcaneus. This is called the tarsal tunnel and it transmits the following structures:

- The tibialis posterior tendon, the flexor digitorum longus tendon, the posterior tibial artery and vein, the tibial nerve and the flexor hallucis longus tendon (from front to back) (Fig 2.23)

ANKLE JOINT

The ankle joint is a synovial hinge joint between the deep recess created by the distal tibia and fibula with their respective malleoli and the talus of the foot.

- Articular surfaces are lined by hyaline cartilage and a fibrous capsule is attached to their margins, extending anteriorly onto the dorsum of the neck of the talus

Ligaments (Fig 2.24)

The ankle joint is strengthened by strong collateral ligaments: the medial and lateral ligaments.

- **Medial (deltoid) ligament** – a large, strong, triangular ligament with deep (anterior tibiotalar) and superficial parts

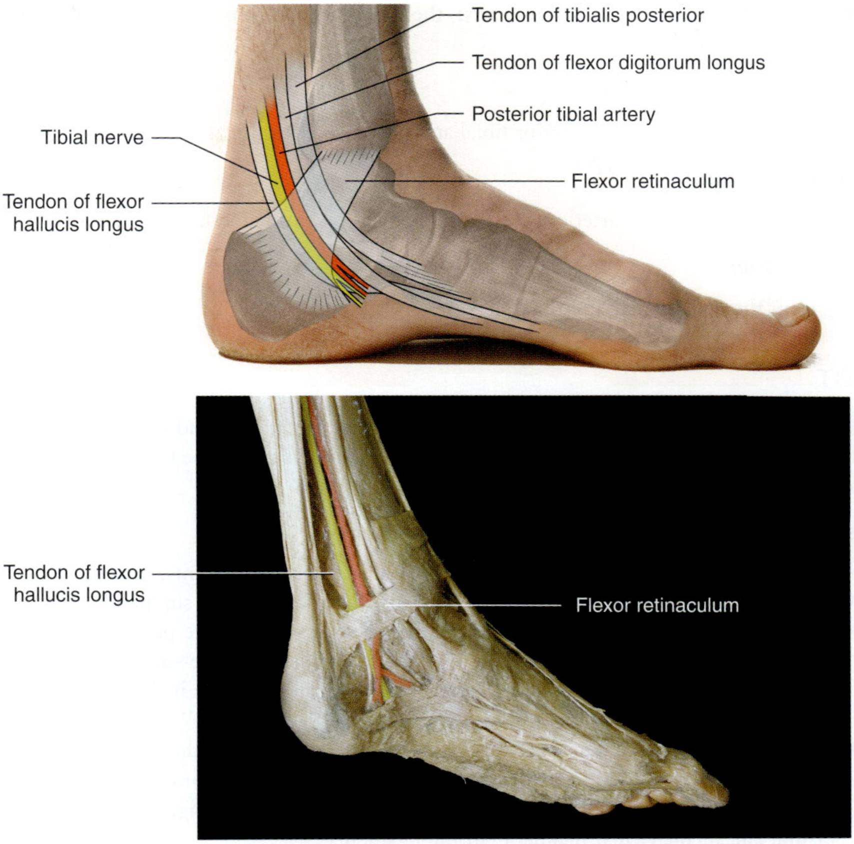

Tendon of tibialis posterior
Tendon of flexor digitorum longus
Posterior tibial artery
Tibial nerve
Flexor retinaculum
Tendon of flexor hallucis longus

Tendon of flexor hallucis longus
Flexor retinaculum

Fig. 2.23 Flexor retinaculum and contents of the tarsal tunnel.

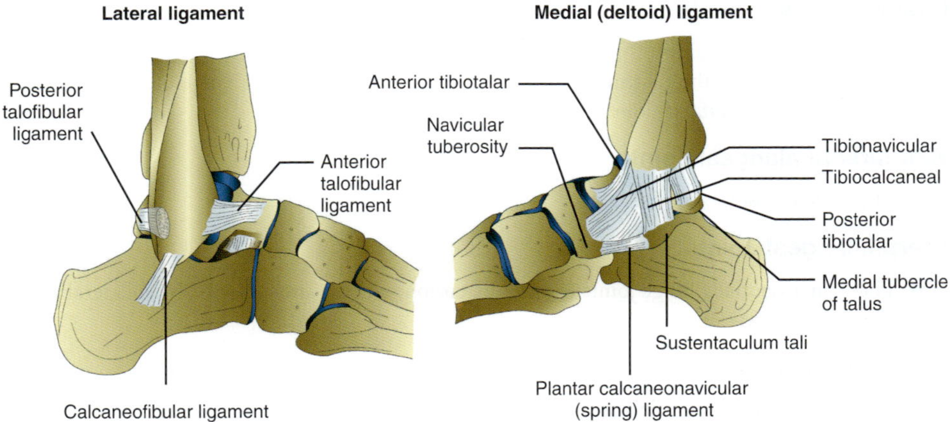

Fig. 2.24 Ligaments of the ankle joint. Left: Lateral view. Right: Medial view.

- **Lateral ligament** – has three parts: the anterior and posterior talofibular and the calcaneofibular

Blood Supply

This is from the anterior and posterior tibial and fibular arteries.

Lymph Drainage

Lymphatics accompany the arteries (deep) and saphenous veins (superficial).

Nerve Supply

This is from the deep fibular and tibial nerves.

FOOT

The foot has three groups of bones (seven tarsal bones, five metatarsals and the phalanges). These are interconnected by numerous joints and an array of ligaments giving the foot structure, flexibility and strength.

Intertarsal joints

These include the subtalar, talocalcaneonavicular and calcaneocuboid joints.

- They are all synovial joints concerned with inversion/eversion and supination/pronation
- The **subtalar joint** (talocalcaneal joint) is between a large concave posterior facet on the undersurface of the talus and a corresponding convex facet on the superior surface of the calcaneus. The joint is stabilised by several talocalcaneal ligaments including an interosseous talocalcaneal ligament
- The **talocalcaneonavicular joint** is between the rounded head of the talus and, from front to back, the navicular and the superior surface of the sustentaculum tali of the calcaneus. Numerous ligaments reinforce the joint, including the bifurcate ligament and the strong plantar calcaneonavicular ligament (spring ligament)
- The **calcaneocuboid joint** is between the anterior surface of the calcaneus and the posterior surface of the cuboid. It is strengthened by the bifurcate ligament and the long and short plantar ligaments

Tarsometatarsal Joints

- These are synovial joints
- The joint between the first metatarsal and the cuboid has a greater range of motion than the other tarsometatarsal joints

Metatarsophalangeal Joints

- These are ellipsoid synovial joints

Interphalangeal Joints

- These are essentially hinge joints (flexion/extension) and are strengthened by collateral and plantar ligaments

Arches of the Foot

The bones of the foot do not lie flat on the ground, but rather are configured into two longitudinal arches and a transverse arch by their shape and supporting ligaments and tendons.

- The medial and lateral longitudinal arches extend between the posteroinferior part of the calcaneus and the heads of the metatarsals. The medial longitudinal arch is higher than the lateral arch and gains additional support from the plantar calcaneonavicular ligament and the tibialis anterior and posterior. The head of the talus is the highest point of this arch. Rupture of the tendon of the tibialis posterior or of the spring ligament may cause a pathologically flat foot (pes planus). The lateral longitudinal arch is supported by the long and short plantar ligaments and the tendon of the fibularis longus. Both arches are reinforced by the plantar aponeurosis and the long and short flexors of the toes

- The transverse arch lies in the coronal plane and is formed by the cuneiforms, the cuboid and the bases of the metatarsals, which are linked together by ligaments. The arch is reinforced by the tendon of the fibularis longus, which passes obliquely across the sole

THORAX

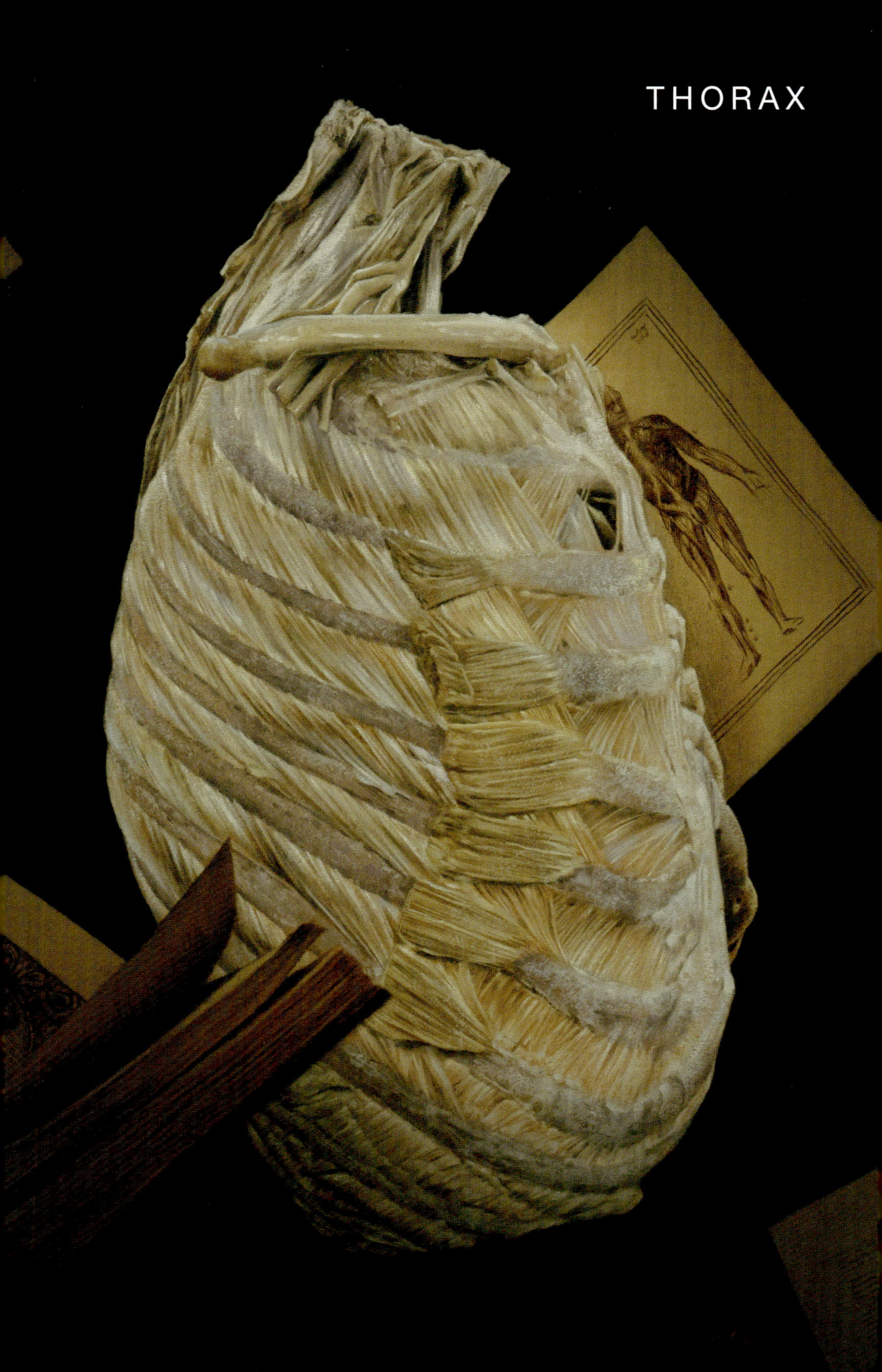

CHAPTER 3

Thorax

CHAPTER OUTLINE

Part 1 Body Wall

SKIN AND SUBCUTANEOUS TISSUE

Subcutaneous fatty tissues over the distensible parts of the body wall are positioned upon a condensation of the underlying fibrous fascia that allows the fatty tissue above to slide freely. It is known as Scarpa's fascia. This fascia fades out posterior to the midaxillary lines and merges superiorly with the posterior capsule of the breast. It is also continuous into the perineum.

BLOOD SUPPLY

This is via the neurovascular plane (between the middle and innermost muscular layers) and via a series of segmental arteries.

VENOUS DRAINAGE

This collects in an anastomosing network draining away from the umbilicus.

LYMPH DRAINAGE

This follows the veins (note that the lymph drainage superficially does not follow arteries).

- From above the umbilicus: anteriorly to pectoral nodes, posteriorly to scapular nodes
- From below the umbilicus: anteriorly to the medial group of superficial inguinal nodes, laterally and posteriorly to the lateral group of nodes

NERVE SUPPLY

- Above the second rib, the skin is supplied by supraclavicular branches of the cervical plexus
- Below this, the skin is supplied as follows:
  - A midline strip is supplied by anterior cutaneous branches (T2–L1)

- A broad lateral strip is supplied by the lateral cutaneous nerves, emerging from the mid axillary line with anterior and posterior branches passing obliquely and supplying skin right down to the buttock
- A posterior strip of the skin is supplied by the posterior rami of the spinal nerves-medial fibres in the upper part and lateral fibres in the lower part

Part 2 Thoracic Wall and Diaphragm

BONES OF THE THORAX

Articulated Thoracic Skeleton

- Ribs slope inferiorly at 45° (from vertebral bodies anteriorly)
- Anterior ends of the ribs fall progressively short; this is supplemented by longer costal cartilages

Sternum

- Consists of the manubrium (with sternal notch or jugular notch) and the body, connected by a secondary cartilaginous joint which rarely ossifies
- Note the demifacet for articulation on the manubrium with the second costal cartilage
- Xiphoid process represents the unossified lower end of the body (it may ossify late in life)
- Ossification of the sternum
  - Variable 1° centres appear in the fifth fetal month in four to five rows and are fused at 25 years

Ribs

- **First rib** (Fig 3.1)
  - Head is small (single facet)

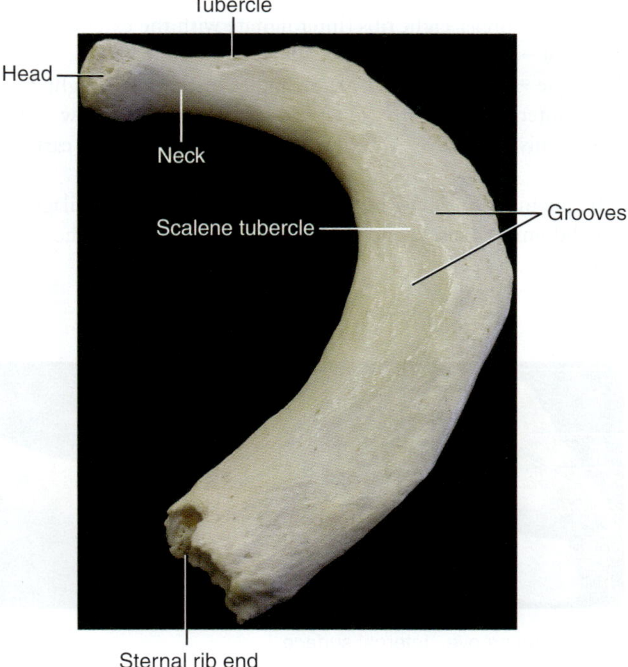

Fig. 3.1 First left rib, anterior view.

- Neck slopes backwards and upwards to join the shaft and structures. The structures which are in contact with the neck of the rib:
  - The anterior ramus of C8 above the neck and of T1 below
  - Other structures include the sympathetic trunk (near the head), supreme intercostal vein and superior intercostal artery
- Tubercle is the highest and most posterior part of the rib
- Over the shaft of the rib pass the **subclavian vein** (anteriorly) and the **subclavian artery** (posteriorly) in their respective grooves, and separated by the **scalene tubercle** in between (attachment for scalenus anterior)
- Forms a primary cartilaginous joint with the manubrium (immovable)

- **Typical ribs (two to ten)** (Fig 3.2)
  - Head is bevelled (two articular facets for own vertebral body and one above)
  - Neck is flattened with the upper border curving up into a thin prominent ridge
  - Tubercle shows two smooth facets (medial and lateral)
    - Medial facet is covered with hyaline cartilage and makes a synovial joint with its own vertebra's transverse process
    - Lateral facet receives lateral costotransverse ligament
  - Shaft contains **costal groove** inferiorly
    - Neurovascular bundle lies within the costal groove. The most superior structure is the vein and the most inferior is the nerve (**v**ein/**a**rtery/**n**erve)
- **11th rib** has a single articular facet
- **12th rib** varies in length, has a single articular facet, but no tubercle, angle or groove

Thoracic Cage

- Multiple muscular attachments
  - Pectoralis major – upper six costal cartilages and anterolateral surface of manubrium and sternal body
  - Serratus anterior – upper eight ribs (interdigitate with the external oblique muscle)
  - Pectoralis minor – ribs three to five
  - External oblique – anterior aspect of the angles of the lower eight ribs, interdigitating with serratus anterior posteriorly (four) and latissimus dorsi below
  - Rectus abdominis muscle – anterior surfaces of the costal cartilages of ribs five to seven
  - Internal oblique muscle – lower borders of the last six costal cartilages
  - Transverse abdominis muscle and diaphragm interdigitate on the inner surface of the lower six ribs

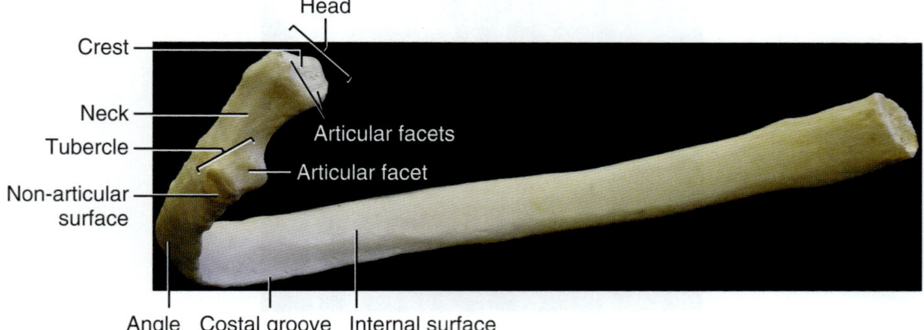

Fig. 3.2 Typical rib (two to ten), posterior view.

  - Serratus posterior superior and inferior are attached just lateral to posterior aspect of the angles of ribs two to five and nine to twelve, respectively
  - Scalene muscles and the quadratus lumborum
  - Intercostal muscles
- Note that the costal cartilages anteriorly are lower than the vertebrae:
  - Sternal notch/jugular notch (1st cartilage): T3
  - Sternal angle (2nd cartilage): T4/5
  - Lower border of sternum (6th or 7th cartilage): T9

THORACIC JOINTS

- Anteriorly, the ribs join the costal cartilages (**costochondral joints**). The upper seven costal cartilages articulate with the sternum, the eighth to tenth articulate with each other and the last two (11th and 12th) are free (floating ribs)
- Posteriorly, ribs articulate at their heads and tubercles with the vertebral bodies and transverse processes (collectively they are called **costovertebral joints**)

Joints at the Head of the Ribs

- Articulate by two articular facets – the lower rib facet articulates with its own vertebral body and the upper rib facet articulates with the vertebral body from the level above. The ridge (crest) between the two is attached to the intervertebral disc by the **intra-articular ligament**
- The front of the capsule of the synovial joints is reinforced by the radiate ligament, which consists of three bands
- First rib articulates with T1 only, and ribs 11 and 12 articulate only with their own vertebrae

Joints at the Tubercles (Costotransverse Joints – Tubercle of a Typical Rib Has Two Facets)

- Medial facet: articulates with a facet near the tip of the transverse process (a small encapsulated synovial joint)
- Lateral facet: gives attachment to the lateral costotransverse ligament
  - Lateral costotransverse ligament – runs from the lateral facet to the transverse process
- Three ligaments help to stabilise the costotransverse joint:
  - Lateral costotransverse ligament
  - Costotransverse ligament – runs between the back of the neck of the rib and the front of the transverse process
  - Superior costotransverse ligament of the neck – runs from the crest of the rib to the undersurface of the transverse process of the vertebra above

Costochondral Joints

- Each rib makes a primary cartilaginous joint with its costal cartilage. This is a deep concavoconvex joint

Interchondral Joints

- Ribs seven/eight, eight/nine and nine/ten are joined together by small synovial joints

Sternochondral Joints

- Rib one articulates with the manubrium via a primary cartilaginous joint. These move together as one, and give increased stability
- Ribs two to seven (via their costal cartilages) articulate with the sternum by a synovial joint

Manubriosternal Joint

- A secondary cartilagenous joint containing an intervening disc of fibrocartilage which rarely ossifies

Xiphisternal Joint

- A fibrocartilaginous disc between cartilage-covered surfaces

THORACIC MUSCLES (Fig 3.3A–C)

Outer Layer

Includes the external intercostals, serratus posterior muscles (supplied segmentally) and levator costae.

- External intercostals – pass obliquely downwards and forwards from the sharp lower border of the rib above to the rounded upper margin of the rib below. Extends from the costotransverse ligament to the costochondral junction blending into the anterior intercostal membrane

Middle Layer

- Internal intercostals run downwards and backwards from the costal groove of the rib above to the upper margin of the rib below and extend from the posterior intercostal membrane as far as the side of the sternum

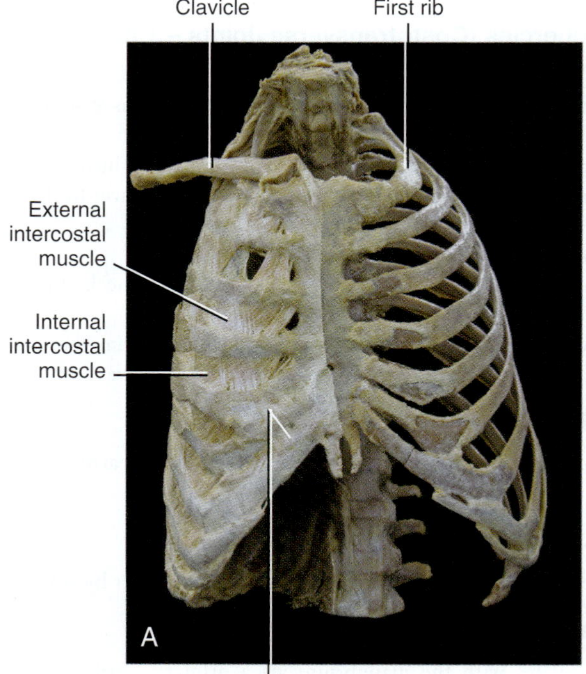

Fig. 3.3 (A) Muscles of the anterior thorax and their relations.

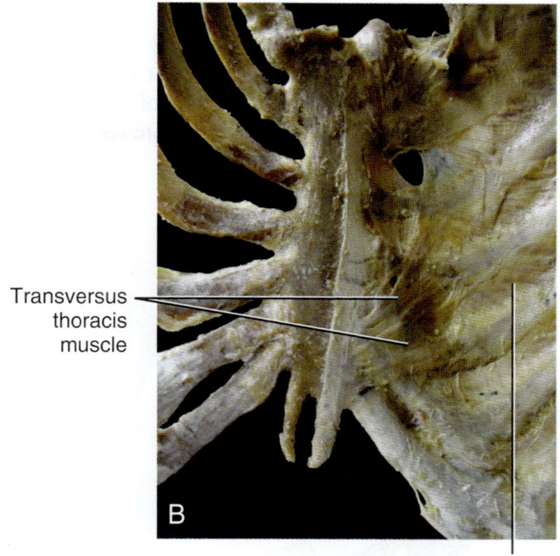

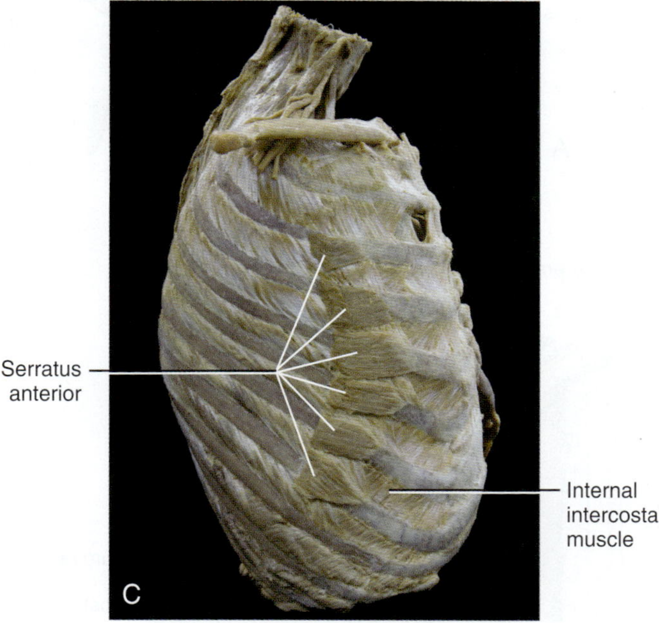

Fig. 3.3, cont'd **(B)** Muscles of the anterior thorax, internal view. **(C)** Muscles of the thorax, lateral view.

Inner Layer (= Transversus Thoracis Group)

- Innermost intercostals lie laterally, and are better developed below than above
- Transversus thoracis
- Subcostal muscles

INTERCOSTAL SPACES (Fig 3.4A and B)

- Running between the middle and innermost **muscular** layers is the neurovascular plane consisting of a vein, an artery and a nerve (superior to inferior) under the protection of the costal groove. Collateral branches run along the lower intercostal space but can generally be ignored

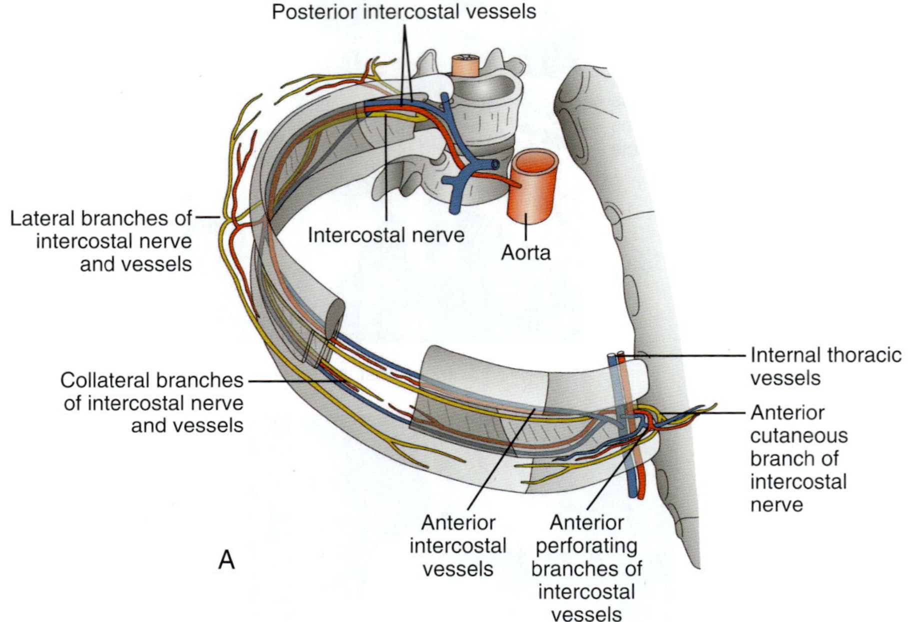

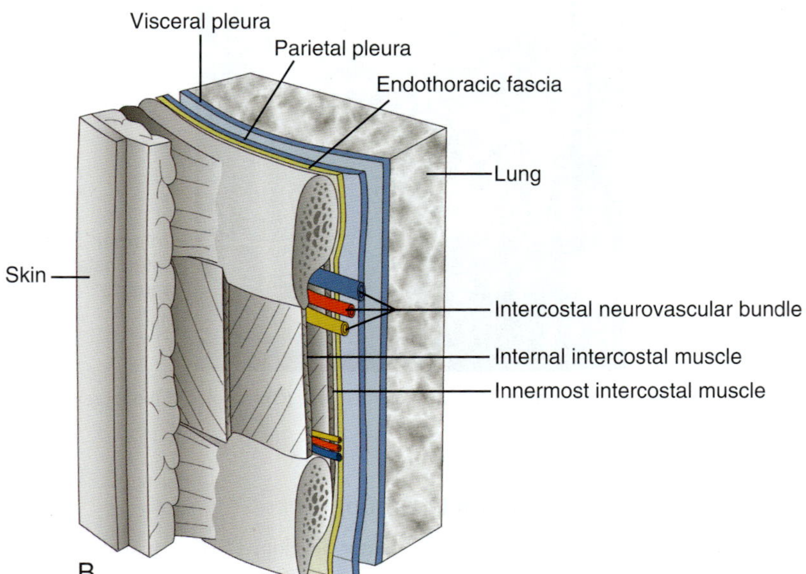

Fig. 3.4 (A, B) Intercostal space and neurovascular structures.

Intercostal Nerves

- The main nerve has a lateral cutaneous branch and a terminal anterior cutaneous branch
  - Lateral branch pierces the overlying muscles, dividing into anterior and posterior branches
  - Anterior cutaneous branch in the upper six spaces passes anterior to the internal thoracic artery and then pierces the muscles to reach the skin
- The lower five intercostal nerves slope downwards before exiting their intercostal rib space to supply the anterior abdominal wall
- The first nerve is very small and supplies no skin
- The 12th nerve (subcostal nerveT12) passes quickly into the abdominal cavity behind the lateral arcuate ligament

Intercostal Arteries (Fig 3.5)

- Arteries enter the intercostal spaces both anteriorly and posteriorly
- Posteriorly:
  - Superior intercostal artery supplies the upper two spaces (from costocervical trunk, subclavian part II)
  - Spaces three to eleven are supplied by posterior intercostal branches from the thoracic aorta, with each giving off a small collateral branch
- Anteriorly:
  - Supplied by the internal thoracic artery (upper six) and musculophrenic artery in the seventh to ninth spaces

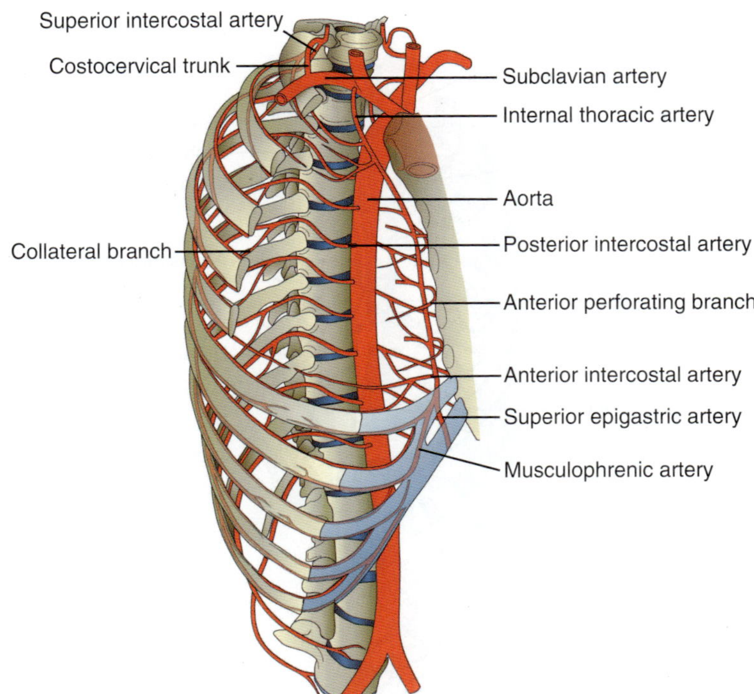

Fig. 3.5 Arterial supply of the thoracic wall.

Intercostal veins (Fig 3.6A and B)

- In each space there is one posterior and two anterior veins that accompany the arteries
- The drainage via posterior veins is not regular
  - The first space is drained by the supreme intercostal vein into the vertebral vein or brachiocephalic vein
  - The second and third spaces drain via the superior intercostal vein into the azygos vein on the right side and into the brachiocephalic vein on the left side
  - The lower eight spaces drain into the azygos system (azygos on the right, hemiazygos and accessory hemiazygos on the left)

Lymph Drainage (Deep Lymphatics Follow Arteries)

- Anteriorly to intercostal/parasternal nodes and posteriorly to intercostal nodes

Internal Thoracic Artery (see Fig 3.5)

- Branch from the subclavian artery (part one): passes vertically down one finger's-breadth lateral to the sternum and divides at the costal margin into the superior epigastric and musculophrenic arteries. Each space receives two anterior arteries or anterior branches from the internal thoracic/musculophrenic arteries
- Perforating branches emerge towards the skin and are especially large in the second and third spaces (to supply the breast)

Suprapleural Membrane

- A dense layer attached to the inner border of the first rib and costal cartilage giving rigidity to the thoracic inlet to prevent distortion (Sibson's fascia)

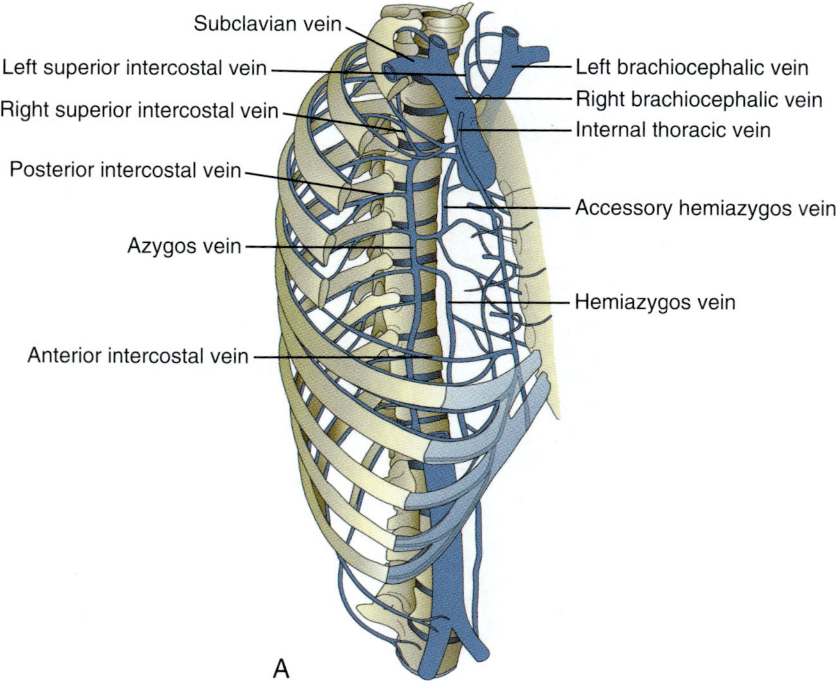

Fig. 3.6 (A) Venous drainage of the thoracic wall.

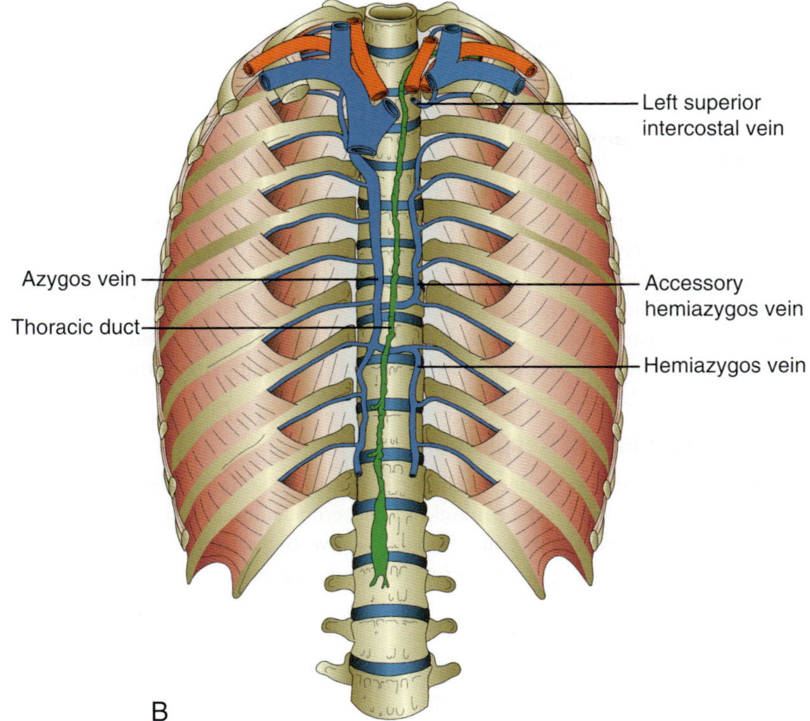

Fig. 3.6, cont'd **(B)** Azygous venous system of the thorax.

DIAPHRAGM

- Thin muscular sheet specialised for respiration
- Two crura anchor the diaphragm to the vertebrae – the right one is larger (L1–3) than the left (L1–2)
- Nerve supply is by the phrenic nerve (C3–5) to each side. Includes parts of crura, one each side. Fibres radiate out in three branches (anterior, lateral and posterior) and contain both motor and sensory fibres
- Median arcuate ligament lies between both crura in front of the aorta at the level of T12
- Medial arcuate ligament is a thickening of the psoas fascia extending from the body of the vertebra (L1) to the transverse process (L1)
- Lateral arcuate ligament is a thickening of the anterior layer of the lumbar fascia extending from the transverse process to the twelfth rib
- Blood supply is mainly by the right and left inferior phrenic arteries. The intercostal arteries (lower five) and subcostal supply the costal margin of the diaphragm.
- The pericardiophrenic artery supplies the phrenic nerve, pluera (mediastinal surface) and pericardium

Diaphragmatic Openings

- T12 – aortic hiatus, behind median arcuate ligament
  - Aorta, azygos vein and thoracic duct (from cisternae chyli)
- T10 – oesophageal opening, usually 2.5 cm to the left of the midline in the fibres of the left crus with fibres from the right forming a sling (supplied by the left)

- Oesophagus, vagal trunks, oesophageal branches of the left gastric vessels
- T8 – vena caval opening lying in the central tendon
  - Vena cava, right phrenic nerve
- Other structures that make their own openings include:
  - Hemiazygos vein passes through the left crus
  - Greater, lesser and least splanchnic nerves pierce the crura
  - Sympathetic trunks pass behind the medial arcuate ligaments
  - Subcostal nerve and vessels pass behind the lateral arcuate ligament
  - Left phrenic nerve pierces the muscular dome
  - Neurovascular bundles of vertebral levels seven to eleven pass between the digitations of the diaphragm and the transversus abdominis
  - Superior epigastric vessels descend to the anterior abdominal wall, crossing the diaphragm in the interval between the sternal and the costal parts of the muscle
  - Extraperitoneal lymph vessels pass directly through

Thoracic Movements and Respiration

In quiet respiration, inspiration is due to the action of the diaphragm, the intercostal muscles adjacent to the sternum and the scalene muscles. The sternocleidomastoid and the external intercostal muscles are accessory. Expiration is largely passive but assisted by the external oblique muscle, internal oblique muscle and transversus abdominis muscles.

Part 3 Thoracic Cavity

DIVISIONS OF THE MEDIASTINUM

- A horizontal plane through the sternal angle (T4/5) (Fig 3.7) divides the mediastinum into superior and inferior. This plane (of Louis) also passes through the **second costal cartilage**.
- Plane passes through:
  - Bifurcation of the trachea
  - Beginning and end of the aortic arch

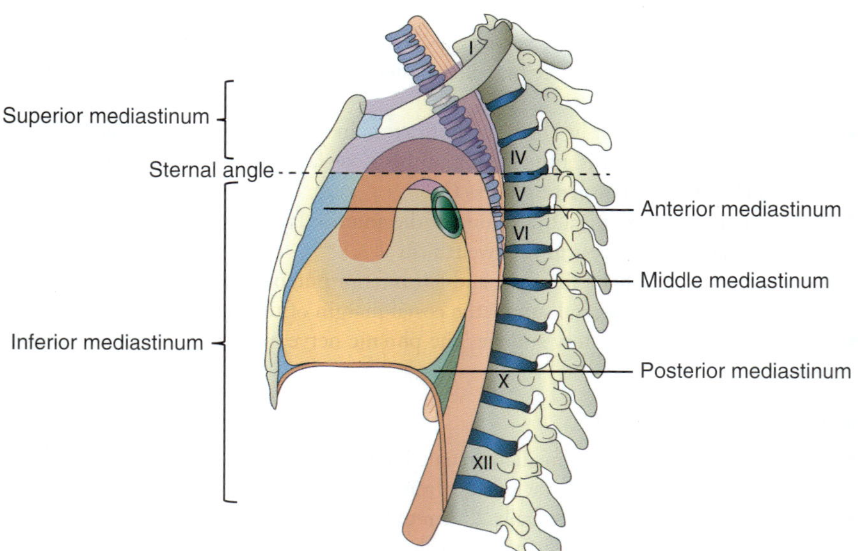

Fig. 3.7 Division of the mediastinum, sternal angle plane.

- Just above the bifurcation of the pulmonary trunk
- Azygos vein entering the superior vena cava
- Where the thoracic duct moves from the left to the right of the oesophagus
- Ligamentum arteriosum
- Superficial and deep parts of the cardiac plexus

Part 4 Superior Mediastinum

GENERAL TOPOGRAPHY

- The superior mediastinum is wedge-shaped, with the anterior boundary being the manubrium and the posterior boundary being the upper four thoracic vertebrae
- Thoracic inlet (Fig 3.8)
  - Midline is wholly occupied by the trachea and oesophagus
  - Apices of the lungs lie laterally
- Within the mediastinum, the veins are on the right and the arteries are on the left; hence there is great asymmetry in the thorax

GREAT VESSELS: ARTERIES (Fig 3.9A and B)

- Aortic arch passes from sternal angle at T4/5 level (front to back and just to the left) over the left bronchus and bifurcation of the pulmonary trunk
  - At the apex (midpoint) it gives off the brachiocephalic, left common carotid and left subclavian arteries
  - Relationships:
    - To the left lie the phrenic (anteriorly) and vagus nerves (posteriorly) and the sympathetic and superficial cardiac plexus supplied by the vagus
    - The left superior intercostal vein passes forwards to the left brachiocephalic vein (superficial to the vagus, deep to the phrenic)

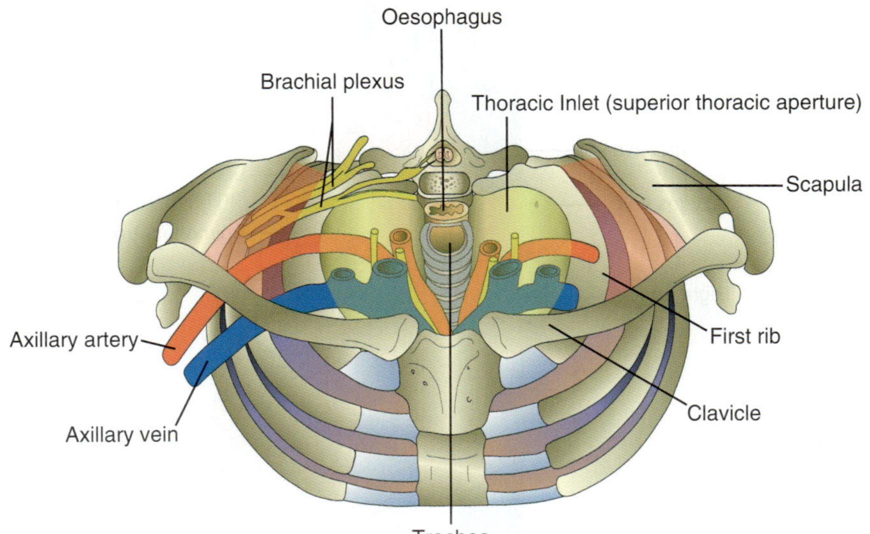

Fig. 3.8 Thoracic inlet, superior view.

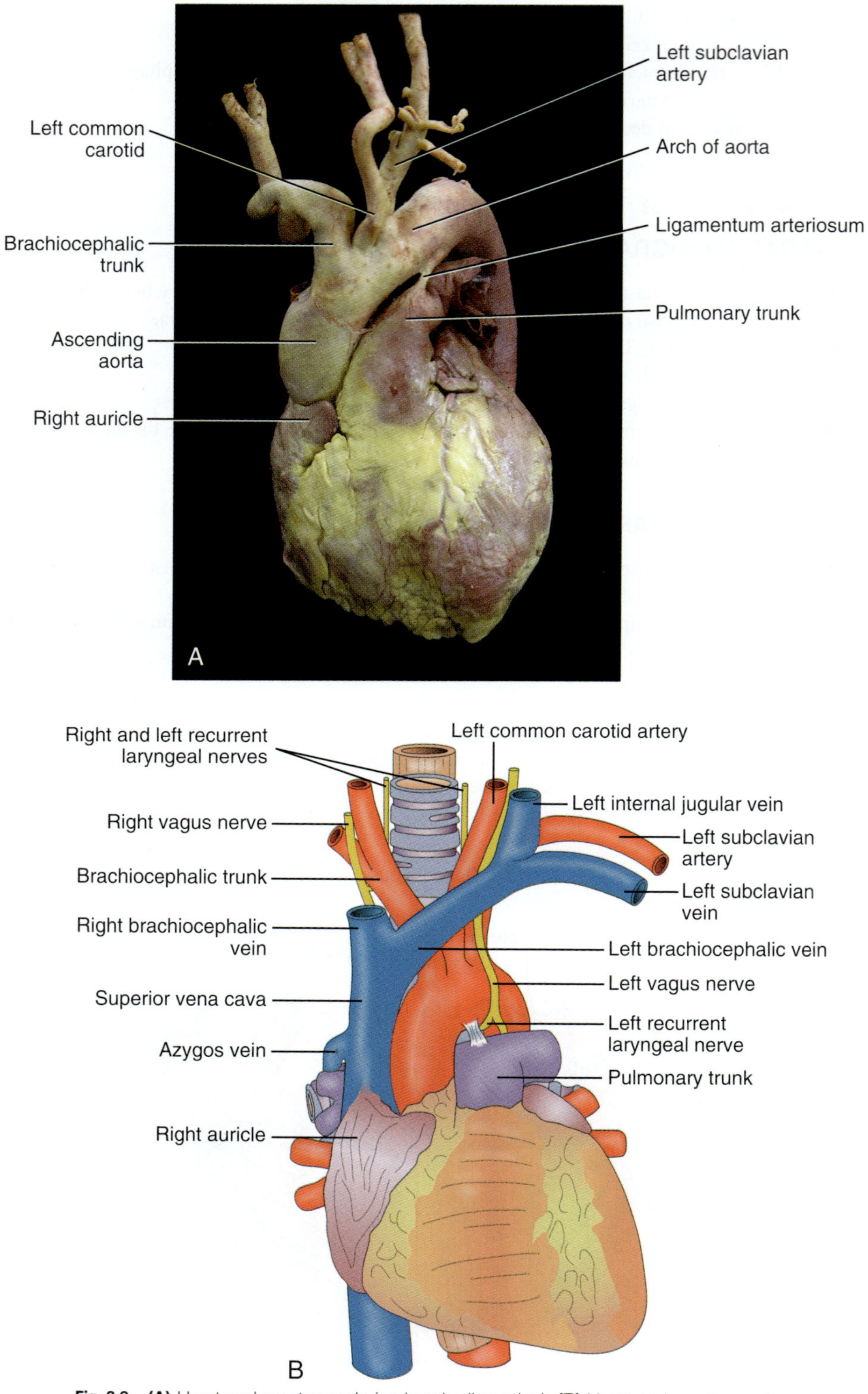

Left subclavian artery
Left common carotid
Arch of aorta
Ligamentum arteriosum
Brachiocephalic trunk
Pulmonary trunk
Ascending aorta
Right auricle
A

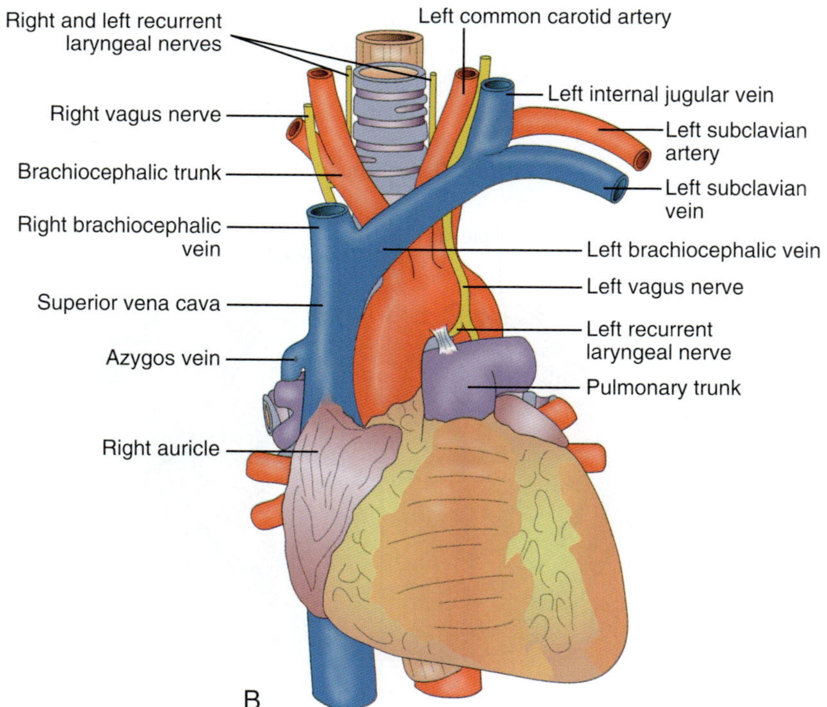

Fig. 3.9 (A) Heart and great vessels (cadaveric dissection). **(B)** Heart and great vessels.

    - The left recurrent laryngeal nerve hooks around the arch of the aorta posterior to the ligamentum arteriosum, passing back up on the right hand side of the aorta
    - The pulmonary trunk bifurcates into the right and left pulmonary arteries in the concavity of the aortic arch
    - The trachea and oesophagus lie on the right side
    - Baroreceptors lie in the adventitial layer (supplied by vagal fibres)
    - Aortic bodies lie under the arch and detect hypoxia (supplied by vagal fibres)
- The brachiocephalic trunk arises a little to the left of the midline, sloping away to the right across the trachea, to divide at the right sternoclavicular joint with no other branches (except for the rare thyroidea ima artery)
- The left common carotid artery arises just behind the braciocephalic trunk and slopes in front of the trachea
- The left subclavian artery arises next, arching over the apex of the lung, parting from the common carotid artery just behind the sternoclavicular joint
- The **ligamentum arteriosum** is the remnant of the **ductus arteriosus** from the left pulmonary artery to the concavity of the aortic arch

GREAT VESSELS: VEINS (see Fig 3.9A and B)

Brachiocephalic Veins

- Brachiocephalic veins are formed behind the sternoclavicular junction from the internal jugular and subclavian veins
    - Internal jugular vein lies lateral to the common carotid artery and in front of the scalenus anterior
    - Subclavian vein lies lateral to and then posterior to the scalenus anterior
    - Right brachiocephalic vein runs vertically downwards and receives the right lymphatic duct, right jugular lymph trunk and subclavian lymph trunks (everything not drained by the thoracic duct)
    - Left brachiocephalic vein passes almost horizontally behind the sternum and joins with the right brachiocephalic vein at the lower border of the first right costal cartilage to form the superior vena cava. At its commencement it receives the thoracic duct, the vertebral vein, the internal thoracic vein, the inferior thyroid plexus of veins, the left superior intercostal veins and the large thymic vein

Superior Vena Cava

- Commences at the lower border of the first right costal cartilage
- Formed by the union of the left and right brachiocephalic veins
- Pierces the pericardium at the third right costal cartilage and receives the azygos vein (T4/5 = sternal angle level)
- Enters the right atrium at the lower border of the third right costal cartilage

Cardiac Plexus (see Fig 3.9A and B)

- Consists of sympathetic, parasympathetic and afferent fibres
- Divided into deep and superficial parts
- Superficial part is formed by the union of the inferior cervical cardiac branch of the left vagus with the cardiac branch of the left cervical sympathetic ganglion. It lies in front of the ligamentum arteriosum under the arch of the aorta
- Deep part is larger, receiving fibres from the right and left vagus, and the right and left recurrent laryngeal nerves of the cervical sympathetic ganglia. This lies to the right of of the ligamentum arteriosum, in front of the left bronchus at the bifurcation of the pulmonary trunk
- Sympathetic fibres are postganglionic

- Parasympathetic fibres are preganglionic
- Afferent fibres run with sympathetic fibres and may be destroyed in a myocardial infarction

TRACHEA

- Commences in the neck below the cricoid cartilage (at C6 level) and bifurcates into the left and right main bronchus just below the sternal angle (T4/5)
- Consists of the cervical part and thoracic part
- The thoracic part is supplied by the inferior thyroid artery and bronchial arteries

PHRENIC AND VAGUS NERVES

Phrenic Nerve (C3–5)

- Right phrenic nerve is in contact with venous structures along its entire course: the right brachiocephalic vein, the superior vena cava, the right atrium and the inferior vena cava. It crosses the diaphragm by passing through the vena caval foramen in the central tendon
- Left phrenic nerve has the left common carotid and the left subclavian arteries on its medial side. It crosses the aortic arch *superficial* to the left superior intercostal vein and then runs laterally down the pericardium over the left ventricle towards the apex. To reach the undersurface of the diaphragm, it pierces the muscular part of the diaphragm

Vagus Nerves (Fig 3.10)

- Right vagus is in contact with the trachea once inside the superior mediastinum, and at the sternal angle plane it passes deep to the ayzgos. It continues behind the root of the lung
- Left vagus is held away from the trachea by the great arteries from the arch of aorta. It crosses the arch *deep* to the left superior intercostal vein. The nerve then continues behind

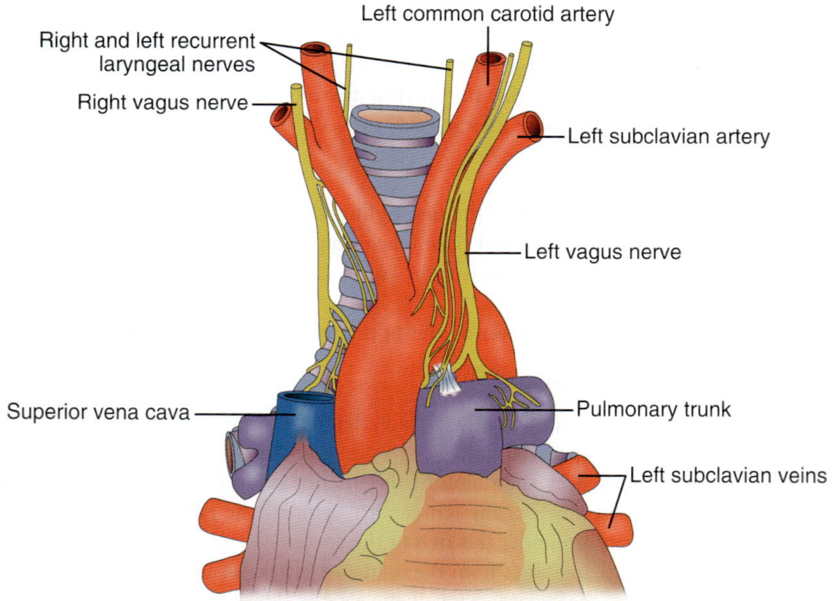

Fig. 3.10 Vagus nerves and their relations.

the lung root and passes into the midline to enter the oesophageal plexus of the lower oesophagus

Part 5 Anterior Mediastinum

- Essentially a potential space, continuous with the superior mediastinum

THYMUS

- Bilobed organ and more prominent in children
- Relationships: anteriorly is the pretracheal fascia, the sternohyoid, the sternothyroid, the manubrium and the upper part of the body of the sternum
- Lobes are overlapped slightly by the pleura
- Blood supply: via the inferior thyroid and internal thoracic arteries
- Lymph drainage: the parasternal, tracheobronchial and brachiocephalic nodes

Part 6 Middle Mediastinum and Heart

PERICARDIUM

Fibrous Pericardium

- A sac enclosing the heart and great vessels (fusing with the vessels except for the inferior vena cava)
  - Broad base which overlies the central tendon of the diaphragm (both originating from the septum transversum)
  - Connected by weak sternopericardial ligaments to the sternum, and supplied by the pericardiophrenic and internal thoracic arteries

Serous Pericardium

- The reflected inner lining deep to the fibrous pericardium; it has two layers: the parietal and visceral layers
  - Between the parietal and the visceral layers are the transverse and oblique sinuses
    - Oblique sinus is a cul-de-sac between the four pulmonary veins and the inferior vena cava; it permits pulsation of the left atria
    - The transverse sinus separates cardiac inflow and outflow
    - Sinuses are separated from each other by a double fold
  - Phrenic nerve supplies fibrous and parietal layers, but the visceral layer is insensitive
    - Myocardial pain is transmitted by sympathetic nerves, and pericardial pain via the phrenic nerve

HEART

Borders

- Right border consists entirely of the right atrium
  - Extends from the lower border of the right third costal cartilage to the right sixth costal cartilage
- Inferior border is mostly right ventricle and a small portion of the left ventricle (apex)
  - Extends from the right sixth costal cartilage to the apex (left fifth intercostal space)
- Left border is mostly left ventricle with the auricle of the left atrium superiorly
  - Extends from the apex to the lower border of the left second costal cartilage

Surfaces

- Anterior (sternocostal) surface consists of the right atrium and right ventricle (plus a narrow strip of the left ventricle)
- Diaphragmatic surface consists of right atrium (receives the inferior vena cava), one-third right ventricle and two-thirds left ventricle
- Posterior surface, or the base, consists almost entirely of the left atrium

Fibrous Skeleton

- Atria and ventricles are attached to a fibrous skeleton lying on the sagittal plane
- Atria lie to the right of the fibous skeleton, and ventricles to the left with no electro-muscular continuity except the atrioventricular conduction bundle
- Membranous part of the interventricular septum (the bases of the cusps of the tricuspid and the mitral valves are attached to the fibrous skeleton)

Heart Chambers

- Right atrium (Fig 3.11)
  - Upper end is prolonged as the right auricle (overlying the commencement of the aorta)
  - Crista terminalis separates the smooth and roughened areas
  - The inferior vena cava opening is protected by a ridge extending up to the coronary sinus
  - Posterior wall forms the interatrial septum (above the coronary sinus) and is where the fossa ovalis is located (lower part)
- Right ventricle
  - Lies to the left of the vertical atrioventricular groove (in which the right coronary artery runs)
  - Walls are thrown into numerous muscular ridges (trabeculae carneae) and form the moderator band and papillary muscles
  - The tricuspid valve separates it from the right atrium and contains anterior, posterior and septal cusps
  - Edges of ventricular surfaces receive the chordae tendineae

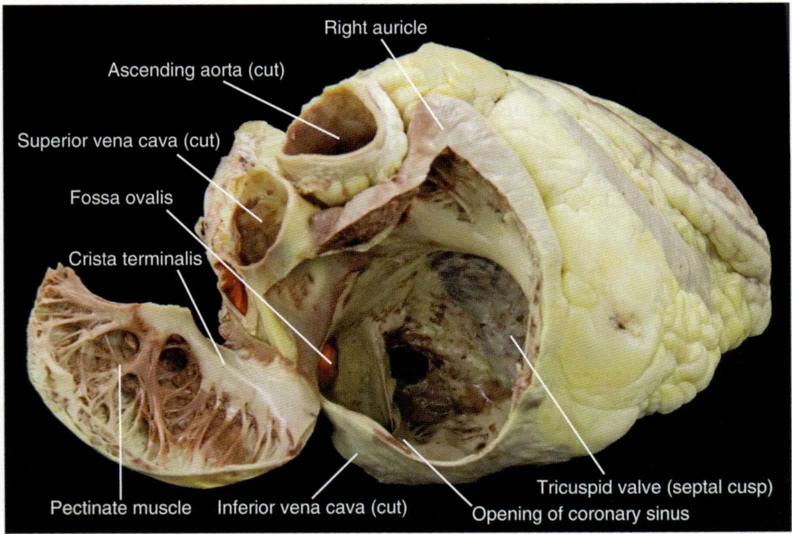

Fig. 3.11 Right atrium (interior view).

- The ventricle funnels up to the pulmonary orifice (where the walls are thin) and the pulmonary valve
- The pulmonary valve contains anterior, left and right cusps and lies near the horizontal plane higher than the aortic orifice

- Left atrium
  - Forms the posterior surface (base) of the heart, with a small auricle projecting upwards
  - Four pulmonary veins enter symmetrically
  - Cavity is smooth-walled apart from the auricle
  - Bicuspid mitral valve contains anterior and posterior cusps
- Left ventricle (Fig 3.12)
  - The walls are three times as thick as the right ventricle, and the cavity bulges into the right ventricle
  - It has well-developed trabeculae carneae with two papillary muscles
  - The aortic valve has posterior, left and right cusps

Conducting System

- The sinoatrial (SA) node (specialised muscle fibres) initiates conduction, which spreads to the atrial cardiac muscle fibres and then to the atrioventricular (AV) node. From there it passes through the bundle of His and then divides into the right and left bundle branches before spreading via subendocardial Purkinje fibres to generate ventricular contraction
- The sinoatrial node is crescent-shaped and 1–2 cm by 5 mm in size
- The atrioventricular node is buried in the muscle of the interatrial septum

Heart Valves

- Structure of heart valves
  - Tricuspid and mitral valves have free edges with a serrated outline. Integrity requires active contraction of the papillary muscles

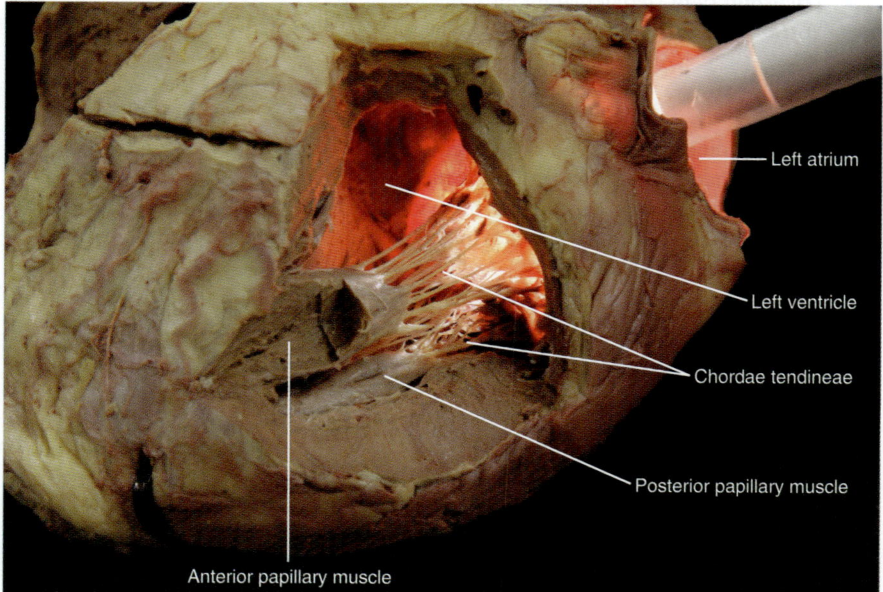

Fig. 3.12 Left ventricle (interior view).

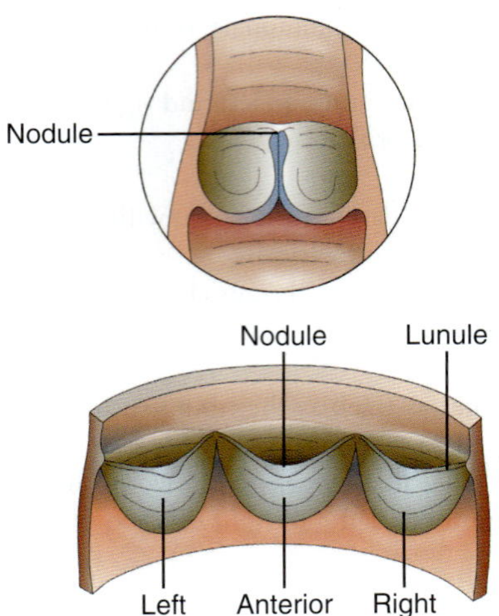

Fig. 3.13 Semilunar valve. Top: valve closed, coronal section. Bottom: detubularised view, showing the three constituent semilunar cusps.

- Pulmonary valve and aortic valve (Fig 3.13) have a free edge containing a central fibrous nodule; their competence is passive, the result of pressure between the cusps and depending on the integrity of the straight edges
- Valves are composed of fibrous tissue with extensive elastic fibres, and are covered with vascular endothelium

- For auscultation:
  - **Aortic:** right sternal margin, second intercostal space
  - **Pulmonary:** left sternal margin, third costal cartilage
  - **Tricuspid:** right sternal margin, fifth intercostal space
  - **Mitral:** site of apex beat (left midclavicular line in the fifth intercostal space)

Vasculature

- Great vessels
  - The ascending aorta is 5 cm long. It gives off the sinuses and then runs to the right of the pulmonary trunk (both within a common sleeve in front of the transverse sinus)
  - The pulmonary trunk is 5 cm long and wide bore; it arches backwards and to the left of the aorta, and gives off its branches upon emerging from the pericardium
- Blood supply (Fig 3.14A and B)
  - The right coronary artery passes between the right auricle and the infundibulum of the right ventricle. It then passes vertically downwards and then posteriorly
    - The SA nodal artery originates from right coronary artery in 60% of cases
    - The right marginal artery originates from the inferior margin
    - The AV nodal artery lies posteriorly
    - The posterior interventricular artery passes along the posterior interventricular groove to the apex (in 90% 'right dominant' cases)
  - Left coronary artery arises behind the pulmonary trunk and divides into the circumflex (continuation of) and the anterior interventricular artery
    - The SA nodal artery originates from the left coronary artery in 40% of cases
    - The circumflex artery passes down the back of the heart and gives off various branches
    - The anterior interventricular artery (also known as the left anterior descending artery) runs down in the posterior interventricular groove to anastomose with the

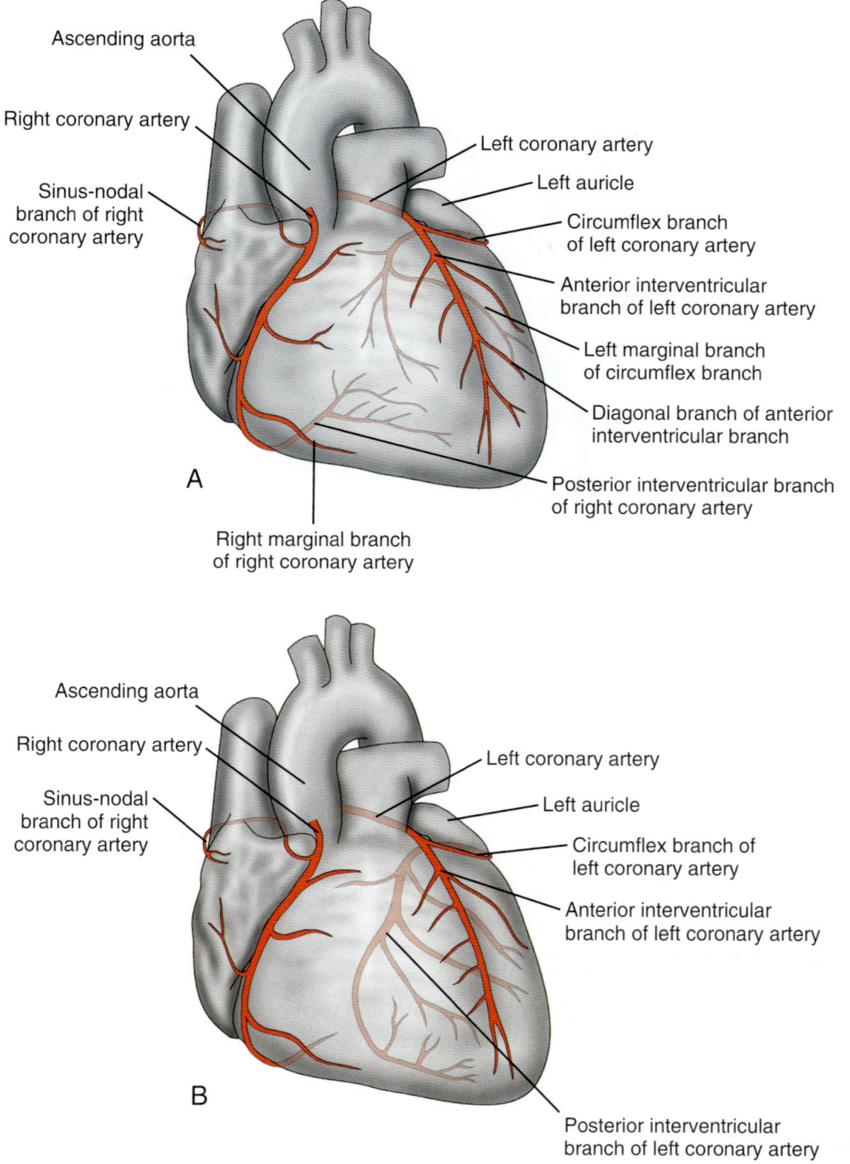

Fig. 3.14 (A) Coronary arteries, right dominant arrangement. **(B)** Coronary arteries, left dominant arrangement.

posterior interventricular artery (in 10% 'left dominant' cases, the posterior interventricular artery is given off by the left coronary artery)

- The coronary sinus (Fig 3.15) lies in the posterior part of the atrioventricular groove and drains into the right atrium
- Mediastinal nodes drain with the arteries

Innervation

- Heart is innervated by the cardiac plexus; note also the presence of baroreceptors

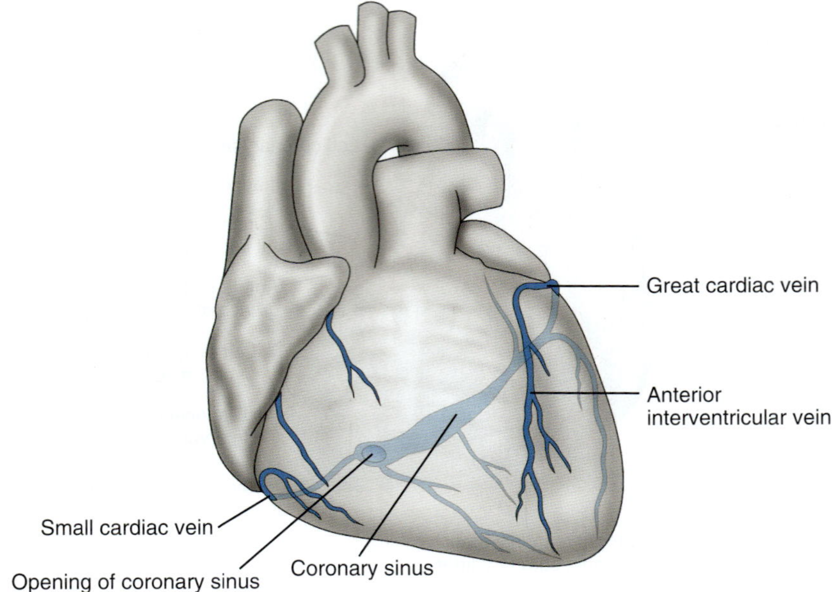

Fig. 3.15 Venous drainage of the heart and coronary sinus.

Part 7 Posterior Mediastinum

GENERAL TOPOGRAPHY

- Posterior to the pericardium and diaphragm, below the superior mediastinum and between the pretracheal and prevertebral fascia
- Bound posteriorly by T4–12 and anteriorly by the pericardium and diaphragm

DESCENDING (THORACIC) AORTA

- Commencing at T4/5 just left of the midline and slanting towards the midline
- Gives off nine posterior intercostal arteries, the subcostal artery, bronchial arteries and small oesophageal vessels

OESOPHAGUS

- Length 25 cm in length, running from the cricoid cartilage (cricopharyngeus) at C6 (midline) to the cardiac orifice of the stomach at T10 (2.5 cm left of the midline)
- Initially in contact with vertebral bodies, it moves forwards so that it is in front of the thoracic aorta
- Intra-abdominal part averages 1–2 cm

Relations

- Crossed by the arch of the aorta on its left side
- Azygos vein is on the right

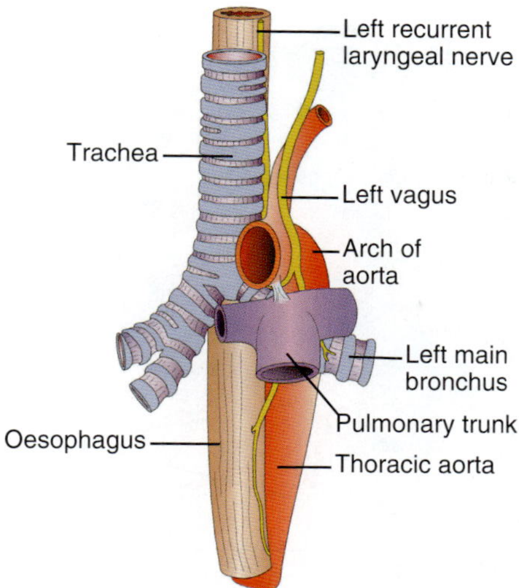

Fig. 3.16 Left main bronchus and its relations.

- Anteriorly: below the tracheal bifurcation it is crossed by the *left* main bronchus (Fig 3.16) and the *right* pulmonary artery
- Posteriorly: the thoracic duct inclines from right to left
- Just above the diaphragmatic opening, firm connective tissue connects it with the aorta

Constrictions

- Narrowest part is the cricopharyngeal sphincter (15 cm from the incisors)
- Slight constriction where it is crossed by the aortic arch (22 cm), the left main bronchus (27 cm) and where is passes through the diaphragm (38 cm)
- Left atrial enlargement can also cause indentations

Blood Supply

- The upper third is from the inferior thyroid artery and venous drainage via the brachiocephalic vein
- The middle third is from the oesophageal branches of the thoracic aorta (Fig 3.17) and venous drainage is via the azygos vein
- The lower third is via oesophagael branches from the left gastric artery and venous drainage via the left gastric vein (into the portal vein)

Lymph Drainage

- Follows the arteries to (1) deep cervical, (2) tracheobronchial and (3) preaortic nodes

Nerve Supply

- Upper part is via the recurrent laryngeal nerve and sympathetic fibres from the middle cervical ganglion
- Lower part is from the greater splanchnic nerves; parasympathetic supply is from the vagus nerves (motor supply)
- Pain fibres run with both the vagal and the sympathetic supply; pain can be referred to the neck, arm and thoracic wall

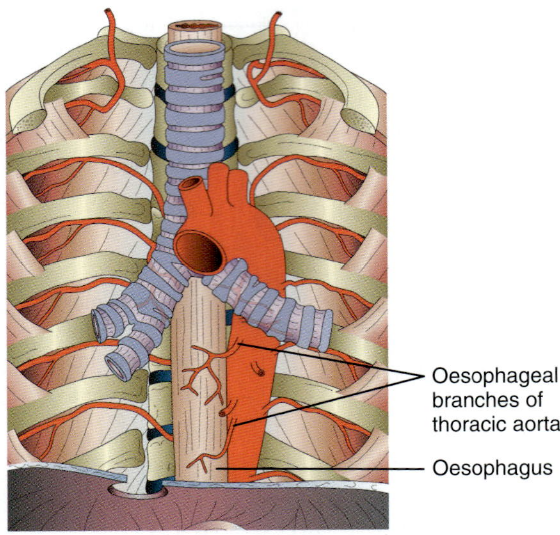

Fig. 3.17 Blood supply of the oesophagus.

Structure

- Inner circular and outer longitudinal layer
- Skeletal muscle (rapid contraction) is in the upper third and visceral muscle is in the lower two-thirds
- The inner circular layer is a direct continuation of the cricopharyngeus muscle, and the lower 5 cm acts as a physiological sphincter (although there is no anatomical demarcation)

LYMPH NODES OF THE THORAX

- Visceral preaortic nodes lie in front of the aorta, draining the middle of the oesophagus
- Somatic para-aortic nodes lie alongside the aorta and drain the intercostal spaces (posterior intercostal group)
  - Upper nodes drain into the thoracic duct or right lymphatic duct and lower ones to the descending intercostal trunk
- Parasternal nodes lie alongside the internal thoracic artery and drain the anterior intercostal spaces
- Anterior, middle and posterior diaphragmatic groups drain the associated areas

THORACIC DUCT (Fig 3.18)

The thoracic duct is the longest lymphatic channel in the body. It originates from the cisterna chyli (T12) and passes upwards to the right of the aorta and the oesophagus. It then moves to the left behind the oesophagus to reach the left of the mediastinum. It lies anterior to the great vessels off the aortic arch and enters the confluence point of the left internal jugular and subclavian veins, as two to three separate branches with *NO* valves.

- Receives lymph from:
  - Lower half of the body
  - Left posterior interclavicular nodes
  - Left jugular and subclavian trunks

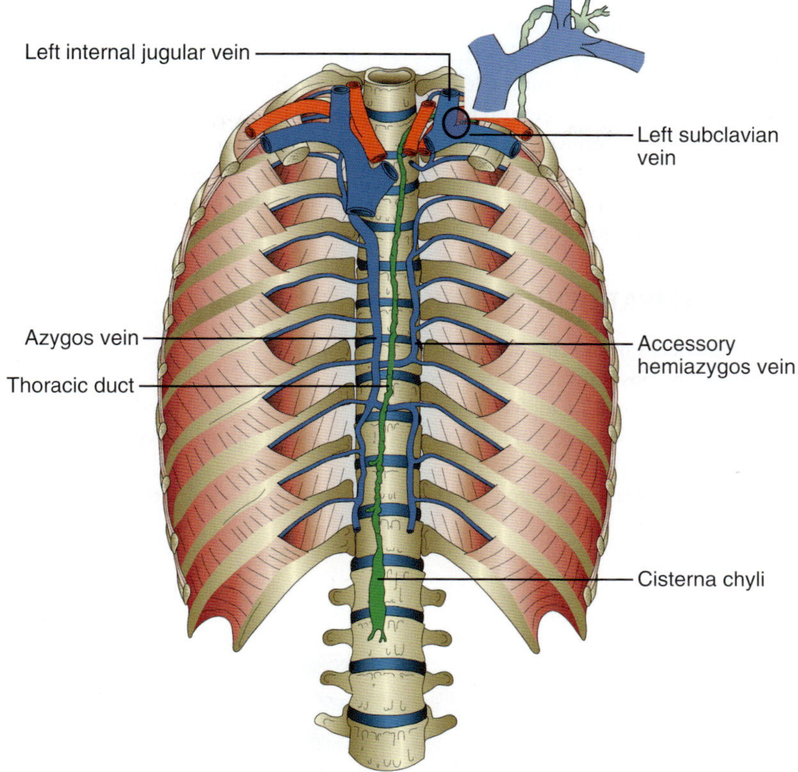

Fig. 3.18 Thoracic duct and its relations.

- The drainage trunks of the right thoracic wall, right upper limb, and right head and neck may join together to drain into the right brachiocephalic vein, or they can remain separate and drain independently into the respective veins

AZYGOS SYSTEM OF VEINS (see Fig 3.6B)

- The thoracic wall and upper lumbar regions are drained by the posterior intercostal and lumbar veins into the azygos system
- The azygos system is made of two longitudinal trunks:
  - Right is a single trunk
  - Left becomes divided
- Right side: azygos vein (persistent right posterior cardinal vein)
  - Begins at the union of the ascending lumbar and subcostal veins
  - Travels through the aortic opening (T12), passes upwards adjacent to the vertebral bodies (on a plane posterior to that of the oesophagus) and arches over the right main bronchus
  - Enters the superior vena cava at T4/5
  - Receives:
    - Lower right posterior intercostal veins
    - Right superior intercostal vein

    - Bronchial veins from the right lung
    - Veins from middle third of the oesophagus
- Left side: hemiazygos vein = lower; accessory hemiazygos vein = upper
  - Each lies longitudinally on the left side of the vertebrae
  - Receives the lowest left eight posterior intercostal veins (four each)
  - Hemiazygos vein receives the lowest left four posterior intercostal veins
  - Accessory hemiazygos vein receives the middle left four posterior intercostal veins, bronchial veins from the left lung, and veins from the middle third of oesophagus
  - The two hemiazygos veins join the azygos system, crossing the midline at T8 and T9

THORACIC SYMPATHETIC TRUNK (Fig 3.19A and B)

- Lies on the necks of the ribs just lateral to the heads
- Anterior to the posterior intercostal vessels
- Typically fewer than 12 ganglia
- Each side receives a white ramus from its corresponding spinal nerve (emerging from the anterior ramus)
- After relay a postganglionic grey ramus is given to each thoracic nerve, which usually lies medial to the white ramus

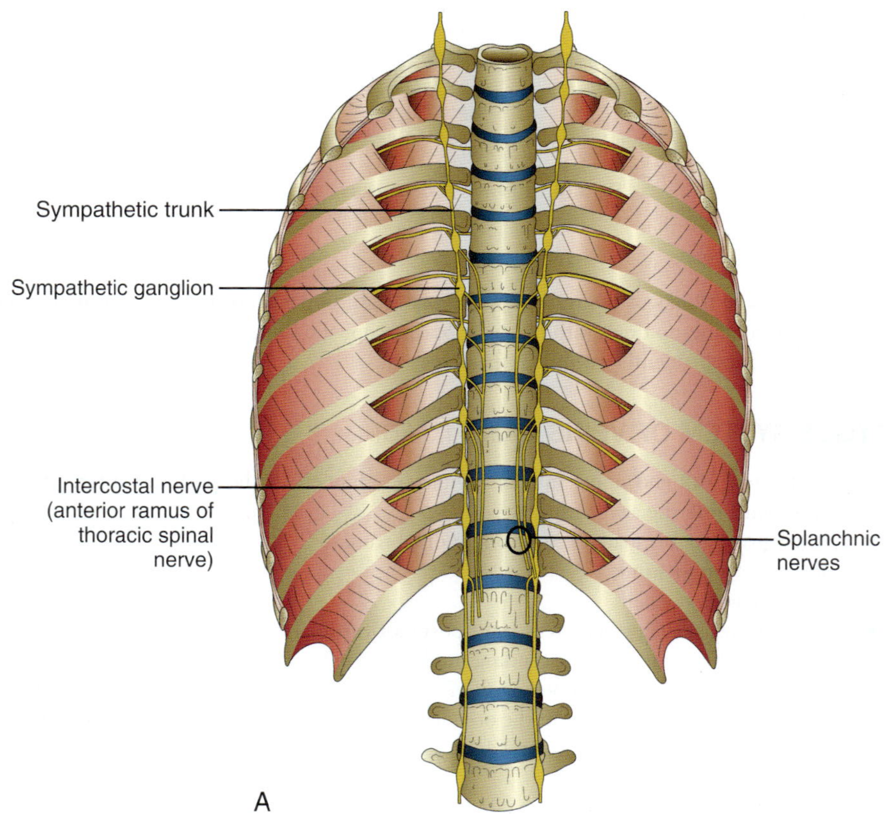

Fig. 3.19 **(A)** Sympathetic trunks.

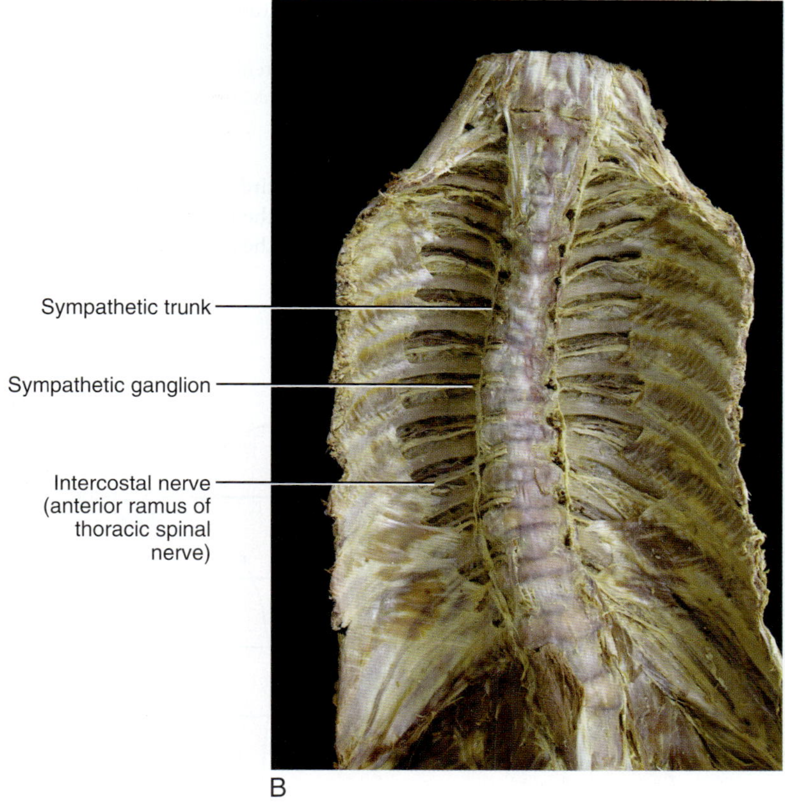

Fig. 3.19, cont'd **(B)** Sympathetic trunks (cadaveric dissection).

- The heart is supplied from the cervical and upper thoracic ganglia (through the cardiac plexus)
- The splanchnic nerves come from the lower eight ganglia

Part 8 Pleura

- Membrane of fibrous tissue covered by a single layer of flat mesothelial cells to reduce friction
- The parietal layer lines the thoracic cavity and is attached by loose areolar tissue. It also covers the diaphragm, pericardium (strong attachment), mediastinum and suprapleural membrane
- From the lung root, a cuff invaginates to form the visceral pleura
  - The visceral layer coats the lungs and extends into the interlobar clefts
  - Its function is to provide low-friction surfaces for breathing movements
- Pulmonary ligaments (double layer of pleura) hang down from the pulmonary hilum, providing dead space for vessel expansion (e.g. inferior pulmonary veins)

NERVE SUPPLY

- Visceral pleura has only autonomic supply (insensate)
- Parietal pleura is supplied segmentally by intercostal nerves over costal elements

- Parietal pleura over the diaphragm is supplied centrally (domes) by the phrenic nerves, and by the intercostal nerves at the peripheries
- The mediastinal parietal pleura is innervated by the phrenic nerve

SURFACE MARKINGS (Fig 3.20A and B)

- Parietal pleura – anteriorly projects above the medial third of the clavicle (nearly 3 cm)
- Surface marking of the dome of the pleura projects to the inner border of the first rib and posteriorly forms a minor bulge in front of the neck of the first rib (beneath the suprapleural membrane)

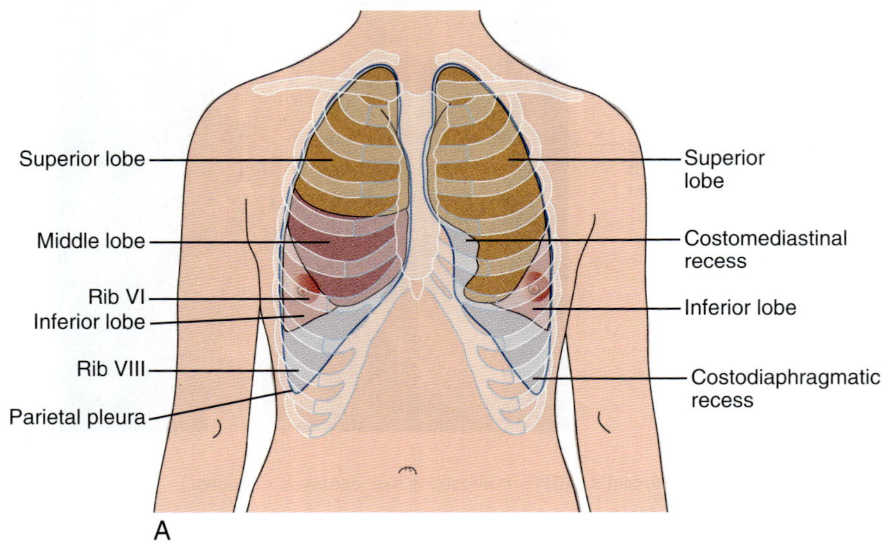

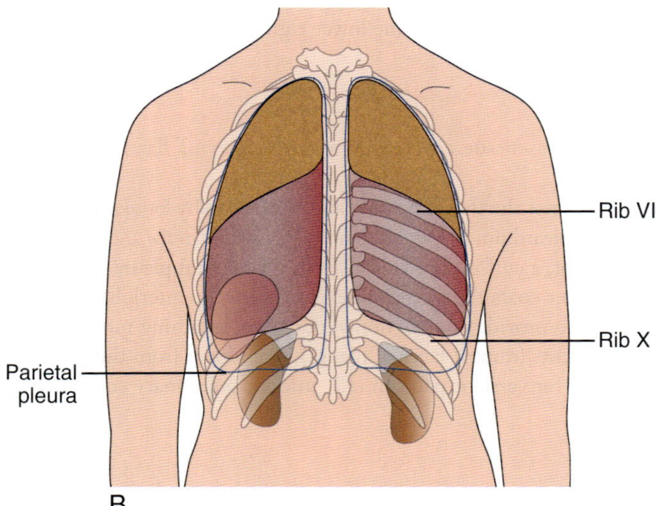

Fig. 3.20 **(A)** Anterior surface markings of the lung and pleura. **(B)** Posterior surface markings of the lung and pleura.

- Line of pleural reflection
  - At the sternoclavicular joint they meet in the midline at the level of the second rib (= sternal angle)
  - Pass vertically down to the fourth costal cartilage, then the right continues vertically and the left descends laterally
  - Each turns lateral at the sixth costal cartilage
  - They cross the midclavicular line at the eighth rib
  - They cross the midaxillary line at the tenth rib (= costodiaphragmatic recess)
  - They cross the 12th rib at the lateral border of the erector spinae

Part 9 Lungs

LUNG ROOTS (Fig 3.21)

- The left lung root contains (enclosed in a sleeve):
  - The left pulmonary artery (superiorly)
  - The left bronchus, sloping away from the trachea (posteriorly and superiorly)
  - Two pulmonary veins, one in front of the other (anteriorly and inferiorly)
  - Bronchial vessels, autonomic nerves, lymph nodes and lymph channels
- Right lung root
  - As above, but the bronchus and pulmonary artery branch to the upper lobe outside the lung
  - Root of the lung lies within the curve of the azygos vein

PULMONARY ARTERIES

- Left pulmonary artery is attached to the inferior surface of the aortic arch by the ligamentum arteriosum
  - It passes anterior to the left bronchus to enter the hilum of the lung
- Right pulmonary artery passes inferior to the carina (anterior to the oesophagus)
  - At the lung root it is anterior to the bronchus
  - It gives off its branch to the upper lobe and then enters the hilum

FISSURES

- Oblique fissure extends from the surface of the lung to the hilum, dividing the lung into upper and lower lobes

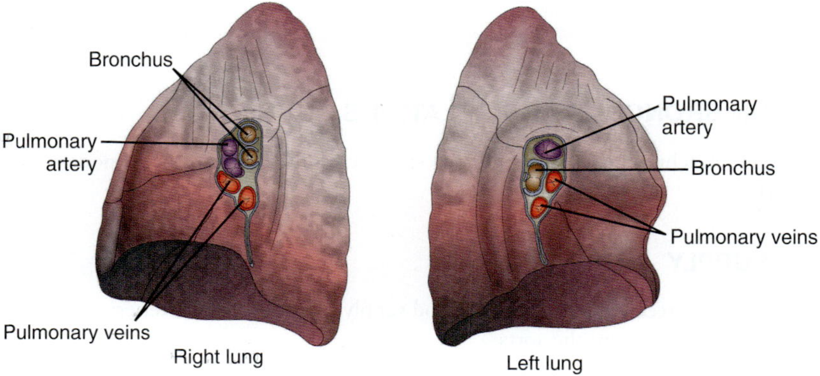

Fig. 3.21 Roots of the lungs.

- Horizontal fissure (right lung only) passes from the anterior margin of the oblique fissure to separate a wedge-shaped middle lobe from the upper lobe (may be incomplete/absent). On the left, a corresponding fissure separates out the lingula lobe, although this is never complete
- The involution of the pleura into the fissures is what provides the slippery surface allowing the lung to expand more easily

SURFACE MARKINGS

- The hila lie approximately behind the third and fourth costal cartilage at the sternal margin (T5–7)
- Surface markings of the lung coincide with the pleura generally – except for the area of cardiac dullness on the left and inferiorly the two ribs above the pleural reflection

LOBAR AND SEGMENTAL BRONCHI

- Each main bronchus is about 5 cm long (right slightly shorter, more vertical and wider). The **carina**, an internal ridge, lies to the left of the midline. Therefore, foreign bodies that fall down the trachea are much more likely to fall into the right main bronchus
- The right main bronchus gives off its upper lobe bronchus outside the lung
- Each lobar bronchus gives rise to segmental bronchi (10 in total)

TABLE 3.1 ■ **Summary of the Bronchopulmonary Segments**

Right		Left	
Upper (3)	Apical	Upper (3)	Apical
	Posterior		Apicoposterior
	Anterior		Anterior
Middle (2)	Lateral	Middle (2)	Superior lingual
	Medial		Inferior lingual
Lower (5)	Apical	Lower (5)	Apical (superior)
	Medial		Medial (cardiac)
	Anterior basal		Anterior basal
	Lateral basal		Lateral basal
	Posterior basal		Posterior basal

LEFT MAIN BRONCHUS AND RELATIONS (see Fig 3.16)

The left main bronchus crosses three structures: the descending aorta, the pulmonary trunk and the oesophagus.

BLOOD SUPPLY

- Bronchial tree receives independent blood supply from bronchial arteries:
  - Two on the left from the aorta
  - One on the right from the third posterior intercostal artery
- Alveoli contain a rich capillary plexus from the pulmonary tree

LYMPH DRAINAGE

- Lymphatic channels run towards the hilum
- From the pleura, they run along the bronchi and pulmonary artery
- Hilar lymph nodes lie just within or beyond the lung

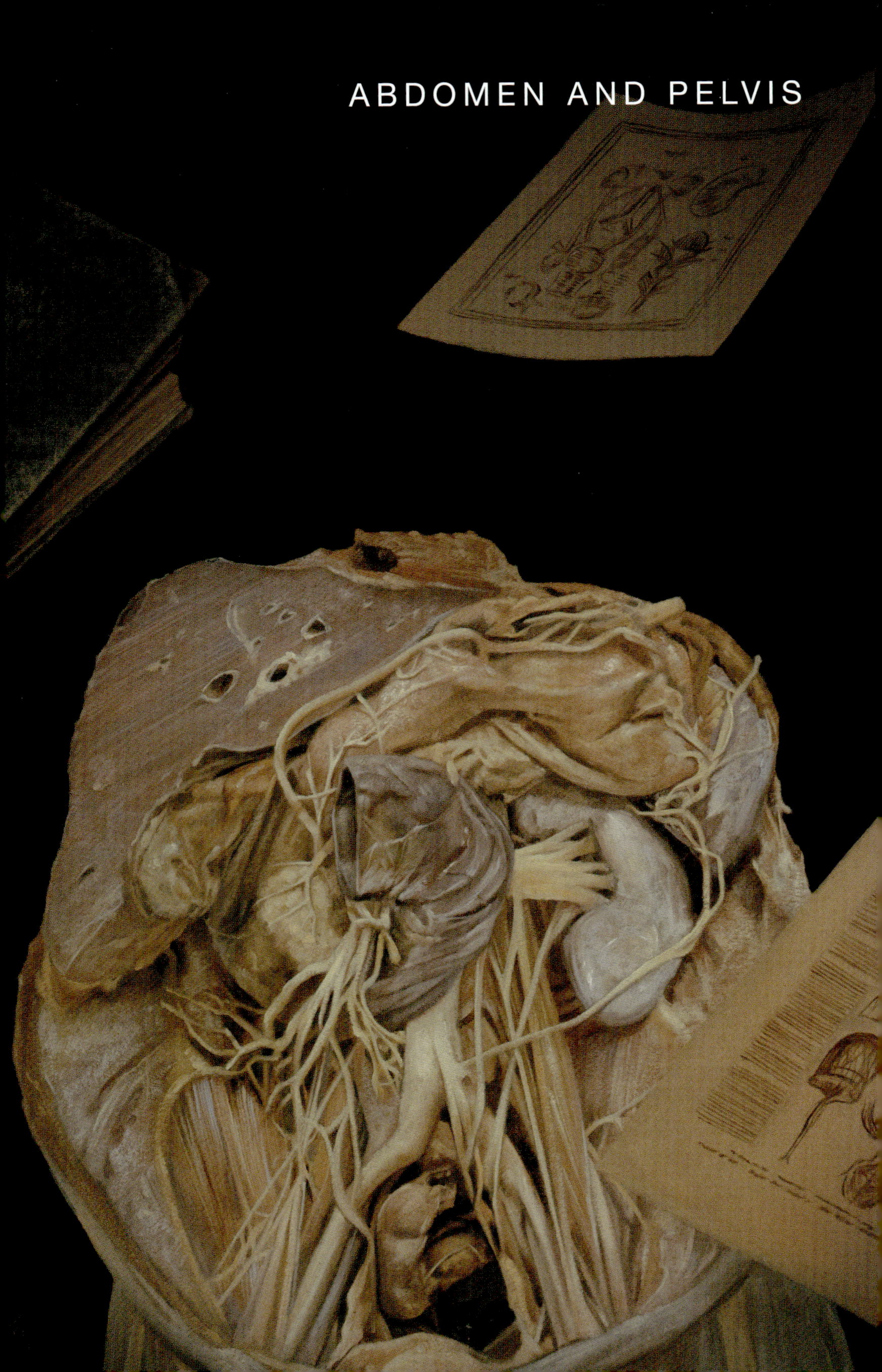

ABDOMEN AND PELVIS

CHAPTER 4

Abdomen and Pelvis

4-1 Abdomen

CHAPTER OUTLINE

Part 1 Anterior Abdominal Wall (Fig 4.1A and B)

SUPERFICIAL FASCIA

- A layer of fatty connective tissue continuous with the superficial fascia in other regions of the body

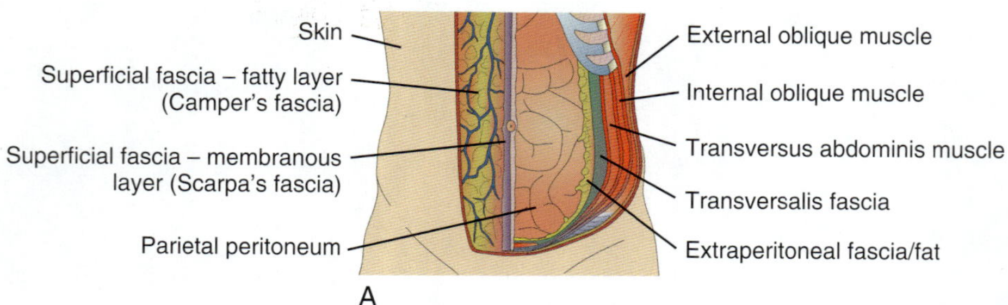

Fig. 4.1 **(A)** Layers of the anterior abdominal wall.

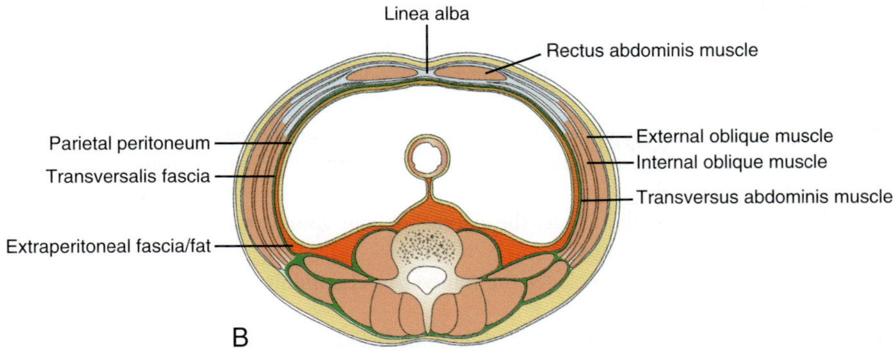

Fig. 4.1, cont'd **(B)** Layers of the abdominal wall, transverse section.

- Below the umbilicus it forms two distinct layers:
  - Superficial fatty layer (Camper's fascia) – continuous with the superficial fascia of the thigh and fuses with the deeper layer in males to form the superficial fascia of the penis
  - Deeper membranous layer (Scarpa's fascia) – thin and membranous and contains little fat. It is continuous with the deep fascia of the thigh (fascia lata) and the dartos fascia of the scrotum, and continues into the anterior perineum to become the superficial perineal fascia (Colles' fascia)

MUSCLES

TABLE 4.1 ■ **Summary of Anterolateral Abdominal Wall Muscles**

Muscle	Superior Attachment	Inferior Attachment	Concentric Action	Innervation
External oblique	Eight digitations from the anterior angles of lower 8 ribs (upper 4 digitations from the middle 4 ribs and serratus anterior, the lower 4 digitations from the lower 4 ribs and latissimus dorsi	Outer half of iliac crest, inguinal ligament, pubic tubercle and crest, aponeurosis of anterior rectus sheath, linea alba and xiphisternum	Compresses abdominal contents and supports the inguinal canal Together – flex the trunk Individually – abduction or rotation	Anterior rami T7–12
Internal oblique	Thoracolumbar fascia, anterior $^{2}/_{3}$ of iliac crest and lateral $^{2}/_{3}$ of inguinal ligament	Costal margin, aponeurosis of rectus sheath, conjoint tendon to pubic crest and pectineal line	Compresses abdominal contents and supports the inguinal canal Together – flexes the trunk Individually – rotation to the same side	Anterior rami T7–12 (conjoint tendon by L1)
Transversus abdominis	Costal margin, lumbar fascia, iliac crest and lateral half of inguinal ligament	Aponeurosis of posterior rectus sheath and conjoint tendon to pubic crest and pectineal line	Compresses abdominal contents and supports the inguinal canal	Anterior rami T7–12 (conjoint tendon by L1)
Rectus abdominis	5th–7th costal cartilages, inferior costal margin and xiphoid process	Pubic crest and pubic symphysis by two heads	Flexes trunk, aids forced expiration and compresses abdominal contents	Anterior rami T7–12
Pyradamidalis	Lower linea alba	Pubic crest	Tenses linea alba	Subcostal nerve T12

Rectus Sheath

- Rectus abdominis and pyramidalis muscles are enclosed in an aponeurotic tendon sheath
- Formed by the aponeuroses of the external oblique, internal oblique and transversus abdominis muscles
- Completely encloses the upper three-quarters of the rectus abdominis
  - The internal oblique aponeurosis splits at the edge of the rectus: half passing anteriorly and half posteriorly
  - Anterior rectus sheath includes the external oblique aponeurosis plus half of the internal oblique aponeurosis
  - Posterior rectus sheath includes the transversus abdominis aponeurosis plus half of the internal oblique aponeurosis
- For the lower quarter of the rectus abdominis below the arcuate line, the rectus sheath covers only anteriorly (all three layers pass anteriorly)
  - The aponeuroses of the internal oblique and transversus abdominis muscles fuse below the arcuate line
- Splitting of the internal oblique forms the semilunar line, a shallow and bloodless groove from the pubic tubercle to the costal margin
- Contains:
  - The ends of the T7–12 nerves and accompanying vessels
  - The superior and inferior epigastric vessels

Vascular Supply

- Superior epigastric artery
- Inferior epigastric artery
- Deep circumflex iliac artery
- Lumbar arteries
- Veins accompanying arteries

Nerve Supply

- The rectus muscle and the external oblique muscle are innervated by the lower intercostal and subcostal nerves (T7–12)
- The internal oblique and transverse abdominis muscles are innervated by T7–12 plus L1 (iliohypogastric and ilioinguinal nerves)

Lymph Drainage

- Superficial lymph drainage is via quadrants. The left and right upper quadrants drain to their ipsilateral pectoral group of axillary nodes, and the left and right lower quadrants drain to their ipsilateral inguinal nodes below the umbilicus
- Deep lymph drainage is into the extraperitoneal tissue: above the umbilicus to the mediastinal nodes and below it to the external iliac and para-aortic nodes

INGUINAL CANAL

- An oblique intermuscular slit (≈ 6 cm long) lying above the medial half of the inguinal ligament
- Commences at the deep ring and ends at the superficial ring
- Transmits the spermatic cord (male) or round ligament (female) and the ilioinguinal nerve

Anterior Wall and Superficial Inguinal Ring

- An external oblique aponeurosis is assisted laterally by the internal oblique muscle
- Fibres of the external oblique aponeurosis run parallel with the inguinal ligament at their lower border

- They diverge to make a V-shaped opening at the superficial inguinal ring:
  - Medial crus to the pubic crest
  - Lateral crus to the pubic tubercle
- Intercrural fibres run perpendicular to and bind the crura
- Fibres from the lateral crus pass upwards behind the medial crus to blend with the rectus sheath and with those from the other side (forming the posterior crus)

Floor

- The rolled-in (gutter-shaped) lower edge of the inguinal ligament is reinforced medially by the lacunar ligament
- Lacunar ligament fills the angle between the inguinal ligament and the pectineal line. It passes upwards from the inguinal ligament to the pubic bone
- The inguinal ligament fuses laterally with the transversalis fascia

Roof

- Formed by the lower edges of the internal oblique and transverse abdominis aponeuroses
- These muscles arch in a concentric fashion and are inserted into the pubic tubercle and the pectineal line
- The ilioinguinal and iliohypogastric nerves supply the lowermost fibres of the internal oblique and transverse abdominis
- The contraction of the tendons of the internal oblique and transverse abdominis muscles tightens the conjoint tendon and lowers the roof of the canal

Posterior Wall and Deep Inguinal Ring

- Posterior wall is formed by the transversalis fascia (laterally) and the conjoint tendon (medially)
- The weak transversalis fascia forms the posterior wall lateral to the conjoint tendon. It is reinforced medially by the conjoint tendon (strong)
- Laterally the wall is thin – covered by weak areolar tissue
- The integrity of the canal depends on the anterior wall laterally and the posterior wall medially
- The interfoveolar ligament consists of the transversus abdominis muscle fibres and constitutes a functional medial edge to the deep ring
- The deep ring lies above the midpoint of the inguinal ligament (halfway between the anterior superior iliac spine and the pubic tubercle)
- The inferior epigastric artery crosses the medial aspect of the deep inguinal ring, giving off the cremasteric branch, and forms the lateral boundary of the inguinal triangle (Hesselbach's triangle)
- Passing through the deep ring are:
  - The genital branch of the genitofemoral nerve
  - The cremasteric artery
  - The ductus deferens and accompanying artery
  - The testicular artery and veins
  - The obliterated remnants of the processus vaginalis
  - Autonomic nerves
  - Lymphatics
  - The ilioinguinal nerve does *NOT* pass through the deep ring despite being a constituent of the inguinal canal (due to it slipping in from the side)

Spermatic Cord (Fig 4.2)

- The ductus deferens and accompanying structures pass through the deep ring, picking up coverings from the layers of the anterior abdominal wall, which then become the spermatic cord

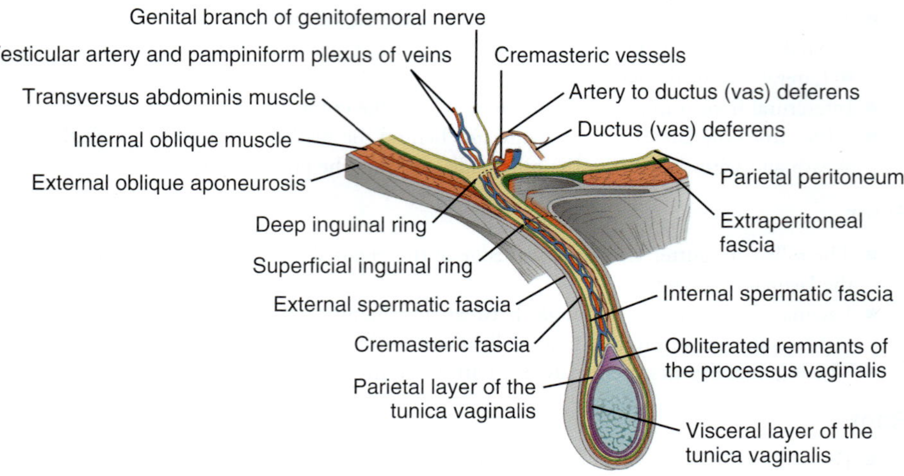

Fig. 4.2 Spermatic cord and its contents.

Coverings

- The internal spermatic fascia – an investment derived from the transversalis fascia
- The cremasteric fascia and muscle – originate from the internal oblique and transverse abdominis aponeurosis and muscles
- The external spermatic fascia – derived from the external oblique aponeurosis

Constituents

1. Ductus (vas) deferens (lies in the lower and posterior part of the cord)
2. Arteries: (a) testicular artery, (b) artery to the ductus deferens, (c) cremasteric artery
3. Veins: pampiniform plexus
4. Lymphatics: (a) deep structures to the para-aortic nodes and (b) superficial structures (from the coverings) to the external iliac nodes
5. Nerves: (a) genital branch of the genitofemoral nerve (supply to the cremaster muscle) and (b) sympathetic fibres which accompany the arteries
6. Obliterated remnants of the processus vaginalis

TESTIS

- Oval-shaped, covered by the tunica albuginea
- Epididymis is on the posterolateral surface
- Ductus deferens is a direct continuation from the lower pole of the epididymis and lies medial to it
- The anterior and lateral parts lie free in the tunica vaginalis (the remnant of the processus vaginalis)
- Testis, epididymis and tunica vaginalis lie in the scrotum surrounded by a thin membrane, adherent to each other
- Right and left testes are separated by the median scrotal septum

Blood Supply

- The testicular artery arises directly from the aorta (via the spermatic cord) and gives off a branch to the epididymis before reaching the back of the testis. It then divides into the medial and lateral branches, which sweep around horizontally within the tunica albuginea

- The pampiniform plexus runs up and acts as a counter-current heat exchange system. The left vein invariably joins the left renal vein, while the right drains directly into the inferior vena cava

Lymph Drainage

- Lymph capillaries lie between the seminiferous tubules
- Lymphatics run back with the testicular artery to the para-aortic nodes (*however, the overlying scrotal skin drains into the inguinal nodes*)

Nerve Supply

- The testes are supplied by sympathetic nerves around the T10 segment. The efferent fibres pass with the greater or lesser splanchnic nerve to the coeliac ganglion where they synapse. The postganglionic grey fibres then reach the testis via the testicular artery
- The sensory fibres share the same pathway as the sympathetic supply
- There is no parasympathetic supply

EPIDIDYMIS AND DUCTUS DEFERENS

- The epididymis is a firm structure, 7 m long, tightly coiled, with a large head, small tail and small sinus between it and the testis
- It is an organ of storage and maturation of spermatozoa
- The ductus deferens is a direct continuation of the epididymis and it passes up medially
- Blood supply is by a branch of the testicular artery
- Venous and lymph drainage are the same as the testis
- The nervous supply is via sympathetic fibres

Part 2 Abdominal Cavity

- Transpyloric plane – midway between the jugular notch and the pubic symphysis. Important relations in this plane are:
  - The tip of the ninth costal cartilage
  - The pylorus of the stomach
  - The fundus of the gall bladder
  - The body of the stomach
  - The lower border of the first lumbar vertebra and the upper border of the second lumbar vertebra (L1/2)
  - The end of the spinal cord (at the conus medullaris)
  - The head, neck and body of the pancreas
  - The superior mesenteric artery leaves the aorta
  - The splenic vein runs in this plane
  - The hilum of kidneys (right just below, left slightly above)
  - Formation of the portal vein

Part 3 Peritoneum

- A serous membrane composed of parietal (well-innervated) and visceral (poorly innervated) parts
- A single layer of flattened mesothelial cells with overlying areolar tissue. Over the expansile parts it is loose, while over the non-expansile parts it is thick
- The retroperitoneal organs (pancreas, duodenum, ascending and descending colon) have firm attachments to the muscular fasciae (comprised of the psoas and iliac fasciae as well as the anterior layer of the lumbar fascia) (Fig 4.3)

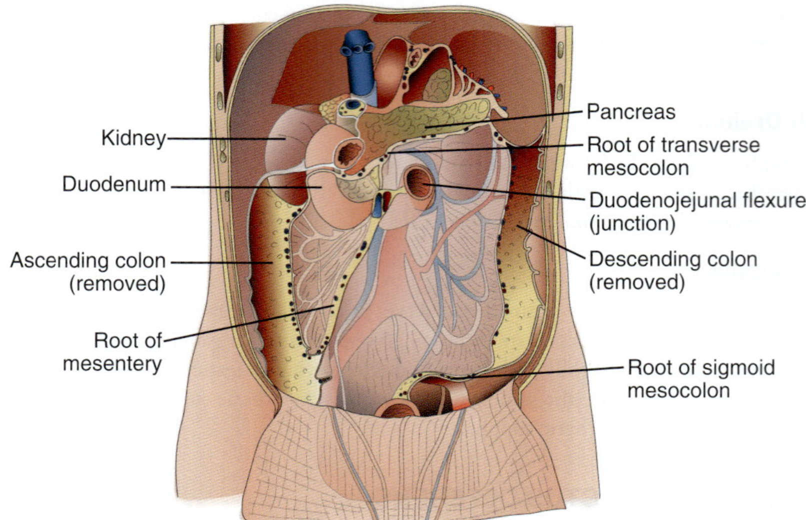

Fig. 4.3 Structures of the retroperitoneum.

- Various folds or reflections of peritoneum connect the viscera to the abdominal walls or to one another (Fig 4.4):
  - Mesentery (mesentery, transverse mesocolon, sigmoid mesocolon and mesoappendix)
  - Omentum (greater and lesser omentum)
  - Ligaments (associated with the liver, stomach and spleen)

Peritoneal Folds of the Anterior Abdominal Wall (Fig 4.5)

- The falciform ligament – passes upwards from the umbilicus towards the xiphisternum. It contains the posterior and crescentic free margin of the ligamentum teres (obliterated remains of the left umbilical vein) and enters the fissure of ligamentum teres on the visceral surface of the liver. After delivering the ligament to the liver, it continues up and to the right of the midline
- The median umbilical fold containing the median umbilical ligament – the obliterated remains of the urachus, in the midline

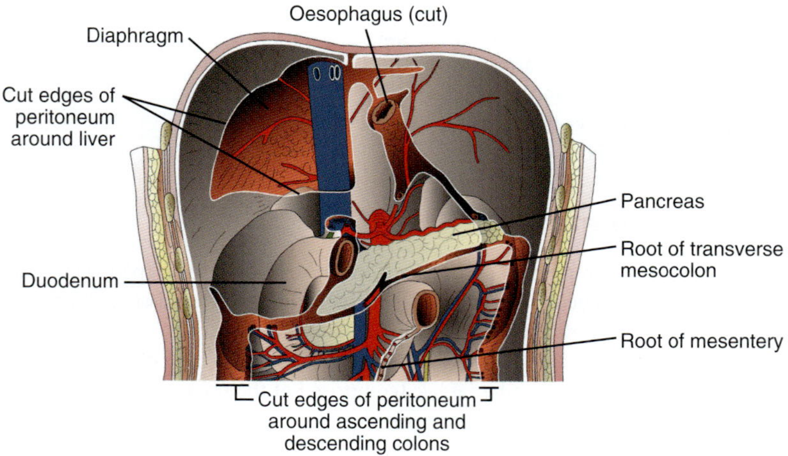

Fig. 4.4 Folds and reflections of the peritoneum.

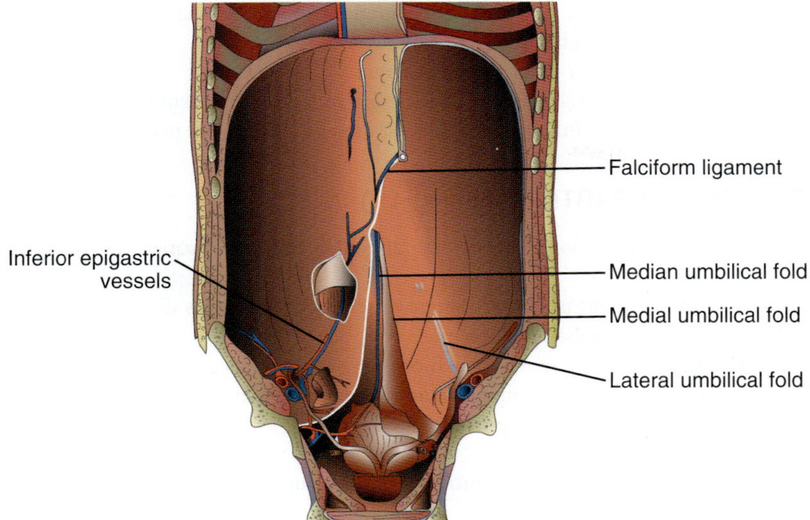

Fig. 4.5 Peritoneal folds of the anterior abdominal wall (posterior view).

- The medial umbilical fold (×2) – obliterated remains of the umbilical artery
- The lateral umbilical fold (×2) – containing the inferior epigastric vessels (these do not reach the umbilicus)

Peritoneal Cavity (Fig 4.6)

- The greater sac is the main cavity, and normally contains only a few millilitres of fluid (for lubrication)
- The lesser sac (omental bursa) is an invagination of the greater sac behind the stomach, through the epiploic foramen
- The greater omentum is a vascular apron originating from the greater curvature of the stomach
- The lesser omentum is the two layers of the peritoneum that extend between the liver and the upper border of the stomach

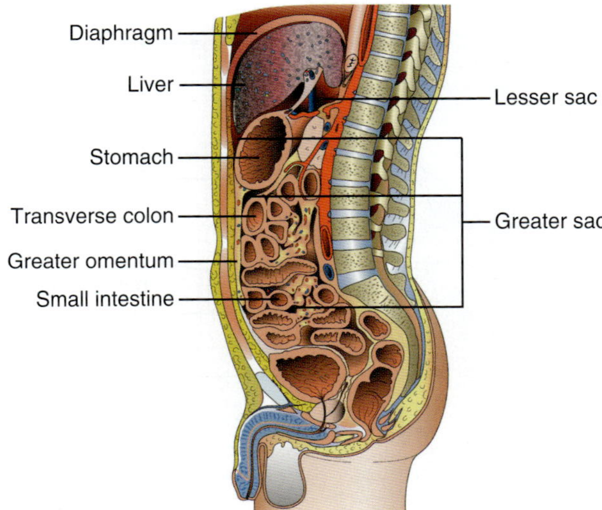

Fig. 4.6 Peritoneal cavity and its contents, sagittal section.

- The epiploic foramen is a 2.5 cm vertical slit and its boundaries are:
  - Upper boundary – caudate process of the liver
  - Lower boundary – first part of the duodenum
  - Anterior boundary – right side of free margin of the lesser omentum
  - Posterior boundary – inferior vena cava covered by the parietal peritoneum

PERITONEAL COMPARTMENTS (Fig 4.7)

- The transverse mesocolon divides the abdomen into the supracolic and infracolic compartments
- Supracolic compartment is above the transverse mesocolon and is divided into four:
  - Right subphrenic – subdiaphragmatic
  - Right subhepatic (hepatorenal pouch of Morison) – between the liver and the kidney; lowest point when in the supine position (where fluid is most likely to accumulate)
  - Left subphrenic – subdiaphragmatic
  - Left subhepatic – lesser sac
- Infracolic compartment is divided into two parts (the upper right and lower left) by the root of the mesentery
  - Upper right compartment:
    - Boundaries – apex: ileocolic junction; right: ascending colon; left: attachment of the mesentery; base: transverse mesocolon
    - Floor – the lower pole of the right kidney, the second part of the duodenum turning to the third part and the duodenojejunal flexure (which lies to the left of the midline on the left psoas muscle at L2); the right colic vessels also cross over the floor
    - Right paracolic gutter lies laterally and is a pathway for fluid spread
  - Lower left compartment:
    - Larger and quadrilateral in shape
    - Boundaries – upper: transverse mesocolon; right: mesentery; left: descending colon; lower: attachment of the sigmoid colon
    - Floor – the fourth part of the duodenum (and duodenojejunal flexure), paraduodenal fossae, inferior pole of the left kidney and the sigmoid mesocolon
    - Left paracolic gutter is limited above by the phrenicocolic ligament

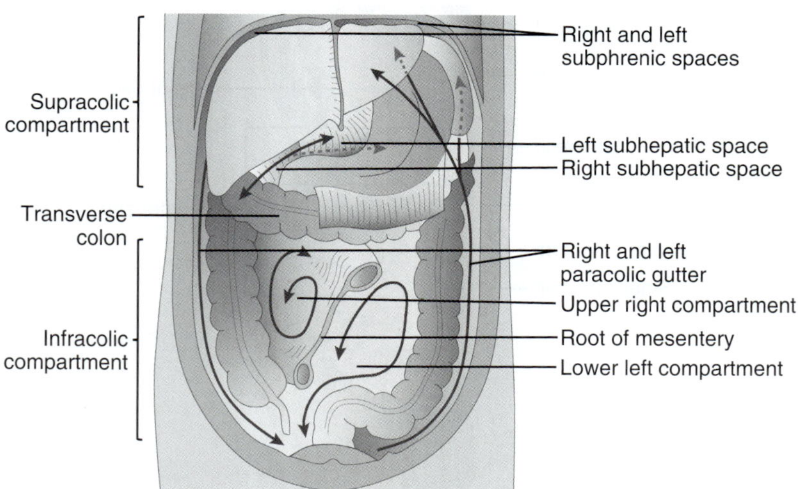

Fig. 4.7 Peritoneal compartments and their communications.

Part 4 Vessels and Nerves of the Gut (Fig 4.8A and B)

BLOOD SUPPLY OF THE FOREGUT

Arterial Supply: Coeliac Trunk (Level T12)

- The trunk divides into its three branches at the upper border of the pancreas:
  - The left gastric artery runs up the left crus, giving off an oesophageal branch (to the lower third) and then enters the lesser omentum

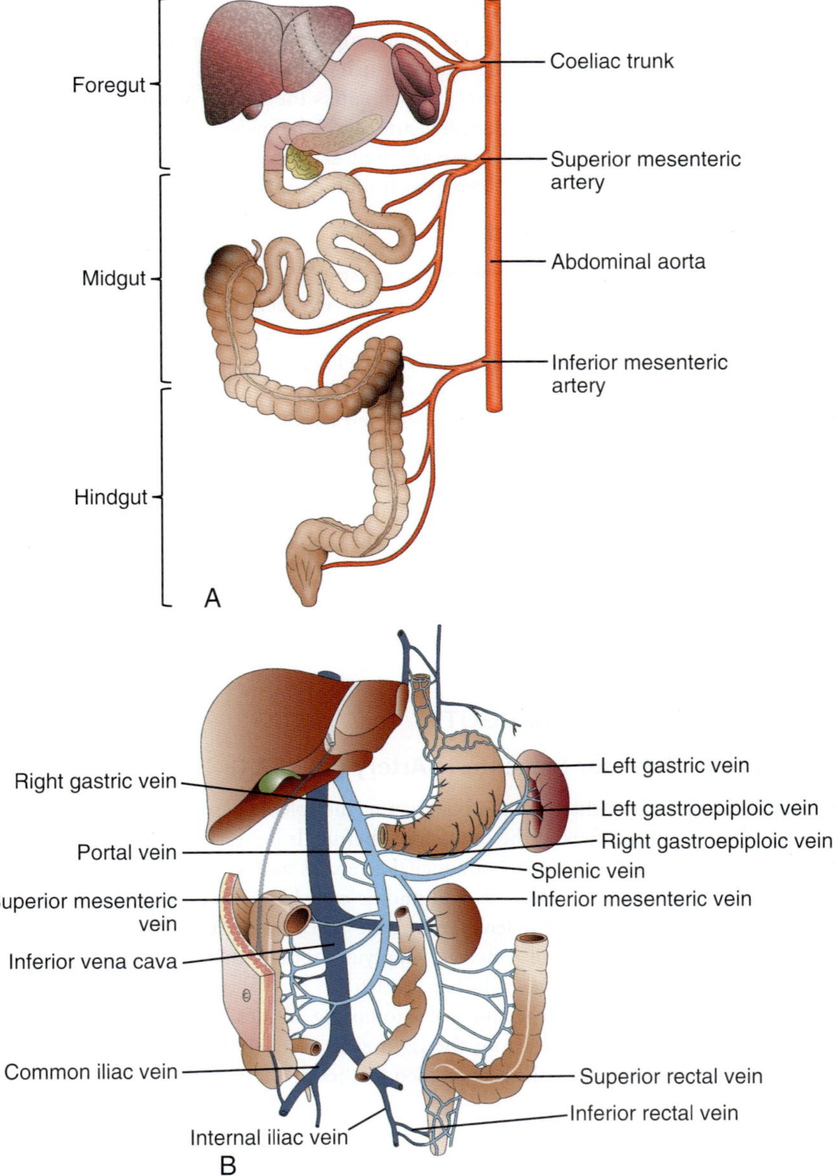

Fig. 4.8 **(A)** Arterial supply of the fore-, mid- and hindgut (schematic). **(B)** Venous drainage of the abdominal viscera.

- The splenic artery runs across the upper border of the pancreas, over the left crus and psoas
  - At the hilum of the left kidney, it turns forwards and runs in the lienorenal (splenorenal) ligament to the hilum of the spleen
  - It is the main supply to the pancreas. It also gives off short gastric arteries (runs in the gastrosplenic ligament) and the left gastroepiploic artery (runs in the greater omentum)
- The common hepatic artery passes over the upper border of the pancreas and then down to the first part of the duodenum
  - It turns forwards at the epiploic foramen to run upwards as the hepatic artery proper (changes its name); it lies to the left of the common bile duct and then bifurcates (Y-shaped) at the porta hepatis
  - It gives off the right gastric artery, which supplies the lesser curve of the stomach
  - It gives off the gastroduodenal artery, which divides into:
    - The right gastroepiploic artery, which enters the greater omentum
    - The superior pancreaticoduodenal artery, which divides into two branches to encircle the head of the pancreas. These anastomose with two branches of the inferior pancreaticoduodenal artery, which arise from the superior mesenteric artery

Venous Drainage of the Foregut

- Similar to the arterial supply, but there is no gastroduodenal vein
- Splenic vein unites with the superior mesenteric vein (behind the neck of the pancreas) to form the portal vein
- Right and left gastric veins (which also drain the lower third of the oesophagus) both drain into the portal vein
- Right and left gastroepiploic veins run with their corresponding arteries. The right gastroepiploic vein joins the superior mesenteric vein at the lower border of the neck of the pancreas. The left gastroepiploic vein joins the splenic vein, as do the short gastric veins
- Splenic vein runs below the artery through the lienorenal ligament and over the left kidney, psoas, sympathetic trunk, left crus, aorta, superior mesenteric artery and inferior vena cava
- Inferior mesenteric vein joins the splenic vein
- Superior pancreaticoduodenal vein runs up in the curvature between the pancreas and the duodenum to enter the portal vein

BLOOD SUPPLY OF THE MIDGUT

Arterial Supply: Superior Mesenteric Artery (Level L1)

- Supplies the gut from the common bile duct to the splenic flexure, over the left renal vein, and is directed to the apex of the physiologic hernia. It lies on the left renal vein
- It gives off the inferior pancreaticoduodenal artery, as well as ileal and jejunal branches, to the left and the ileocolic, right colic and middle colic branches to the right
  - The inferior pancreaticoduodenal artery: the first branch runs in a curve between the duodenum and the head of pancreas, supplying both. It may originate from the jejunal branch and may give off the right hepatic artery
  - The jejunal and ileal branches form anastomosing arcades
  - The ileocolic branch arises from the right side relatively low down and gives off ileal and colic branches. The colic branch then further divides into the anterior and posterior caecal arteries
  - The right colic branch originates from the root of the mesentery and crosses the right psoas, gonadal vessels, ureter, genitofemoral nerve and quadratus lumborum. It divides near the left side of the ascending colon into ascending and descending branches

- The middle colic branch arises from the lower border of the neck of the pancreas and then passes between the layers of the transverse mesocolon. It lies to the right of the midline and, upon reaching the transverse colon, divides into the left and right branches. The left branch anastomoses with a branch of the left colic artery (from the inferior mesenteric artery) at a watershed area

Venous Drainage of the Midgut

- Each branch of the superior mesenteric artery is accompanied by a vein; all of them drain into the superior mesenteric vein

BLOOD SUPPLY OF THE HINDGUT

Arterial Supply: Inferior Mesenteric Artery (Level L3)

- Supplies the gut from the splenic flexure to the upper third of the anal canal
- It is a smaller artery than the superior mesenteric artery and runs obliquely down in the left infracolic compartment to the pelvic brim
- It crosses the pelvic brim at the bifurcation of the left common iliac vessels, passing over the sacroiliac joint, and then converges with the ureter
- It lies on the aorta, left psoas, sympathetic trunk, common iliac artery and hypogastric nerve
- Beyond the pelvic brim, it continues along the wall as the superior rectal artery
- It does not cross the ureter, but all of its branches do
  - The left colic artery passes up to the splenic flexure, dividing into ascending and descending branches
    - The ascending branch crosses the left psoas, gonadal vessels, ureter, genitofemoral nerve and quadratus lumborum. It then divides into the upper and lower branches, each of which further divides into ascending and descending branches
    - The descending branches pass laterally and downwards, dividing above the pelvic brim into 3–4 branches
  - The sigmoid arteries consist of 3–4 branches forming anastomotic loops

Venous Drainage of the Hindgut

- The superior rectal vein runs up in the root of the sigmoid mesocolon (to the left of the artery) and becomes the inferior mesenteric vein, receiving tributaries identical to the branches
- It runs for some distance left of the artery, and it is not until the duodenojejunal flexure that it arches to the right, raising a ridge and creating the paraduodenal recess
- It passes along the lower border of the pancreas in front of the left renal vein to enter into the splenic vein
- Alternatively it may enter the superior mesenteric vein

LYMPH DRAINAGE OF THE GASTROINTESTINAL TRACT

- Filtration starts with the lymphoid follicles (mucous membrane), which aggregate in the terminal ilium's antimesenteric border as Peyer's patches
- Lymph passes through the muscle layer to the nearby nodes:
  - The first group lies in the peritoneum adjacent to gut as juxtaintestinal nodes (small intestine) and paracolic nodes (large intestine)
  - The second groups lie along the main blood vessels
- Pre-aortic groups are at the base of coeliac trunk, superior mesenteric artery and inferior mesenteric artery
  - The lymph then moves upwards eventually to the cisterna chyli
- Note: the large intestine has additional epicolic nodes

NERVE SUPPLY TO THE GASTROINTESTINAL TRACT

- All parts are supplied by sympathetic (postganglionic – inhibitory) and parasympathetic (preganglionic – excitatory) nerves
- These nerves travel with the gut arteries
- Most come from the coeliac plexus, but the inferior hypogastric plexus contributes the parasympathetic fibres to the hindgut (S2–4)
- From the midoesophagus to the rectum, nerve cells and fibres that supply muscles, blood vessels and glands are concentrated in two plexuses:
  - Myenteric plexus (Auerbach's), which is situated between the two muscle layers of the gut
  - Submucous plexus (Meissner's), which is submucosal
- These function without an extrinsic nerve supply (enteric nervous system)
- The system receives sympathetic and parasympathetic inputs
- Note: other transmitters include vasoactive intestinal peptide and substance P

Part 5 Gastrointestinal Tract

OESOPHAGUS

(See the Oesophagus section in Chapter 3 for further information.)

- Passes through diaphragm at T10, 2.5 cm left of the midline, and is bound firmly by the phreno-oesophageal ligament
- The anterior and posterior vagal trunks are related to their respective surfaces on the oesophagus
- Enters the stomach at the cardiac orifice
- Factors that guard against gastro-oesophageal reflux are:
  - The sphincter actions of the lower oesophageal muscle fibres
  - The fibres of the right crural 'sling' around the oesophagus
  - The mucosal flap of the stomach forming a 'rosette'
  - The difference between the negative intrathoracic pressure and the positive intra-abdominal pressure

STOMACH (FIG 4.9)

- The most dilated part of the gastrointestinal tract
- It is a muscular bag, relatively fixed at both ends but mobile in the middle
- The main parts are the fundus, body, pylorus and greater and lesser curvatures
- It is completely invested by peritoneum
- The fundus is the part which projects above the level of the cardia and is usually full of gas
- The body extends from the fundus to the angular notch (incisura anularis)
- The pylorus extends from the angular notch to the gastroduodenal junction (right of the midline, around L1). It consists of the proximal pyloric antrum, which narrows distally at the pyloric canal and includes the circular muscle at the distal end, which is thickened to form the pyloric sphincter
- The stomach consists of outer longitudinal and inner circular muscle layers reinforced by the innermost oblique layer
- The mucosa of the body is parietal (acid secreting) and gives way to pyloric-type G cells (gastrin-secreting) in the pylorus
- Behind the stomach is the stomach bed

- It is covered by the peritoneum from the anterior wall of the lesser sac
- The bed consists of the left crus, the diaphragmatic dome and the upper part of the left kidney overlaid by a triangle of structures: the pancreas (transversely), the spleen (superior and laterally) and the suprarenal gland (superior and medially)
- The transverse mesocolon slopes down from the lower border of the pancreas; above its upper border is the splenic artery
- To the right of the lesser curve lies the aorta, coeliac trunk and its branches with their associated lymph nodes

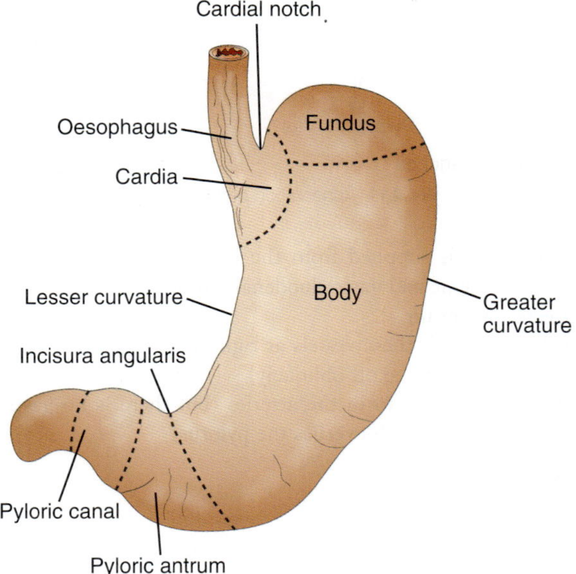

Fig. 4.9 Stomach.

Blood Supply (Fig 4.10)

- The lesser curvature is supplied via the left and right gastric arteries (which anastomose and may be double). The right gastric artery is usually a branch of the hepatic or gastroduodenal arteries
- The fundus is supplied by short gastric arteries from the splenic artery

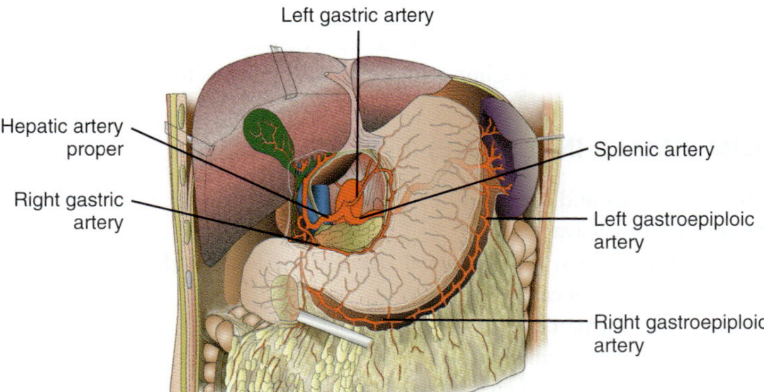

Fig. 4.10 Blood supply of the stomach.

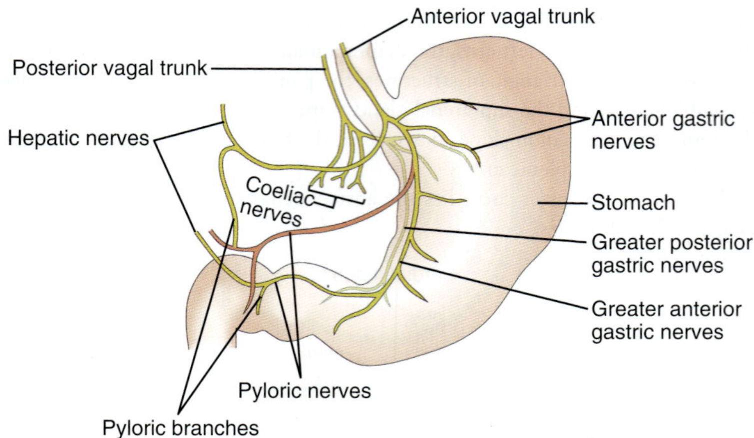

Fig. 4.11 Innervation of the stomach.

- The greater curvature is supplied from the left and right gastroepiploic arteries, which originate from the splenic and gastroduodenal arteries. These arteries anastomose and also supply the greater omentum
- Gastric branches come off these vessels at right angles (in contrast to branches from the vagal nerve trunk, which come off obliquely)
- Venous drainage is identical to in the arteries (but there is no gastroduodenal vein, and there is a prepyloric vein, which overlies the pylorus)

Lymph Drainage

- To the coeliac nodes
- Lymph vessels anastomose freely within the stomach wall
- In rare cases of gastric carcinoma, the left supraclavicular nodes may become palpably enlarged (Troisier's sign)

Nerve Supply (Fig 4.11)

- Sympathetic fibres run with the arteries (vasomotor) accompanied by afferent (pain) fibres
- Parasympathetic supply (vagal) controls motility and secretion
- Anterior vagal trunk runs down the lesser omentum near the lesser curvature, giving branches to the anterior stomach and a hepatic branch, which in turn gives off a pyloric antrum branch
- Posterior vagal trunk runs in the lesser omentum behind the anterior trunk and gives off a large branch to the coeliac ganglion and numerous branches to the posterior stomach

DUODENUM (SMALL INTESTINE) (Fig 4.12)

- A C-shaped tube around the head of the pancreas, curved over the convexity of the aorta and the inferior vena cava
- The first 2 cm is between the peritoneal layers of the lesser and greater omentum and the remainder is retroperitoneal
- It is divided into four parts:
  - First part (superior) – 5 cm long at the level of L1, runs to the right, upwards and backwards
    - The first 2 cm lies between peritoneal folds (intraperitoneal part) and lies on the liver pedicle
    - The next 3 cm lies on right crus, right psoas and medial border of the right kidney

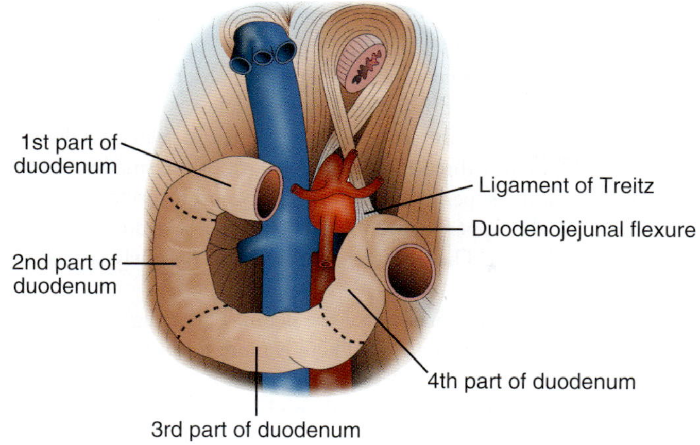

Fig. 4.12 Divisions of the duodenum.

- Second part (descending) – 7.5 cm long at the level of L2, runs alongside the head of the pancreas and curves downwards over the hilum of the right kidney
  - It lies in both the supracolic and the infracolic compartments
  - The hepatopancreatic ampulla (of Vater) opens into the posteromedial wall at the major duodenal papilla
  - The accessory pancreatic duct drains into the minor papilla 2 cm proximal to the minor duodenal papilla
- Third part – 10 cm long at the level of L3, curves forwards from right to left and lies on the aorta at the commencement of the inferior mesenteric artery
  - It is crossed by the superior mesenteric vessels
  - It lies in both the left and the right infracolic compartments
- Fourth part (ascending) – 2.5 cm long at the level of L2; ascends to the left of the aorta on the left psoas and sympathetic trunk
  - It breaks free from the posterior abdominal wall and curves forwards as the duodeno-jejunal flexure, pulling a double sheet of peritoneum from the posterior abdominal wall (mesentery of the small intestine)
  - The duodenojejunal flexure is fixed to the left psoas by fibrous tissue and also the suspensory muscle of the duodenum (ligament of Treitz)

- The superior and inferior duodenal recesses and the paraduodenal recess are formed from the inferior mesenteric vein
- The blood supply is from the superior and inferior pancreaticoduodenal arteries
  - The first 2 cm may receive supply from a variety of sources (important in duodenal ulceration): the hepatic artery, common hepatic artery, gastroduodenal artery, superior pancreaticoduodenal artery, right gastric artery and right gastroepiploic artery
  - Veins correspond to arteries
- Lymph drainage is via channels that accompany arteries to coeliac and superior mesenteric nodes

JEJUNUM AND ILEUM (SMALL INTESTINE)

- Jejunum:
  - Wider bore with thicker walls
  - Lies in the upper part of the infracolic compartment
  - It is approximately two-fifths of the length of the small intestine

- Ileum:
  - Narrower bore with thinner walls
  - The more distal segments have an antimesenteric border of elongated whitish plaques which are aggregated lymphoid follicles (Peyer's patches)
  - It lies in the lower part of the infracolic compartment and then runs down into the pelvis
  - It comprises approximately three-fifths of the length of the small intestine
- The blood supply is via the superior mesenteric artery and it forms arterial arcades
  - A single arcade for the upper jejunum, and two for lower down. These then give off straight arteries to the gut. These arteries are long and narrowly spaced for the jejunum (high, narrow windows)
  - Three to five large arcades are present for the ileum. The straight arteries are shorter and more spread out (low, broad windows). There is more fat in this part of the mesentery
  - Veins correspond to arteries
- Lymph drainage is via the superior mesenteric nodes
- Nerve supply:
  - The parasympathetic supply travels via vessels and normally augments the peristaltic activity
  - The sympathetic supply is vasoconstrictor, inhibits peristalsis and transmits pain that is usually felt in the umbilical region (T9, 10)

LARGE INTESTINE (Fig 4.13)

Caecum

- A blind pouch projecting down below the ileocaecal junction
- It is covered on the front and sides with peritoneum
- The retrocaecal space may be shallow or deep, and may have folds forming retrocaecal recesses
- Taeniae coli are positioned one anteriorly, one posteromedially and one posterolaterally

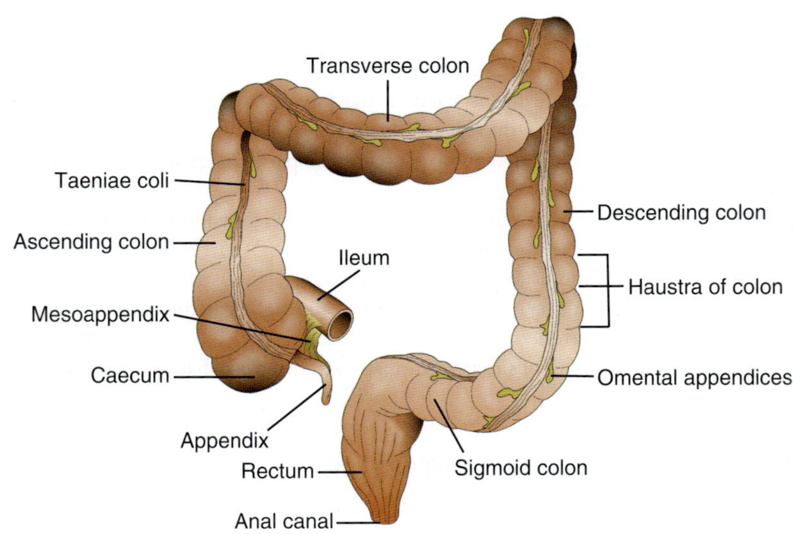

Fig. 4.13 Large intestine.

- The blood supply is via the anterior and posterior caecal vessels (terminal from the ileocolic artery). The posterior caecal vessel is usually larger and gives off the appendiceal artery
- Retrocaecal recesses – three parallel folds of peritoneum form the two ileocaecal recesses:
  - The ileocaecal recess is the space behind the peritoneal fold (vascular fold of caecum), which is formed between the base of the mesentery and the anterior wall of the caecum. It contains the anterior caecal artery
  - The inferior ileocaecal recess is the space behind the ileocaecal fold (bloodless fold of Treves), which is formed between the terminal ileum and the appendix

Appendix (Fig 4.14)

- A blind-ending tube 2–25 cm in length originating from the posteromedial wall of the caecum, 2 cm below the ileocaecal valve
- Its base is at the point of convergence of the taeniae
- Its lumen may obliterate in old age
- Its commonest position in operations is retrocaecal and retrocolic
- The mesoappendix is a triangular fold and a prolongation of the inferior terminal ileum mesentery
- The appendicular artery arises from the posterior caecal artery and has no collateral supply
- Venous drainage corresponds with the arteries
- Lymph drains through nodes associated with the ileocolic artery

Ascending Colon

- 15 cm in length from the ileocaecal junction to the hepatic flexure
- It lies on the iliac fascia and the anterior layer of the lumbar fascia
- The front and sides possess a serous coat
- The paracolic gutter lies laterally
- Embryonic mesentery is retained in 10% of adults
- Taeniae coli are positioned one anteriorly, one posteromedially and one posterolaterally and the wall is sacculated between them

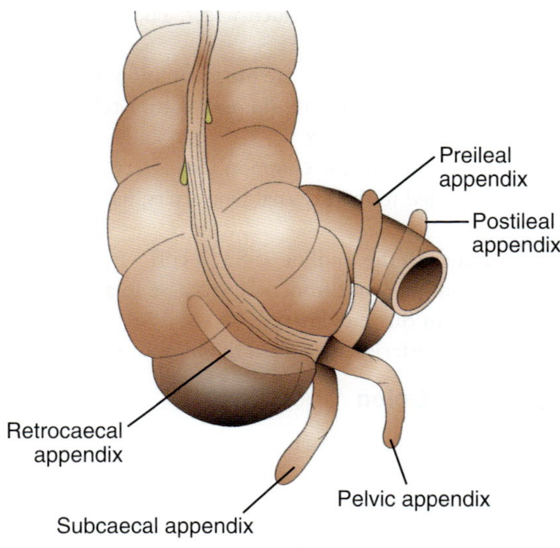

Fig. 4.14 Various positions of the appendix.

- Omental appendices epiploicae project from the serous coat; blood vessels to these perforate the muscle wall, through which the mucous membrane may herniate – (diverticulosis)
- The blood supply is via the ileocolic and right colic arteries from the superior mesenteric artery

Transverse Colon

- 45 cm in length from the hepatic to the splenic flexure
- It hangs down to a variable extent. It is in contact with the anterior abdominal wall and is completely invested in peritoneum (transverse mesocolon)
- The transverse mesocolon is attached from the right kidney, the second part of the duodenum, the pancreas and the inferior pole of the left kidney
- The splenic flexure is higher than the hepatic flexure
- Taeniae coli rotate 180°: the anteriorly positioned from the ascending colon becomes posterior and the other two lie anteriorly
- Appendices epiploicae are larger and more numerous
- The blood supply: the proximal two-thirds is via the right and middle colic arteries from the superior mesenteric artery and the distal third is via the left colic artery from the inferior mesenteric artery

Descending Colon

- 30 cm in length from the splenic flexure to the pelvic brim
- It is plastered down to the posterior abdominal wall (retroperitoneum)
- It lies on the lumbar and then the iliac fascia
- Taeniae coli are positioned as they are for the ascending colon
- Appendices epiploicae are numerous and diverticulosis is common
- The blood supply: via the left colic branch from the inferior mesenteric artery

Sigmoid Colon

- Up to 45 cm from the pelvic brim to commencement of the rectum at S3
- It hangs on the sigmoid mesocolon
- Sacculations persist but taeniae coli are much wider. The distal sigmoid colon has a complete longitudinal coat
- Appendices epiploicae and diverticulosis are most common in this part of the bowel
- The sigmoid mesocolon is hinged but did not completely fuse and distally forms a Λ-shaped base with the limbs diverging
  - The apex is at the bifurcation of the common iliac artery over the sacroiliac joint
  - The lateral limb is attached to the external iliac artery, half way to the inguinal ligament (5 cm)
  - The medial limb extends to the midline at S3 (5 cm)
  - The sigmoid mesocolon spans out from a 10 cm base to a 40 cm border
  - The sigmoid vessels lie in this mesentery
- The blood supply: sigmoid arteries arise from the inferior mesenteric artery

Vessels and Nerves of the Colon

- The arterial supply is as detailed above (Fig 4.15)
- Venous drainage parallels arterial supply
- Lymph drainage follows the arteries (Fig 4.16)
- Nerve supply:
  - Parasympathetic fibres up to the splenic flexure are via the vagal nerve; beyond the splenic flexure the supply is via the pelvic splanchnic nerves (S2–4)

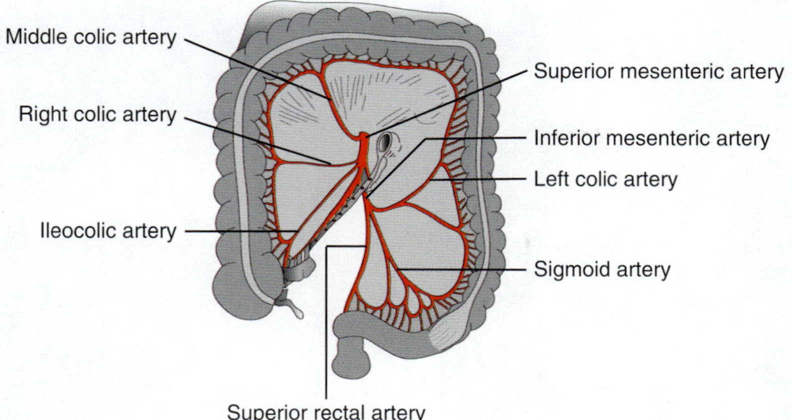

Fig. 4.15 Arterial supply of the colon.

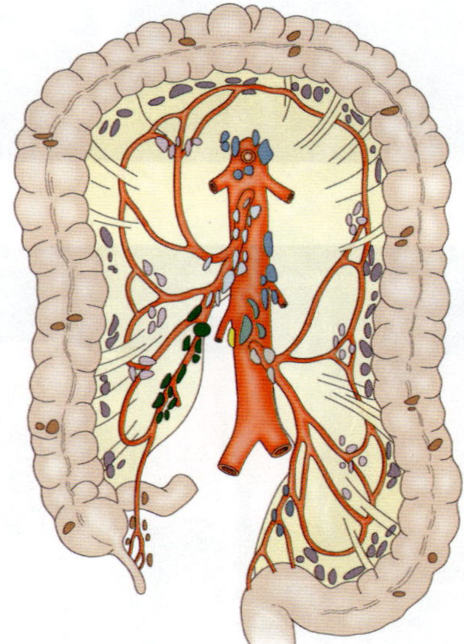

Fig. 4.16 Lymphatics of the colon.

- Sympathetic fibres originate from spinal cord segments T10–12, and pain fibres give peri-umbilical pain from midgut derivatives and hypogastric pain from the hindgut derivatives

Part 6 Liver and Biliary Tract

LIVER (Fig 4.17A–C)

- The largest gland in the body, weighing ~1500 grams
- It has a diaphragmatic and a visceral surface
- The diaphragmatic (superior) surface is divided into anterior, superior, posterior and right surfaces

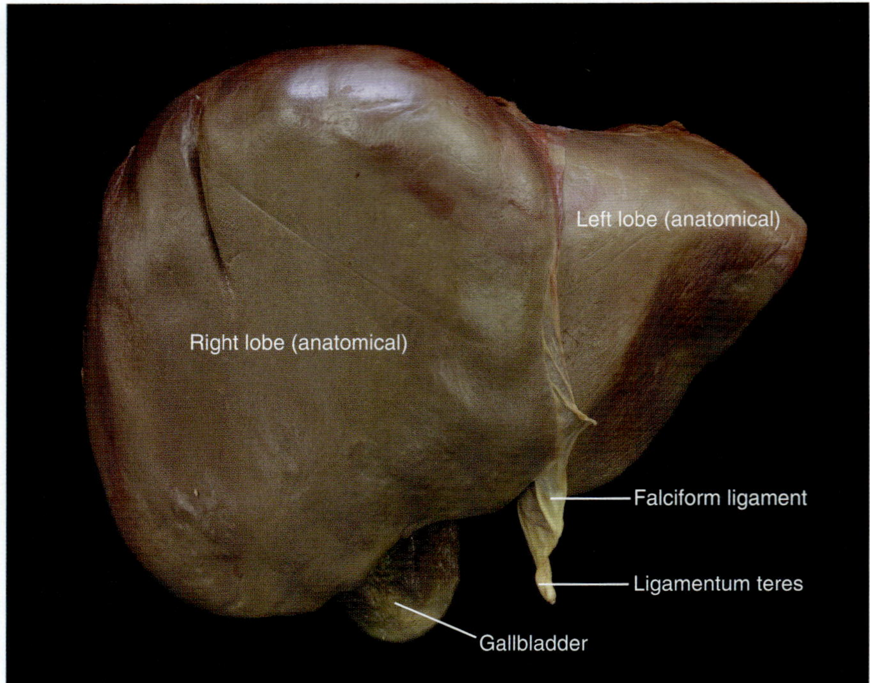

A

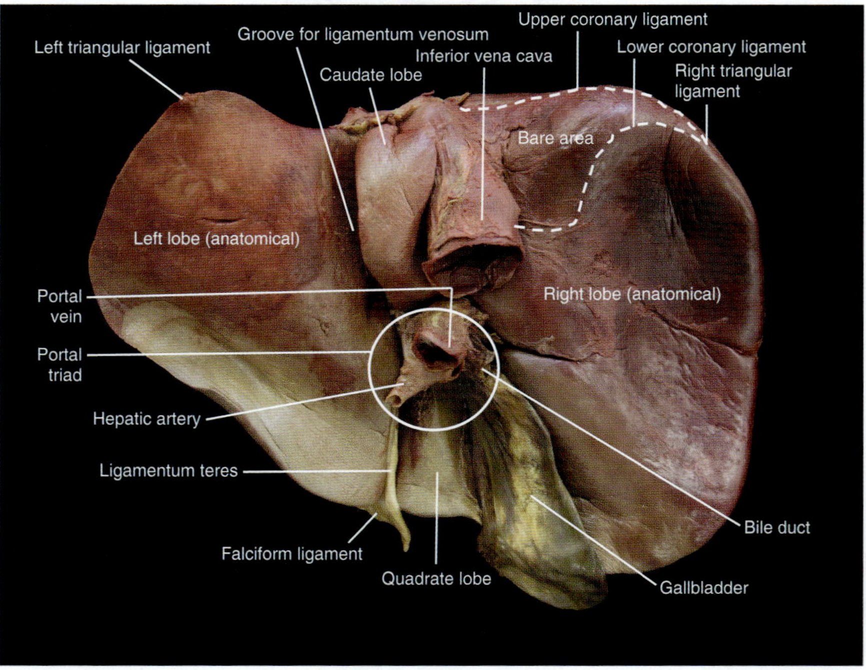

B

Fig. 4.17 Liver. **(A)** Anterior view. **(B)** Posterior view.

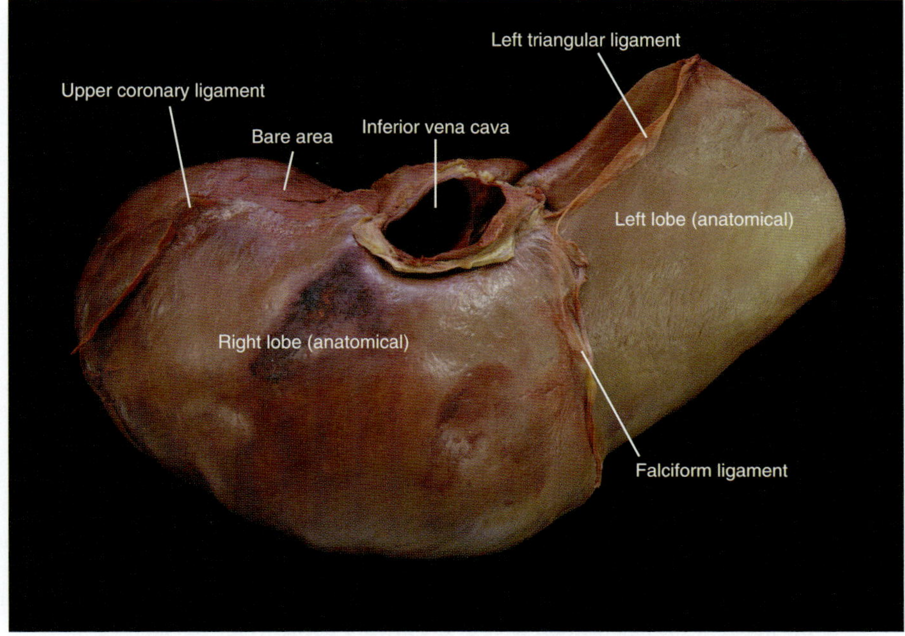

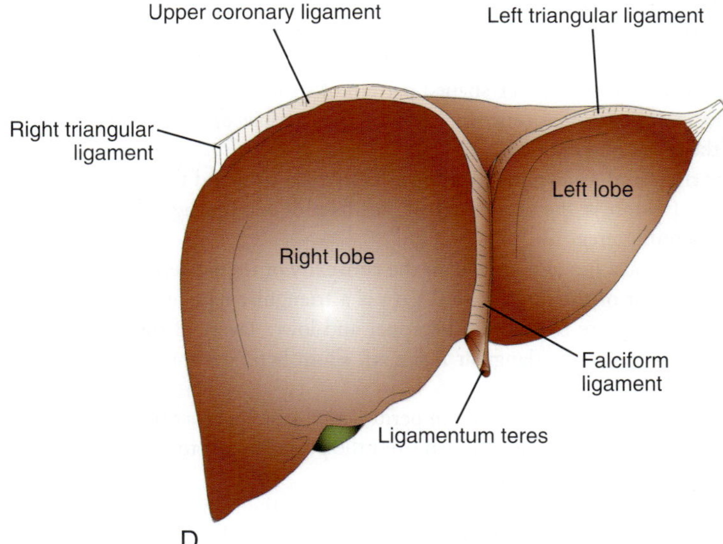

Fig. 4.17, cont'd **(C)** Superior view. **(D)** Ligaments.

- It is covered mostly by peritoneum (Fig 4.18), peeling off in places to join the diaphragm
- The anterior surface is related to the diaphragm, lungs, pleura and ribs, and curves back to join the superior surface
- The superior surface is related to the heart and pericardium centrally, and the lung and pleura laterally

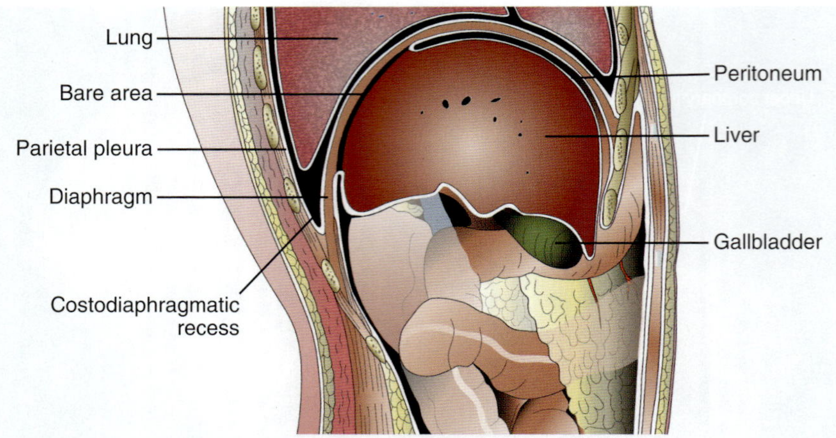

Fig. 4.18 Peritoneal coverings of the liver, parasagittal section.

- The inferior (lower) border slopes up from the right costal margin and then across the epigastrium
- Over the anterior surface, the falciform ligament is attached from near the centre down to the notch of the ligamentum teres in the inferior border (Fig. 4.17D)
- The upper attachment of the falciform divides and sweeps to the left (left triangular ligament) and to the right (upper layer of coronary ligament)
- The right surface extends from ribs seven to eleven

- The visceral (inferior) surface: slopes downwards, forwards and to the right
  - The main feature is an H-shaped pattern of structures
  - The porta hepatis lies centrally (forming the crosspiece), enclosed between the two layers of the lesser omentum
  - The right limb (incomplete) is the inferior vena cava and the gall bladder
  - The left limb is the continuity of the fissures for the ligamentum venosum and the ligamentum teres
  - The vena cava lies in a groove on the convexity of the posterior surface
  - To the right of the inferior vena cava is a triangular bare area. The vena cava forms its base; its sides are formed by the upper and lower layers of the coronary ligament. The apex is at the right triangular ligament. From here, peritoneum sweeps down over the right kidney
  - The visceral surface is covered in peritoneum, which peels off as the lesser omentum
  - The lesser omentum passes down from the porta hepatis to enclose the stomach and the first 2 cm of the duodenum
- The porta hepatis is a transverse slit perforated by the right and left hepatic ducts and the right and left branches of the hepatic artery and portal vein (order = vein, artery, duct, with ducts in front). The cystic duct lies in loose contact with the right end of the porta hepatis

Lobes

- The liver is divided anatomically into the left, caudate, quadrate and right lobes
- The falciform ligament divides the anatomical left and right lobes
- The caudate lobe lies between the inferior vena cava and the fissure for the ligamentum venosum, and it is connected to the right lobe via the caudate process

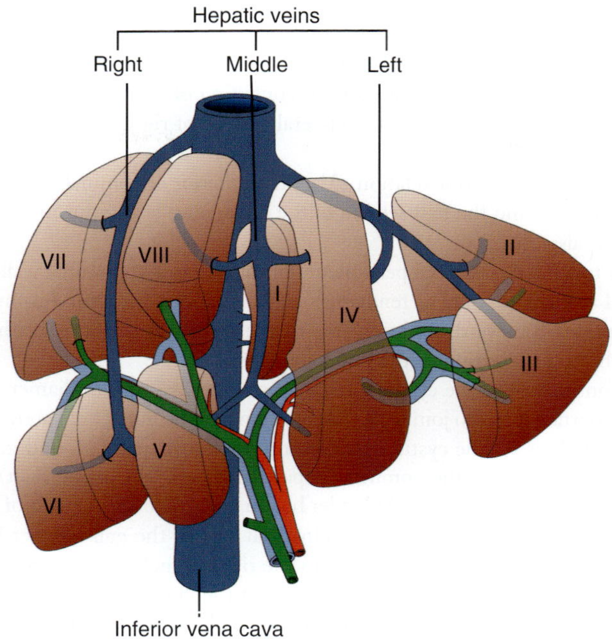

Fig. 4.19 Segments of the liver (Couinaud classification).

- The quadrate lobe lies between the gall bladder fossa and the fissure for the ligamentum teres

Segments (Fig 4.19)

- Typically it is divided into eight segments using the Couinaud classification:
  - Segment I – caudate
  - Segment II – superior left lateral
  - Segment III – inferior left lateral
  - Segment IV – left medial
  - Segment V – inferior right anterior
  - Segment VI – inferior right posterior
  - Segment VII – superior right posterior
  - Segment VIII – superior right anterior

Blood Supply

- From two sources: the hepatic artery (30%) and the portal vein (70%)
- The arterial division (hepatic artery) is Y-shaped and the portal vein division is T-shaped

Lymph and Nerve Supply

- Lymph drainage is to the nodes at the porta hepatis that drain down the hepatic artery and into the retropyloric and coeliac nodes. From the bare area of liver, communication with the extraperitoneal lymphatics perforates the diaphragm and drains into the posterior mediastinum
- The nerve supply is via the sympathetic coeliac ganglia and vagal (anterior/left vagal trunk) pathways

BILIARY TRACT

Gall Bladder

- A globular (pear-shaped) organ of ≈50 mL consisting of a fundus, body and neck
- It lies in the gall bladder fossa on the visceral surface of right lobe of the liver adjacent to the quadrate lobe
- The liver is its main anterior relation. Also, the anterior abdominal wall is anterior to the gall bladder fundus and the first section of the duodenum is anterior to its body. The transverse colon is also anterior
- The fundus touches the parietal peritoneum of the anterior abdominal wall at the tip of the ninth costal cartilage – a site of tenderness in gall bladder disease (Murphy's sign)
- The body passes backwards and upwards to the right end of the porta hepatis and is in contact with the first section of the duodenum
- The neck continues into the cystic duct (2–3 cm long/2–3 mm in diameter), which travels towards the porta hepatis to join with the common hepatic duct (1 cm above the duodenum)
- The blood supply is via the cystic artery (from the right hepatic), found in Calot's triangle (boundaries are the liver, the common hepatic duct and the cystic duct). It can also be sustained by a supply from the gall bladder bed in cases with thrombosis of the cystic artery
- Venous drainage is via multiple small veins that run in the gall bladder bed to the liver. Rarely do cystic veins run from the neck to the right branch of the portal vein
- Lymph drainage is to the porta hepatic nodes, to the cystic node (in Calot's triangle) and to a node located at the anterior border of the epiploic foramen. These then drain to the coeliac group of preaortic nodes
- Mucus is secreted by columnar epithelium (not goblet cells) and only in the neck

Common Hepatic Duct

- The right and left hepatic ducts for completion emerge from the porta hepatis, uniting on the right side in a Y-shaped manner to form the common hepatic duct
- It is 4 cm long and 4 mm in diameter
- The cystic duct usually unites on the right side of the common hepatic duct about 1 cm above the duodenum, but there is significant variation

Bile Duct

- It is 8 cm long and 8 mm in diameter
- It consists of three parts:
  - Upper (supraduodenal) – lies in the free edge of the lesser omentum, anterior to the portal vein and right of the hepatic artery
  - Middle (retroduodenal) – runs behind the first section of the duodenum and slopes down to the right (away from the portal vein)
  - Lower (paraduodenal) – slopes further to the right behind the head of the pancreas and the second part of the duodenum, joining the pancreatic duct at the hepatopancreatic ampulla (of Vater)
- The blood supply is via branches from the cystic, hepatic and gastroduodenal arteries
- The parasympathetic supply (via the hepatic branch) stimulates contraction of the gall bladder and relaxation of the ampullary sphincter. Sympathetic fibres inhibit contraction
- Hormonal control is much more important than neural
- Biliary pain is usually felt in the right hypochondrium and epigastrium, but it may also radiate to the back and infrascapular region

PORTAL VEIN (see Fig 4.8A and B)

- An upward continuation of the superior mesenteric vein, once it combines with the splenic vein (behind the neck of the pancreas)
- The portal vein lies in front of the inferior vena cava, passing up behind the pancreas and the first section of the duodenum through the free edge of the lesser omentum
- It divides at the porta hepatis in a T-fashion into right and left branches
- It receives tributaries from the superior mesenteric vein, splenic vein, right and left gastric veins, superior pancreaticoduodenal veins, cystic vein (to the right branch) and periumbilical veins (with the ligamentum teres joining the left branch)
- Portal–systemic anastomoses (portocaval anastomosis) occur at the:
  - Lower oesophagus
  - Upper end of the anal canal
  - Bare area of the liver
  - Periumbilical region
  - Retroperitoneal region

Part 7 Pancreas (Fig 4.20)

- A composite gland with exocrine (acini) and endocrine (islets of Langerhans) functions
- It is shaped like a hook, lying sideways with the hook on the right turned downwards
- Its length is approximately 15 cm
- It has a firm consistency and is finely lobulated
- It lies immediately behind the peritoneum of the posterior abdominal wall, with the transverse colon attached to the anterior surface just above the inferior border
- It curves around the first lumbar vertebra, inferior vena cava and aorta
- It consists of a head and uncinate process, neck, body and tail
  - Head:
    - The broadest part, moulded into the C-shaped concavity of the duodenum
    - It lies on the inferior vena cava and the right and left renal veins at L2
    - Its posterior surface is indented by the bile duct

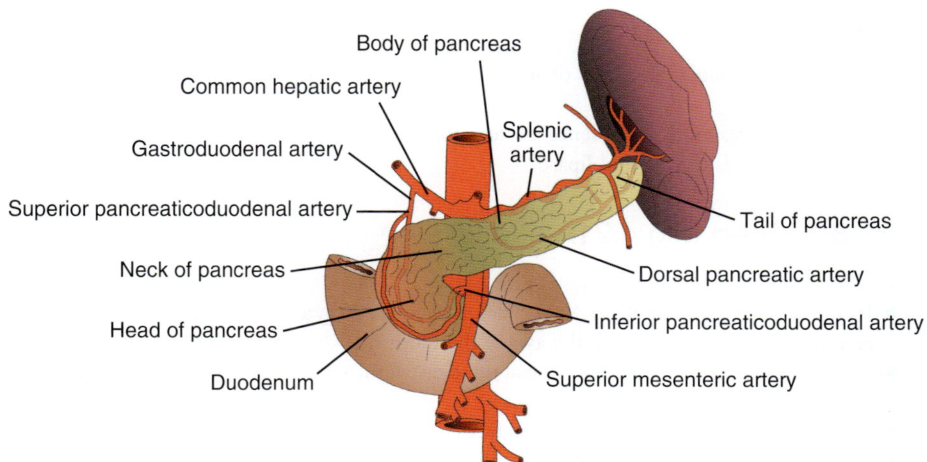

Fig. 4.20 Pancreas, its relations and blood supply.

    - The uncinate process is the prolonged lower, wedge-shaped part and it lies behind the superior mesenteric artery and vein and in front of the abdominal aorta
  - Neck:
    - A narrow band in front of the formation of the portal vein and formation of the SMA
    - The superior mesenteric vein passes between the neck and the uncinate process
    - The transverse mesocolon is attached to the lower border of the neck
  - Body:
    - Passes from the neck to the left, sloping up across the left renal vein, aorta (at coeliac trunk origin), left crus, left psoas and lower pole of the left suprarenal gland to the hilum of the left kidney
    - The coeliac trunk gives off the splenic artery, which passes along the upper border of the body
    - The lower border crosses the origin of the superior mesenteric artery
    - The splenic vein lies closely opposed to the posterior surface
  - Tail:
    - Passes from the anterior surface of the left kidney through the two layers of the lienorenal ligament (accompanying the splenic vessels) to the hilum of the spleen
- The pancreatic duct passes from tail to head. It is joined by the bile duct and enters the second section of the duodenum at the hepatopancreatic ampulla, 2 cm downstream from the accessory duct (draining the uncinate process)

Vascular Supply (see Fig 4.20)

- The arterial supply is primarily from the splenic artery. The superior and inferior pancreaticoduodenal arteries also supply the head
- Venous drainage is by the splenic and superior pancreaticoduodenal veins (into the portal vein) and via the inferior pancreaticoduodenal vein (into the superior mesenteric vein)

Lymph Drainage and Nerve Supply

- Lymphatics follow the arterial course
- The parasympathetic vagal fibres stimulate secretion and are supplied by a posterior branch originating from the coeliac plexus carrying vagal fibres
- The sympathetic vasoconstrictor supply (T6–10) travels via the splanchnic nerves, which also carry pain fibres

Structure

- It consists of lobulated glands of serous acini (exocrine) and islets of Langerhans (endocrine).
- Acinar cells respond to presence of secretin and cholecystokinin by secreting digestive enzymes such as trypsin and lipase

Part 8 Spleen (Fig 4.21A and B)

- The largest lymphoid organ
- Its dimensions are ≈2.5 × 7.5 × 12.5 cm, it weighs 200 g, and it lies between ribs nine and eleven; its long axis lies along the axis of the tenth rib
- It develops in the left leaf of the dorsal mesogastrium, and ends up at the left margin of the lesser sac
- The visceral peritoneum invests all surfaces (gastric, diaphragmatic, colic and renal)
- The hilum makes contact with the tail of the pancreas – which lies in the lienorenal ligament

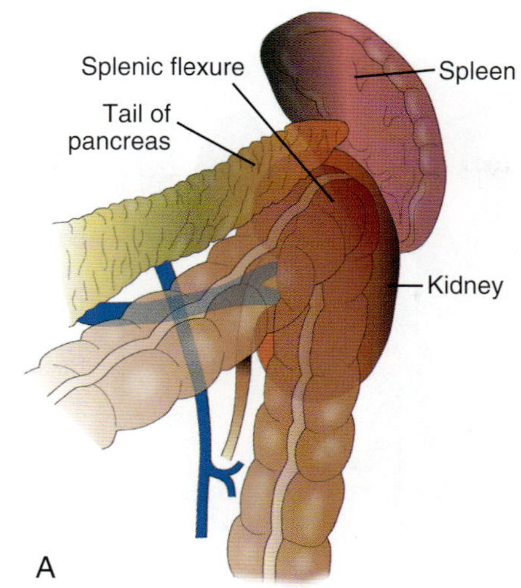

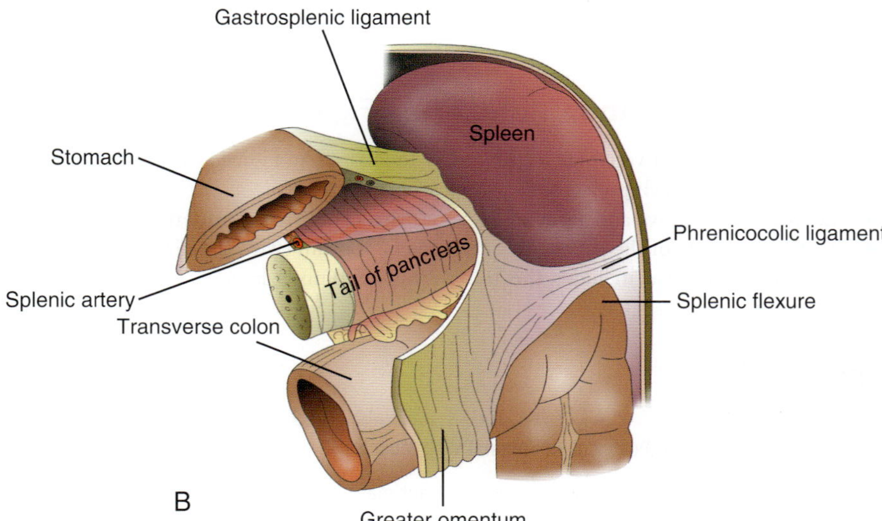

Fig. 4.21 **(A)** Spleen and its relations. **(B)** Spleen and related ligamentous structures.

- The spleen is in contact with the diaphragm and the anterior abdominal wall
- The splenic artery passes between the layers of the lienorenal (splenorenal) ligament, which at the hilum divides into T- or Y-shaped patterns
- Lymph drains from several nodes at the hilum to the retropancreatic nodes and then to the coeliac nodes
- The spleen is supplied by sympathetic fibres only from the coeliac plexus
- Development causes the dorsal mesogastrium to divide into the lienorenal (splenorenal) and gastrosplenic ligaments
- Accessory spleens are common in ≈1/10 individuals

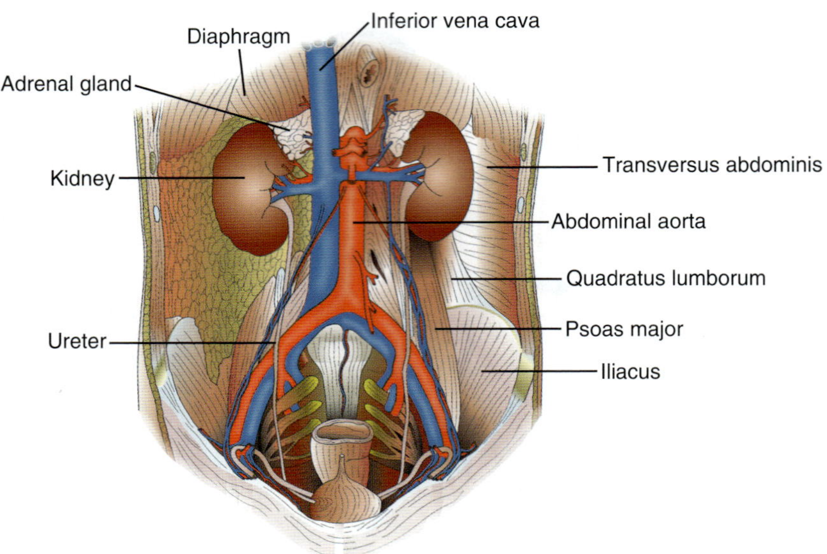

Fig. 4.22 Structures of the posterior abdominal wall.

Part 9 Posterior Abdominal Wall (Fig 4.22)

- Contains five lumbar vertebrae (separated by thick discs and joined by an anterior longitudinal ligament), which project forwards creating a convexity
- The inferior vena cava and aorta are in front, with paravertebral gutters on either side
- The floor consists of the psoas and quadratus lumborum (with the iliacus below the iliac crest). The wall also includes the transversus abdominis laterally and the diaphragm superiorly

MUSCLES

TABLE 4.2 ■ **Summary of Posterior Abdominal Wall Muscles**

Muscle	Proximal Attachment	Distal Attachment	Concentric Action	Innervation
Psoas major	Transverse process of L1–5, bodies of T12–L5 and intervertebral discs of T12–L4	Lesser trochanter of femur	Flexes hip	Anterior rami of L1–3
Psoas minor	Bodies of T12–L1	Pectineal line of pubis and psoas fascia	Weak flexor of lumbar spine	Anterior rami of L1
Quadratus lumborum	Transverse process of L5, iliolumbar ligament and iliac crest	Transverse process of L1–4 and the inferior border of rib 12	Fixes the 12th rib during respiration and laterally flexes the trunk	Anterior rami of T12–L3
Iliacus	Iliac fossa, anterior sacroiliac and iliolumbar ligaments	Lesser trochanter of the femur	Flexes the hip	Femoral nerve L2–4

FASCIA

- The muscles of the posterior abdominal wall are covered by a dense and unyielding fascia, which provides a firm fixation for the peritoneum and underlying viscera
- The psoas fascia invests the surface of the psoas muscle and is attached to the vertebral bodies, fibrous arches and transverse processes. It extends along the pelvic brim attached to the iliopubic eminence at the margins of the muscle. There is a thickening of this fascia from the L1 body to the transverse process, which forms the medial arcuate ligament
- The iliac fascia covers the iliacus muscle. It is attached to bone at the margins of the muscle and to the inguinal ligament. It contributes to the floor of the abdominal cavity. It is prolonged as the femoral sheath, but otherwise does not extend into the thigh
- The lumbar fascia (strictly speaking, the lumbar part of the thoracolumbar fascia) is in continuity with the thoracic fascia. It comprises three layers of fascia enclosing two muscle compartments. The anterior and middle layers occupy only the lumbar region, whereas the posterior layer extends up to the lower part of the neck and below to the dorsal surface of the sacrum
    - Quadratus lumborum occupies the anterior compartment
    - Erector spinae occupies the posterior compartment

ABDOMINAL AORTA AND ITS BRANCHES

- Originates as the thoracic aorta passes behind the median arcuate ligament and diaphragmatic crura at T12
- It inclines slightly to the left and bifurcates at L4 (at the level of the supracristal plane)
- The left sympathetic trunk lies on its left margin
- Between the coeliac trunk and the superior mesenteric artery, the aorta is crossed by the splenic vein and the body of the pancreas
- Between the superior and inferior mesenteric arteries, it is crossed by the left renal vein, the uncinate process of the pancreas and the third section of the duodenum
- Below the duodenum, it is covered by parietal peritoneum

Branches

- Median sacral artery
- Single (unpaired) ventral arteries:
    - Coeliac trunk
    - Superior mesenteric artery
    - Inferior mesenteric artery
- Paired visceral branches:
    - Suprarenal arteries:
        - Arise from between the inferior phrenic and renal branches and run laterally across the crus of the diaphragm
        - The right artery runs between the crus and the inferior vena cava, and then behind the bare area of the liver
        - The left artery lies behind the posterior wall of the lesser sac in the stomach bed
    - Renal arteries:
        - Arise from the aorta at the lower border of L1
        - Each artery gives off a small suprarenal branch and ureteric branches
        - The right renal artery is longer, crossing the right crus and the psoas behind the inferior vena cava

- Gonadal arteries:
  - Arise from near the front of the aorta inferior to the renal arteries
  - They run steeply downwards over the psoas and cross the ureter (supplying its middle third)
  - They are crossed by the colic vessels and peritoneum of the floor of the infracolic compartment
  - They reach the pelvic brim half way between the sacroiliac joint and the inguinal ligament:
    - Male – the testicular artery passes along the pelvic brim above the external iliac artery to enter the deep inguinal ring
    - Female – the ovarian artery crosses the pelvic brim and enters the suspensory ligament to the ovary and fallopian tubes

- Paired branches to the anterior abdominal wall:
  - Subcostal arteries:
    - Branches from the thoracic aorta entering beneath the lateral arcuate ligament
    - They run beneath the subcostal vein and nerve, supplying the anterior abdominal wall
  - Inferior phrenic arteries:
    - Originate just below the aortic hiatus sloping upwards over the crus to the diaphragm, which they supply
    - They give off a number of small suprarenal branches
  - Lumbar arteries (four in number):
    - Originate from the abdominal aorta opposite the vertebral bodies of L1–4, passing beneath the lumbar sympathetic trunks
    - Each branch gives off posterior and spinal branches passing laterally through the psoas
    - The artery of L5 is the iliolumbar, which ascends from the internal iliac artery
  - Common iliac arteries:
    - Are formed by the bifurcation of the aorta at L4, to the left of the midline
    - They pass to the front of the sacroiliac joint to bifurcate into the external and internal iliac arteries
    - The ureter lies in front of the bifurcation into internal and external branches
    - Each common iliac artery is crossed by sympathetic contributions to the superior hypogastric plexus
    - The left common iliac artery is also crossed by inferior mesenteric vessels
  - External iliac arteries:
    - Are a continuation of the common iliac arteries
    - They pass beneath the inguinal ligament to enter the femoral sheath as the femoral artery
    - The inferior epigastric artery is a branch given off near the inguinal ligament and is a key relation for the deep inguinal ring
    - The deep circumflex iliac artery runs above the inguinal ligament
  - Internal iliac arteries are described in the second half of this chapter

INFERIOR VENA CAVA AND ITS TRIBUTARIES

- Begins opposite L5 (below the bifurcation of aorta at the level of the intertubercular plane) and enters the thoracic cavity at T8 by piercing the central tendon of the diaphragm
- It runs to the right of the aorta, lying on the lumbar vertebral bodies
- It overlaps the sympathetic trunk, and crosses the right renal artery
- Inferiorly the tributaries lie posteriorly, while superiorly the tributaries lie anteriorly
- In the infracolic compartment, it lies behind the peritoneum and is crossed by the root of the mesentery and the third part of the duodenum

- In the supracolic compartment, it lies behind the portal vein, head of the pancreas, the common bile duct and the posterior slit of the epiploic foramen to the bare area of the liver
- Its tributaries are not analogous to the arterial branches; blood from the gastrointestinal tract, pancreas and spleen are collected into the portal venous system

Tributaries

- Common iliac vein:
  - Formed in front of the sacroiliac joint by the external and internal iliac veins, and traveling up behind the arteries.
  - The left is longer than the right
  - Each receives iliolumbar +/− lateral sacral vein
  - The left usually receives the median sacral artery
- Lumbar veins:
  - Draining the lateral and posterior abdominal wall (accompanying lumbar arteries and running behind the sympathetic trunks)
  - The third and fourth lumbar veins drain into the inferior vena cava
  - The first and second lumbar veins drain into the ascending lumbar vein
    - Each ascending lumbar vein unites common iliac and iliolumbar veins, passing upwards behind the psoas and in front of the lumbar transverse processes
    - The right ascending lumbar vein passes through the aortic opening
    - The left ascending lumbar vein perforates the left crus
    - Each joins the subcostal veins to form the azygos (right) and hemiazygos (left) veins
- Gonadal veins:
  - These are usually paired (vena comitantes) and unite superiorly on the psoas
  - On the right, the right renal vein usually enters the inferior vena cava (but may enter the renal vein)
  - The left drains into the left renal vein
- Renal veins:
  - Lie in front of the renal artery
  - Join the inferior vena cava at L2
  - The left is three times as long as the right, crosses in front of the aorta and receives the suprarenal, gonadal +/− inferior phrenic veins. It is also connected with the left lumbar azygos and ascending lumbar veins
- Right lumbar azygous vein:
  - Small vessel (may be obliterated) connecting the posterior surface of the inferior vena cava with the azygos vein
  - It lies at the level of the renal vein, behind the psoas
- Right suprarenal vein:
  - A short, stout vessel entering the inferior vena cava behind the bare area of the liver (here the suprarenal gland lies in contact with the liver and inferior vena cava)
- Inferior phrenic veins:
  - Accompany arteries and join the inferior vena cava just below the diaphragm
- Hepatic veins:
  - The left, central and right veins enter the vena cava as it lies in its groove in the back of the liver (central vein drains both halves)

LYMPH NODES AND LYMPH TRUNKS

- Lymph from the alimentary tract, liver, gall bladder, biliary tract, spleen and pancreas passes along the coeliac and superior and inferior mesenteric arteries to the preaortic nodes around the vessel origins

- Lymphatics pass back via paired aortic branches (visceral and somatic) to the para-aortic nodes, which lie alongside the aorta
- The pelvic viscera drain to the nodes along the internal iliac artery
- Lower limbs drain to the deep inguinal nodes and then into the femoral canal and lymph nodes along external iliac artery
- Lymphatics from the iliac arteries drain into para-aortic nodes (note the common iliac artery is considered a paired tributary)
- From the highest of the aortic nodes along with the intestinal and lumbar lymph trunks, the cisterna chyli is formed in front of L1/2. Its upper end becomes continuous with the thoracic duct

SOMATIC NERVES

Nerves supplying the anterior abdominal wall are the subcostal, iliohypogastric and ilioinguinal nerves.

Subcostal Nerve (T12)

- Originates from the thorax and passes behind the lateral arcuate ligament
- It runs below the vein and artery to the tip of the 12th rib and then passes through the transversus abdominis muscle to lie in the neurovascular plane
- It supplies the anterior abdominal wall musculature, the lower part of the rectus abdominis and the pyramidalis muscle
- The lateral cutaneous branch pierces the oblique muscles and supplies the skin over the anterior part of the buttock

Lumbar Plexus

This is formed from the anterior rami of L1–4.

- Iliohypogastric and ilioinguinal (L1) nerves:
  - Lie in front of quadratus lumborum and both divide from a common stem
  - The ilioinguinal nerve represents the collateral branch of the iliohypogastric nerve
  - They emerge from the lateral border of the psoas, behind the lumbar fascia and pass behind the kidney before piercing the fascia and transversus abdominis to reach the neurovascular plane
- Iliohypogastric nerve:
  - Gives off a lateral cutaneous branch to the upper part of the buttock
  - It slopes down in the neurovascular plane until it pierces the aponeurosis of the external oblique, 2.5 cm above the superficial ring, and supplies the skin over the lower rectus and mons pubis
- Ilioinguinal nerve:
  - Pierces the lower border of the internal oblique muscle and enters the inguinal canal from the side (not via the deep ring)
  - At the superficial ring, it pierces the external spermatic fascia to become subcutaneous and supplies the anterior third of the scrotum, the root of the penis, and the upper and medial parts of the groin
  - It gives off muscular branches to the internal oblique and transverse abdominis muscles. These strengthen the conjoint tendon
- Lateral femoral cutaneous nerve (L2, 3):
  - Emerges from the lateral border of psoas on the iliacus muscle (beneath the fascia) and then passes below/through the inguinal ligament into the anterior thigh
  - It supplies the parietal peritoneum of the iliac fossa and the skin of the lateral thigh

- Femoral nerve (L2–4):
  - Emerges from the lateral border of psoas
  - It runs inferiorly deep in the gutter between the psoas and the iliacus
  - It then enters the thigh by passing below the inguinal ligament lateral to the femoral sheath
- Genitofemoral nerve (L1, 2):
  - Emerges from the anterior surface of psoas, running down on the muscle (deep to the psoas fascia)
  - Immediately superior to the inguinal ligament, it perforates the psoas fascia and divides:
    - The genital branch passes through the transversalis fascia (at the deep ring) into the spermatic cord and supplies motor innervation to the cremasteric muscle
    - The femoral branch passes down in front of the femoral artery, pierces the femoral sheath and supplies the skin to the groin below the middle inguinal ligament (femoral triangle)
- Obturator nerve (L2–4):
  - Emerges from medial border of psoas major to enter the pelvis

AUTONOMIC NERVES

Sympathetic Supply

- Arises from the lumbar part of the sympathetic trunk and via the coeliac plexus (from the thoracic sympathetic trunk)
- The **lumbar sympathetic trunk** supplies the somatic branches and the pelvic viscera
  - It receives preganglionic fibres descending from the lower thoracic trunk (which enter by passing behind the medial arcuate ligament on the psoas major and the vertebral border) and from L1, 2
  - The ganglia give off regular somatic and visceral branches, and the trunk passes down to become the sacral part
  - It lies on the left alongside the aorta and right behind the inferior vena cava
  - It lies in front of the segmental vessels; note that branches of the common iliac vessels also lie in front
  - Conventionally there are four lumbar ganglia:
    - Somatic branches pass from the lumbar ganglia to all five lumbar nerves (grey rami) and accompany the vessels
    - The visceral branches arise from all of the lumbar ganglia to join the coeliac, aortic and superior hypogastric plexuses
    - The third and fourth ganglia branches loop around the iliac vessels and, with fibres from the aortic plexus, form the superior hypogastric plexus. This breaks into the right and left hypogastric nerves, which enter the pelvis to form the inferior hypogastric plexus
- The **coeliac plexus** supply is entirely visceral, including gonads
  - The greater and lesser splanchnic nerves enter ganglia which lie at origin of the coeliac trunk
  - Fibres from the plexus then form a postganglionic mesh on the aorta (coeliac plexus) and pass to all of the abdominal viscera along the arteries
  - The fibres are vasomotor, motor to the sphincters, inhibitory to peristalsis and carry sensory information from all of the viscera supplied
  - The suprarenal gland has a second supply (preganglionic) directly from one of the splanchnic nerves (without a relay)

Parasympathetic Supply

- Vagal and pelvic splanchnic nerves supply the parasympathetic fibres
- The vagus is motor and secretomotor to the gut and glands until the splenic flexure
  - It does not supply the gonads, suprarenals or the spleen
- Pelvic splanchnic nerves provide parasympathetic supply from the splenic flexure to the rectum
  - They arise from S2–4 and join the inferior hypogastric plexus to supply the pelvic viscera
  - On the left, fibres travel up to join the inferior mesenteric artery for the hindgut supply

Part 10 Kidneys, Ureters and Suprarenal Glands (see Fig 4.22)

- The kidneys and suprarenal glands lie high on the posterior abdominal wall behind the peritoneum, partly under the cover of the costal margin
- Lie obliquely, with the long axis running parallel with the lateral border of the psoas
- The renal pelvis is a funnel-shaped commencement of the ureter and normally runs posteriorly (anterior to posterior: vein, artery, pelvis). It receives two to three major calyces
- The normal kidney measures 12 × 6 × 3 cm and weighs about 130 grams
- The hila lie around the level of the transpyloric plane (L1/2) – the right hilum lies just below and the left just above it
- The kidney is encapsulated, with perinephric fat surrounding the capsule
- The renal fascia (Gerota's) surrounds the perinephric fat and separates the kidney from the suprarenal gland

RELATIONS OF THE KIDNEY

Posteriorly

- Diaphragm, the quadratus lumborum and laterally the transversus abdominis
- Costodiaphragmatic recess
- Subcostal vessels, the iliohypogastric and ilioinguinal nerves

Hilum

- Right kidney: second part of the duodenum
- Left kidney: tail of the pancreas

Anteriorly

- Superior:
  - Right kidney: peritoneum of the hepatorenal pouch
  - Left kidney: peritoneum of the lesser sac
- Lateral inferior pole – colonic flexures:
  - Right kidney: hepatic flexure
  - Left kidney: splenic flexure
- Medial inferior pole – colic artery:
  - Right kidney: ascending right colic artery
  - Left kidney: upper left colic artery

BLOOD SUPPLY

- Renal arteries have a supply rate of approximately 1 L/min
- At the hilum, the renal artery divides into anterior and posterior divisions, which then further divide into segmental vessels. Each of these is the sole supply to one of the five segments, with no collateral flow:
  - The anterior division supplies the apical, upper, middle and lower segments
  - The posterior division supplies the posterior segment
- Veins communicate with one another and form renal veins at the hilum

LYMPH AND NERVE SUPPLY

- Lymph drainage is to the para-aortic nodes (the upper pole may drain to the posterior mediastinum)
- Sympathetic fibres arise from T12 to L1, which join the thoracic and lumber splanchnic nerves. These form the coeliac, renal and superior hypogastric plexuses, which innervate the kidney
  - These are vasomotor in function
  - Pain fibres accompany the sympathetic fibres
- Parasympathetic supply is present but its function is unclear

URETERS

- Each ureter is 25 cm in length, with a narrowing at the pelviureteric junction, the pelvic brim and the vesicoureteric junction
- It passes over the psoas major and crosses the genitofemoral nerve
- It is crossed by the gonadal vessels
- It leaves the psoas at the bifurcation of the common iliac artery at the sacroiliac joint and passes into the pelvis
- The blood supply is from vessels in the vicinity (e.g. renal artery, vesical arteries)
- Lymphatics drain to the para-aortic nodes

SUPRARENAL GLANDS

- Lie asymmetrically:
  - The right gland is pyramidal and lies on the upper pole of the kidney between the inferior vena cava and the crus. It is in contact with the bare area of the liver
  - The left gland is crescentic and lies more over the medial border of the left kidney, with the lower pole being covered by the pancreas and splenic artery
    - It lies on the left crus, with the left inferior phrenic artery adjacent
- Both glands receive arterial vessels from the renal arteries, the aorta and the inferior phrenic arteries
- Drainage usually occurs by just one vein; the left drains into the renal vein and the right into the inferior vena cava
- The main nerve supply is via myelinated preganglionic sympathetic fibres
- No parasympathetic supply

4-2 Pelvis

Part 11 Pelvic Cavity

BONY PELVIS

- The hip (pelvic) bone, sacrum and coccyx articulate to enclose the pelvic cavity, with the ala of each ilium forming the iliac fossa
- Each pelvic bone is formed by three elements: the ilium, pubis and ischium (Fig 4.23A and B)

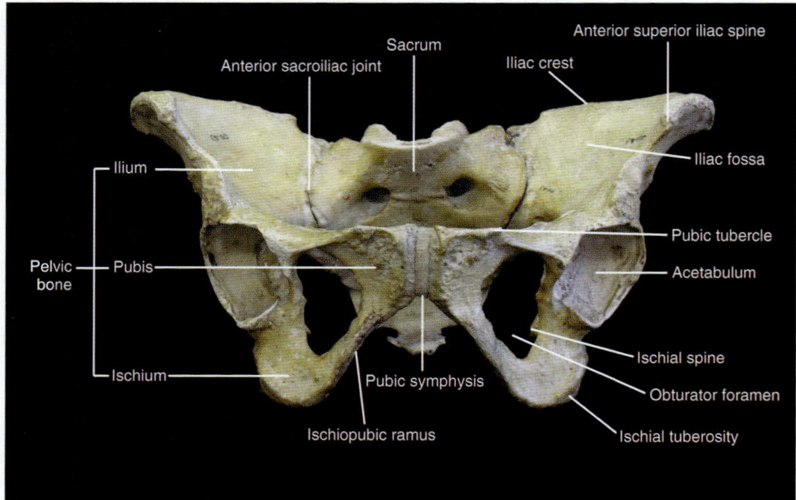

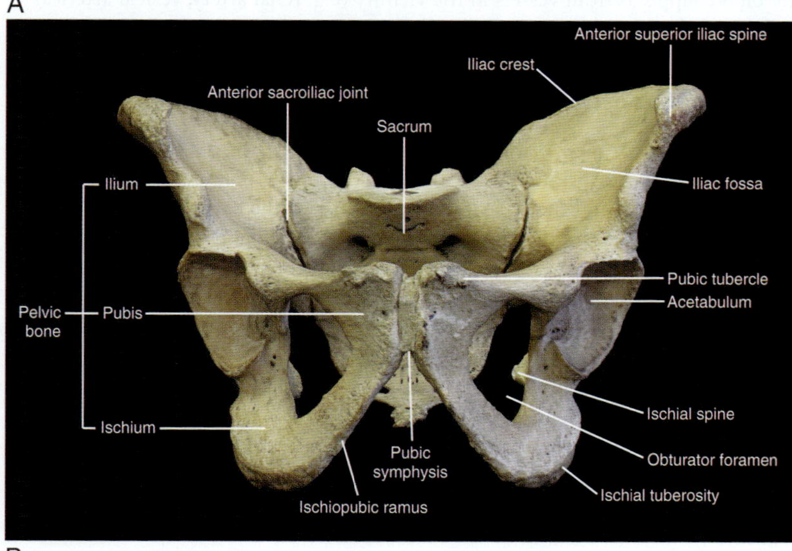

Fig. 4.23 **(A)** Female bony pelvis. **(B)** Male bony pelvis.

- The pelvic brim (the pelvic inlet) is formed by the pubic crest, pectineal line of the pubis, the arcuate line, the ala of the ilium and the promontory of the sacrum (Fig 4.24A–E)
  - It lies obliquely at 60° to the horizontal plane and parallel to the vagina
  - Female: broader with a wide subpubic angle (80°–85°) and less sacral indentation
  - Male: narrower with an acute subpubic angle (50°–60°) and a heart-shaped sacral promontory projecting forwards
- Orientation of the pelvis (anatomical position)
  - The anterior superior iliac spine lies in the same vertical plane as the pubic symphysis
  - The symphysis pubis, ischial spine, tip of the coccyx and appendix of the greater trochanter all lie in the same horizontal plane (the ovaries and seminal vesicles are also in this plane)

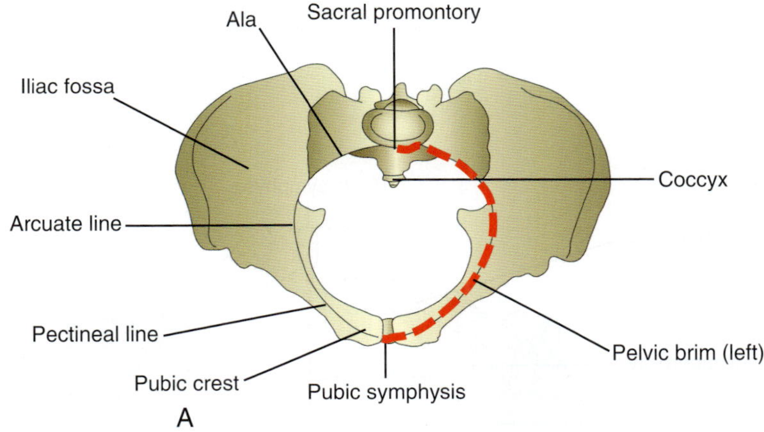

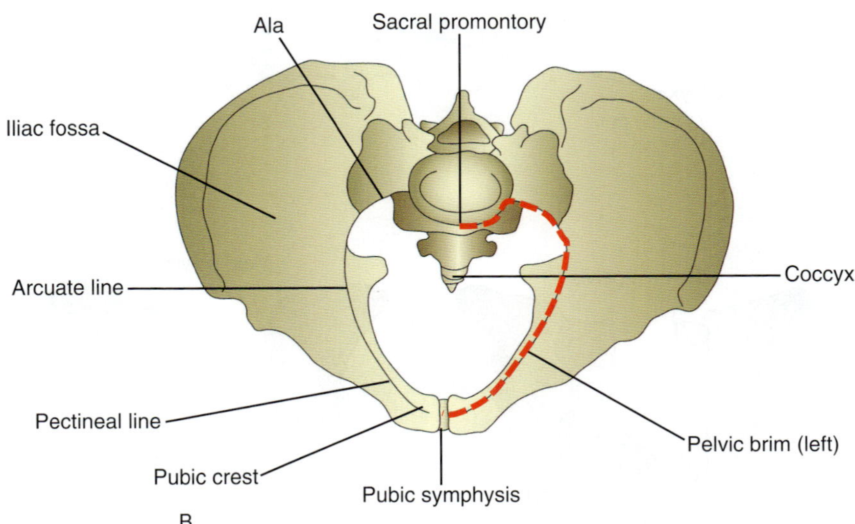

Fig. 4.24 **(A)** Female bony pelvis, superior view. **(B)** Male bony pelvis, superior view.

Continued on following page

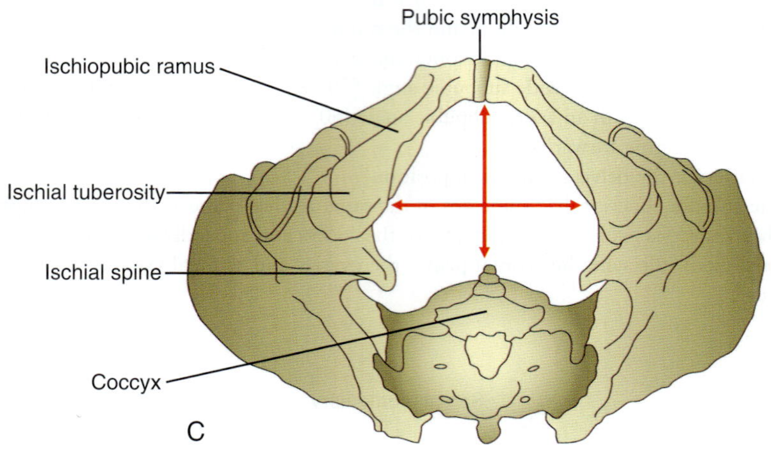

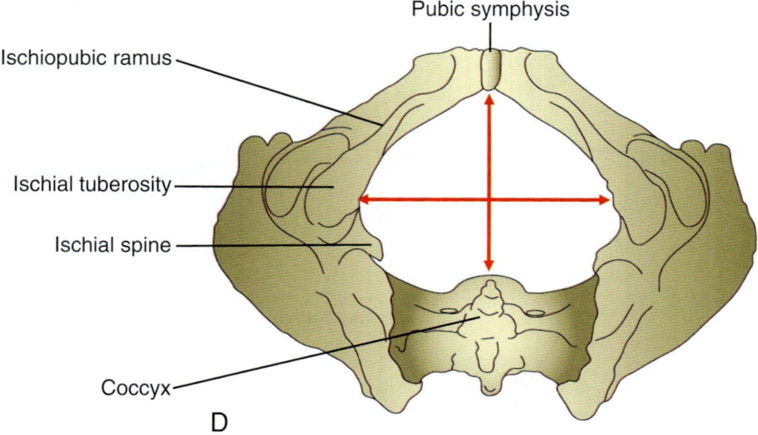

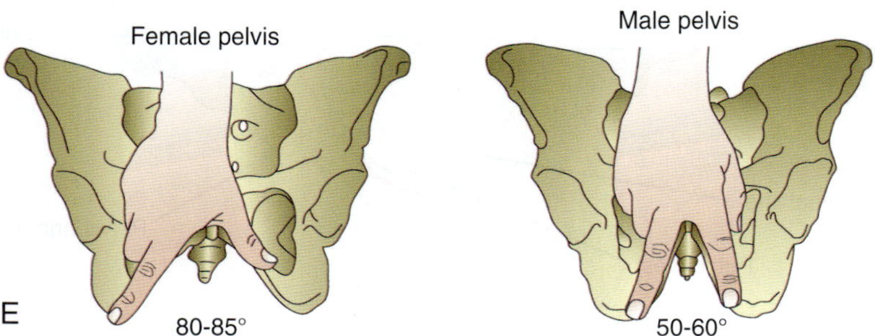

Fig. 4.24, cont'd **(C)** Male bony pelvis, inferior view. **(D)** Female bony pelvis, inferior view. **(E)** Differences in the subpubic angle between females (left) and males (right).

PELVIC WALLS (Fig 4.25A and B)

The pelvic brim divides the false pelvis (above) from the true pelvis or pelvic cavity (below). The muscles of the pelvis are defined as the muscles of the lateral pelvic walls and the muscles of the floor.

Muscles of the Lateral Pelvic Walls

Two muscles, the obturator internus and the piriformis, contribute to the lateral wall of the pelvic cavity.

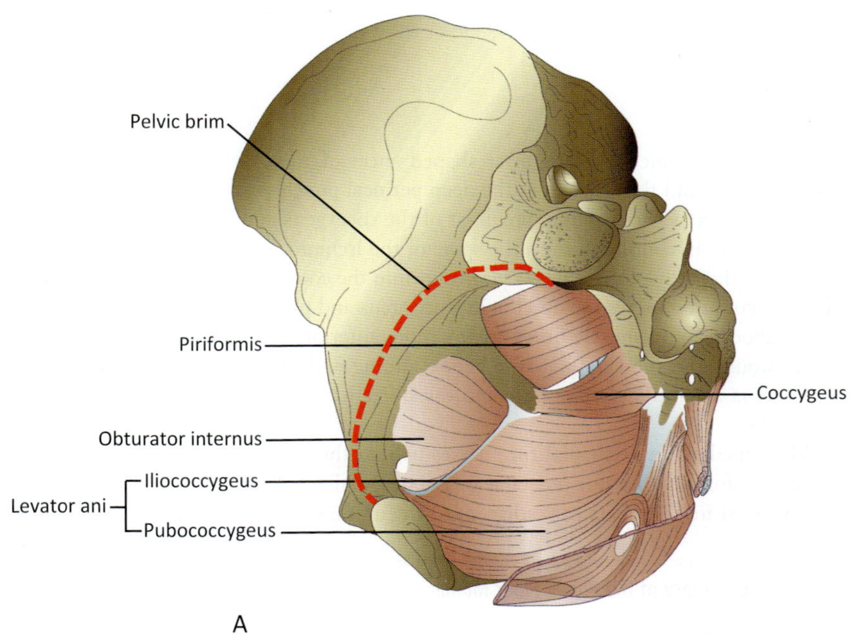

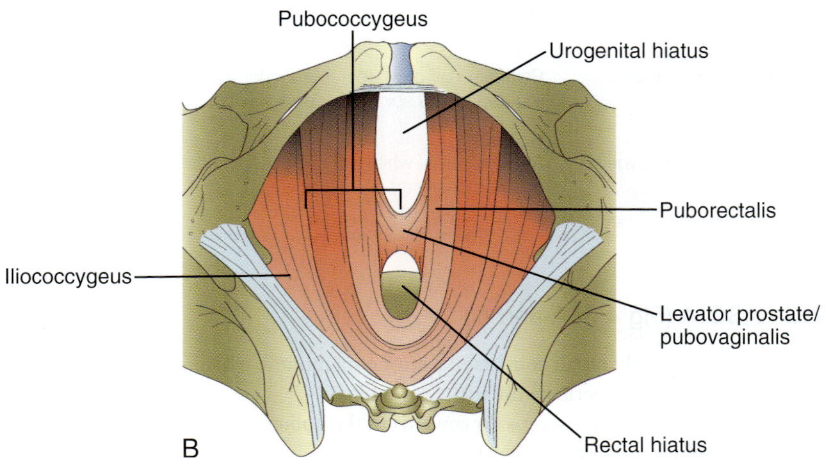

Fig. 4.25 **(A)** Muscular wall of the pelvis. **(B)** Pelvic floor, inferior view.

TABLE 4.3 ■ **Summary of the Lateral Pelvic Wall Muscles**

Muscle	Proximal Attachment	Distal Attachment	Concentric Action	Innervation
Obturator internus	Inner surface of obturator membrane, rim of the pubis and the ischium bordering it	Middle part of medial aspect of greater trochanter of femur	Laterally rotates and stabilises hip	Nerve to obturator internus (L5, S1, 2)
Piriformis	S2–4 costotransverse bars of the anterior sacrum between the sacral foramina	Anterior and medial aspect of the greater trochanter of the femur	Laterally rotates and stabilises hip	Nerve to piriformis (S1, 2)

PELVIC FLOOR

The pelvic floor is formed by the gutter-shaped sheet of muscles; the pelvic diaphragm, the perineal membrane and the muscles in the deep perineal pouch.

- Muscles of the pelvic diaphragm consist of the coccygeus and the levator ani
- Muscles arise in continuity from the spine of the ischium, the white line over the obturator fascia and the body of the pubis. They insert into the coccyx and the anococcygeal ligament
- The levator ani muscles include the iliococcygeus and pubococcygeus
- The pubococcygeus muscle fibres arising more anteriorly swing further medially and inferiorly around the anorectal junction before joining with their opposite muscles fibres
  - There is no midline raphe here and the fibres form a U-shaped sling called the puborectalis
  - More medially, a U-shaped ring passes behind the prostate or vagina into the perineal body to form the levator prostatae or pubovaginalis, respectively
  - The most medial fibres pass adjacent to the urethra and have some sphincteric action

TABLE 4.4 ■ **Summary of the Pelvic Floor Muscles**

Muscle	Subdivision	Attachment	Action	Innervation	
Coccygeus	N/A	Sacrospinous ligament and ischial spine	Anococcygeal body and coccyx	Supports pelvic viscera	S4, 5
Levator ani	Iliococcygeus	Posterior half of white line and ischial spine	Anococcygeal body	Supports pelvic viscera	S3, 4
	Pubococcygeus	Anterior half of white line and posterior part of pubis	Anococcygeal body	Supports pelvic viscera	S3, 4

PELVIC FASCIA (Fig 4.26A and B)

- The fascia of the pelvic wall consists of a strong membrane which covers the pelvic muscles and is attached to the periosteum at their margins
  - The fascia of Waldeyer sweeps downwards in the hollow of the sacrum. The spinal nerves are external to it, while the vessels are internal
  - The sacral plexus lies between the fascia and the piriformis

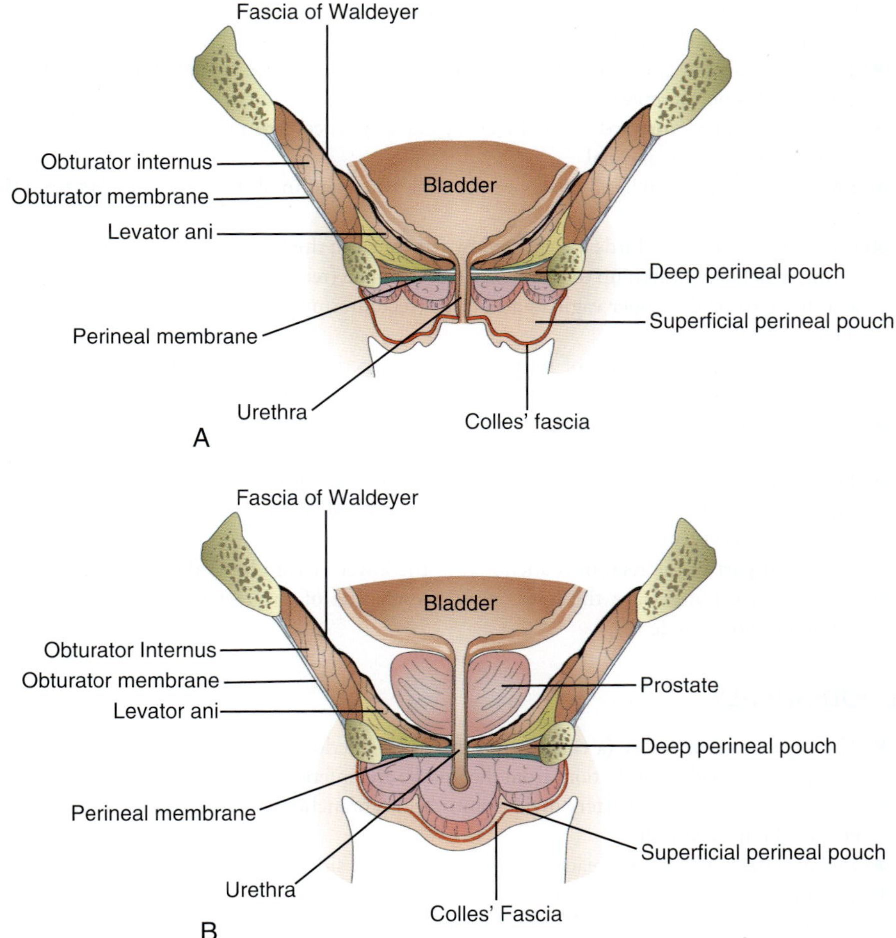

Fig. 4.26 **(A)** Pelvic fascia, coronal section (female). **(B)** Pelvis fascia, coronal section (male).

- The fascia of the floor is really only an epimysium (loose areolar tissue) and the space between the viscera of the pelvis contains so-called ligaments, which are of two types:
  - There are condensations of areolar tissue around the neurovascular bundles (e.g. the lateral ligaments of the uterus and bladder)
  - There are also ligaments in their own right (e.g. the puboprostatic and pubovesical)
- The fascia of the pelvic viscera is loose or dense in conformity with the distensibility of the organ

Part 12 Rectum

- It is 12 cm long, and continuous with the sigmoid colon. It begins at the S3 level proximally and ends distally where the muscle coats are replaced by the anal canal sphincters
- The lowest part is slightly dilated as the rectal ampulla
- It follows the posterior concavity of the sacrum, but also has three lateral flexures (the upper and lower ones curve to the right, while the middle one curves to the left)

    - The resultant folds (of Houston) are produced from the circular muscle in the wall and help to separate flatus from faeces
- The three taeniae come together so there are no sacculations or appendices epiploicae. There is also no mesentery
- From S3 it curves forwards over the coccyx and anococcygeal raphe, behind the perineal body and into the anal canal
- The anorectal junction lies 3 cm above the cutaneous margin of the anus and 5 cm from the coccyx
- Front: the upper two-thirds are covered by peritoneum; the lower third is below the peritoneum, which is reflected up to the bladder in the male (rectovesical pouch, 7.5 cm from the anal margin) or the upper vagina and uterus (rectouterine pouch of Douglas, 5.5 cm from the anal margin)
    - In males, a condensation of retrovesicular connective tissue (Denonvilliers') intervenes between this part of the rectum and the anterior structures
- Sides: the upper third is covered by peritoneum. Retroperitoneal tissue around the middle rectal vessels constitutes the lateral ligaments of the rectum
- The posterolateral relations include S3–5, the coccyx, piriformis, levator ani, coccygeus, anterior rami of the lower three sacral and coccygeal nerves, sympathetic trunk, pelvic splanchnic nerves and rectal vessels
- The lower part of the rectum is anchored to the lower sacrum by Waldeyer's fascia
- Some muscle fibres leave the lower part of each side of the rectal ampulla to form the rectourethralis muscle

BLOOD SUPPLY

- The superior rectal artery (a continuation from the inferior mesenteric artery) is the primary arterial supply, with contributions from the middle and inferior rectal and median sacral arteries
- At S3 the superior rectal artery divides into various branches which supply the whole thickness of the muscle wall
- The middle rectal arteries reach the rectum from the sides via the lateral rectal ligaments
- The inferior rectal arteries penetrate the walls from the anal canal below the level of the levator ani and they can supply up to the level of the peritoneal reflection
- Veins correspond to arteries but anastomose freely, forming the internal and external rectal plexuses
- The superior and inferior rectal veins are the most significant, with drainage occurring into both the portal and the systemic circuits

LYMPH DRAINAGE

- Lymph passes back with the superior and middle rectal arteries and the median sacral artery
- After passing through the lymphoid follicles, it travels to the preaortic lymph nodes via the median sacral artery (in the hollow of the sacrum), the middle rectal artery (on the side wall of the pelvis) or the inferior mesenteric artery

NERVE SUPPLY

- The sympathetic supply arises directly from the hypogastric plexus and also fibres accompanying vascular vessels from the coeliac plexus
- The parasympathetic supply is from S2 and 3 by the pelvic splanchnic nerves
- Pain fibres appear to accompany both the sympathetic and the parasympathetic tracts

Part 13 Urinary Bladder and Ureter in the Pelvis

URINARY BLADDER (Fig 4.27)

- The bladder consists of smooth muscle arranged in whirls and spirals, giving a trabeculated appearance. This is lined with a loose mucous membrane that has a transitional epithelium surface
- No glands or muscularis mucosae are present
- The distended bladder is globular/ovoid (internally smooth) while the non-distended bladder is flattened by the overlying intestines (internally folded), forming a three-sided pyramid
- The sharp apex points to the pubic symphysis and has the remains of the urachus attached to it, forming the median umbilical ligament
- The triangular base faces backwards and forms the posterior surface
  - Male
    - Only the upper part (above the rectovesical pouch) is covered by the peritoneum
    - The ductus deferens medially and the seminal vesicle laterally are attached to this surface. The ureter enters the surface of the bladder at the upper outer corner
  - Female
    - The base is firmly connected with the anterior vaginal wall and uterine cervix, and has no peritoneal covering
- Two inferolateral surfaces slope downwards and medially, and are cradled by the levator ani
  - These surfaces meet behind the pubic bones forming the retropubic space, which contains condensations that form the pubovesical ligaments (in females) and puboprostatic ligaments (in males)
- The neck is the lowest part of the bladder (in the male it lies against the prostate and in the female against the pelvis fascia) and is pierced by the urethra
- The superior surface of the bladder is covered by peritoneum which sweeps upwards on the anterior abdominal wall
- The trigone is triangular in shape and exists between the urethral and the ureteric orifices (2.5–5 cm depending on distension)
  - It is the least mobile part of the bladder
  - The ureters enter obliquely
  - In males, there may be an indentation from the prostate (uvula vesicae)

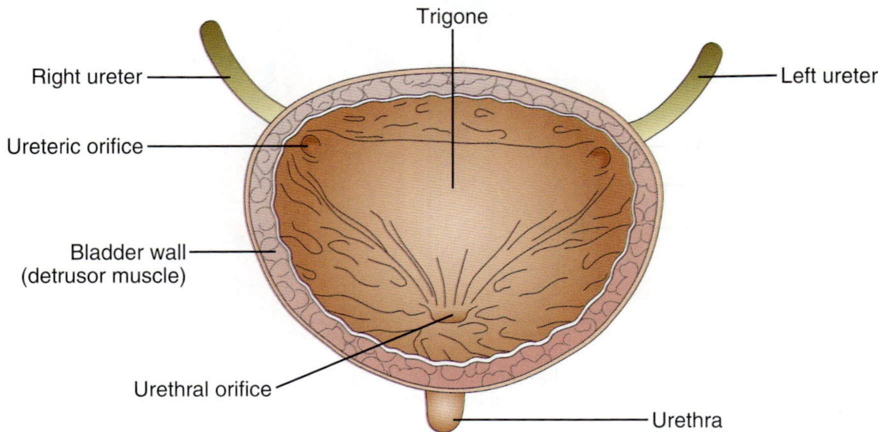

Fig. 4.27 Urinary bladder, coronal section.

- At the male urethral orifice, the circular smooth muscle fibres form a sphincter which is continuous with in the prostate; this helps to avoid retrograde ejaculation

Blood Supply

- Arterial supply is principally from the superior and inferior vesical arteries, with contributions to its lower aspect from the obturator, inferior gluteal, uterine and vaginal arteries
- Veins do not follow the arteries, but rather form a plexus which drains back across the pelvic floor to the internal iliac veins

Lymph Drainage

- Lymphatics follow the arteries back to the internal and external iliac nodes

Nerve Supply

- The sympathetic supply is from L1–2 via the superior hypogastric and pelvic plexuses. It is largely vasomotor but also innervates the superficial trigone muscle and the internal urethral sphincter (in males)
- The parasympathetic fibres are supplied via the pelvic splanchnic nerves and are mainly motor
- Normal bladder sensation is transmitted with the parasympathetic system via the gracile tract, but bladder pain reaches the spinal cord via both tracts and then travels in the lateral spinothalamic tract

PELVIC URETER (Fig 4.28A and B)

- The pelvic part is normally half of the 25 cm length
- It crosses the pelvic brim at the bifurcation of the common iliac artery, and passes over the external iliac vessels and then in front of the internal iliac artery
- It crosses the obturator nerve, the obliterated umbilical artery and the obturator artery and vein
- At the ischial spine, it turns forwards and medially to enter the bladder at the upper lateral angle
  - Males: the ductus deferens crosses the ureter and then runs down medially to it

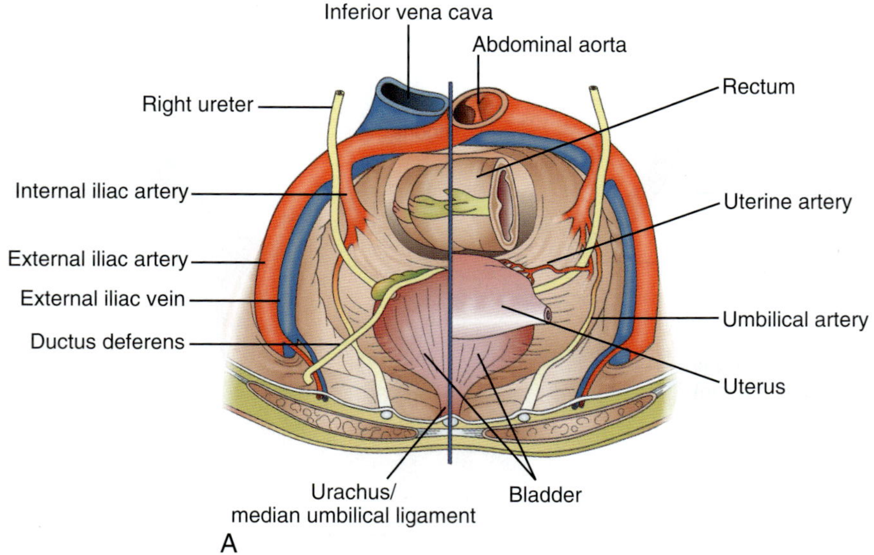

Fig. 4.28 **(A)** Relations of the pelvic ureter. Left: Male. Right: Female.

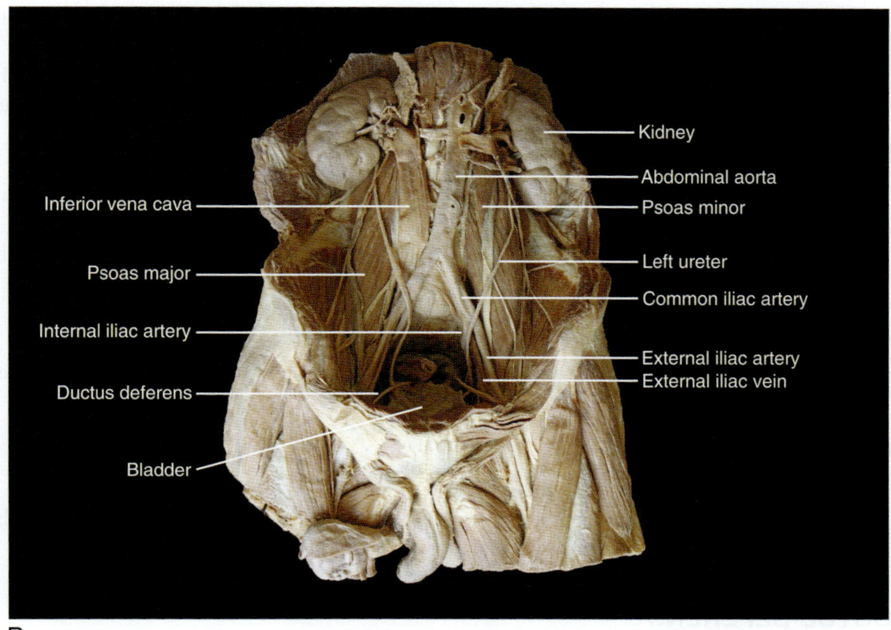

Fig. 4.28, cont'd **(B)** Abdominal and pelvic course of the ureters (male).

- Females: the ureter lies in the base of the broad ligament on the posterior peritoneal layer. It is crossed superficially by the uterine artery and crosses the lateral vaginal fornix 1–2 cm from the cervix
- Only the ductus deferens or the uterine artery lies superior to the ureter in the pelvis

Part 14 Male Internal Genital Organs

PROSTATE

- It lies between the bladder and the urogenital diaphragm, usually broader than it is long with dimensions of 4 × 3 × 2 cm
- It provides about 30% of the seminal fluid
- Base – the upper surface is adjacent to the bladder, and fuses with the neck of the bladder
- Apex – is blunt and forms the lowest part of the prostate. The prostatic urethra becomes the membranous urethra upon its emergence
- Anterior surface – is the back of the retropubic space, and is connected by puboprostatic ligaments
- Inferolateral surface – is clasped by the levator prostatae part of the levator ani
- Posterior surface – accepts the ejaculatory ducts
- It is contained by a thin, inner, 'true' capsule and a condensation of pelvic fascia known as the 'false' capsule. A venous plexus runs between these layers
- The prostate is considered to be in five lobes:
  - Anterior lobe – functionally unimportant
  - Middle lobe – the ejaculatory ducts and urethra pass through this lobe, and enlargements can cause obstruction

  - Posterior and lateral lobes (right and left) – are important because they are the commonest sites of enlargement and cancerous changes
  - The prostatic urethra is the widest part. It has a posterior urethral crest onto which the ejaculatory ducts open. The crest also has a small seminal colliculus (uterus homologue)

Blood Supply

- The arterial supply is primarily via the prostatic branch of the inferior vesical artery. Contributions may also come from the middle rectal and internal pudendal arteries
- A venous plexus exists between the two capsules and receives the deep dorsal vein of the penis before draining into the internal iliac veins

Lymph Drainage

- Lymph drainage passes across the pelvic floor to the internal iliac and sacral lymph nodes. Some may also reach the external iliac nodes

Nerve Supply

- Parasympathetic nerves supply the acini via the pelvic splanchnic nerves
- Sympathetic fibres originating from the inferior hypogastric plexus supply the muscular stroma, which contracts to empty the glands during ejaculation

DUCTUS DEFERENS

- A very thick-walled structure, lined with pseudostratified epithelium and stereocilia
- It is a continuation of the epididymis. It enters the abdomen at the deep inguinal ring and hooks around the interfoveolar ligament and inferior epigastric artery
- It crosses the external iliac artery and vein, the obliterated umbilical artery and the obturator nerve, artery and vein
- It curves medially and crosses the ureter, approaching its opposite counterpart. While both ducts are running side by side, they dilate into the ampullae (storehouse of spermatozoa), which lies medial to the seminal vesicles
- These structures form the ejaculatory ducts, which then pass obliquely to open at the side of the urethral crest

Blood Supply

- Arises from the artery to the ductus deferens, a branch of the superior vesical artery, and anastomoses with the testicular artery

Nerve Supply

- Smooth muscle innervation is from the pelvic plexus
- Sympathetic fibres provide motor input and are important in ejaculation; their division produces sterility

Lymph Drainage

- Accompanies blood vessels to the nearest iliac nodes

SEMINAL VESICLE

- It is thin-walled, consisting of only two layers (inner circular and outer longitudinal)
- It is an elongated sac and produces ≈60% of the seminal fluid

Blood Supply

- Arises from the inferior vesical and middle rectal arteries

Nerve Supply

- Smooth muscle innervation is from the pelvic plexus
- Sympathetic fibres provide motor input and are important in ejaculation; their division produces sterility

Lymph Drainage

- Accompanies blood vessels to the nearest iliac nodes

Part 15 Female Internal Genital Organs and Urethra

UTERUS

- A muscular organ (8 × 5 × 3 cm) consisting of a fundus, body and cervix
  - Fundus – the part above the entrance of the tubes, 5 cm across and 3 cm thick, covered by peritoneum
  - Body – tapers downwards from fundus and is flattened anteroposteriorly. It is covered by peritoneum which becomes the broad ligament laterally
  - Cervix – tapers below the body and protrudes into the vagina. The ureters pass about 1–2 cm from the cervix
    - The canal of the cervix is continuous with the body. It starts at the internal orifice and extends down to the external orifice
- The bulk of the uterus is smooth muscle, organised into three ill-defined layers.
- The endometrium has a lining of columnar epithelium that undergoes regular shedding to facilitate menstruation. This does not take place at the cervix, however, where there is a transition zone to stratified squamous epithelium, the same as the lining of the vagina
- 80% of uteri are anteverted (bent forwards in relation to the long axis of the cervix)
- Uterine support:
  - The most fixed part is the cervix, owing to its attachments to the back of the bladder and vaginal fornix. The vagina is supported via the pubovaginalis and the perineal body
  - The broad ligament is a lax double fold of peritoneum lying laterally between the side wall of the uterus and the pelvis
    - Its lateral attachment crosses the obturator nerve, obliterated umbilical vessels and obturator vessels
    - The upper border has a free edge and contains the uterine tube within the mesosalpinx. The lateral quarter forms the suspensory ligament of the ovary and contains the ovarian veins and lymphatics
    - The posterior layer has the ureter adhering to it
    - The anterior layer is bulged forwards by the round ligament
  - The round ligament extends from the uterus/tube junction to the deep inguinal ring, and then through the inguinal canal to the labia majora
    - It holds the uterus in anteflexion and anteversion
    - It lies in the anterior layer of the broad ligament
    - It is continuous with the ovarian ligament – forming the gubernaculum
  - The lateral ligament consists of thickenings from the cervix to the wall of the pelvis
  - The uterosacral ligaments extend from the cervix, embracing the rectouterine pouch and gubernaculum

Blood Supply

- By the uterine artery (from the internal iliac artery, through the base of the broad ligament); it also supplies the cervix and vagina

- Veins course below the artery at the lower edge of the broad ligament, forming a plexus on the pelvic floor to the internal iliac vein

Lymph Drainage

- Mainly to the external iliac nodes (although drainage to the inguinal nodes is possible). The cervix drains to the external and internal iliac nodes (but not the inguinal nodes)

Nervous Supply

- Via branches of the pelvic plexus, but much of the control is hormonal

UTERINE TUBES

- Are each 10 cm in length
- Each consists of four parts:
  - Intramural part – proximal 1 cm, embedded in the uterine wall
  - Isthmus – lies in the upper edge of the broad ligament (straight and narrow)
  - Ampulla – a dilation
  - Infundibulum – final part which opens into the pelvic cavity with a fimbriated end
- It is formed by two layers of visceral muscle (the inner circular, the outer longitudinal), with the mucous membrane thrown into folds which increase towards the ampulla. The surface epithelium is a mixture of ciliated and non-ciliated columnar epithelium

Blood Supply

- Via a tubal branch of the ovarian artery (the artery runs below the tube)
- The venous drainage is via the tubal veins and enters into the ovarian veins

OVARY (Fig 4.29A–C)

- Ovoid-shaped organ composed of fibrous tissue with embedded ova
- It consists of a fibrous stroma covered by a cuboidal epithelium
- It is attached to the posterior leaf of the broad ligament by the mesovarium (double folded peritoneum). The mesovarium is attached equatorially around the ovary, but does not invest into the organ

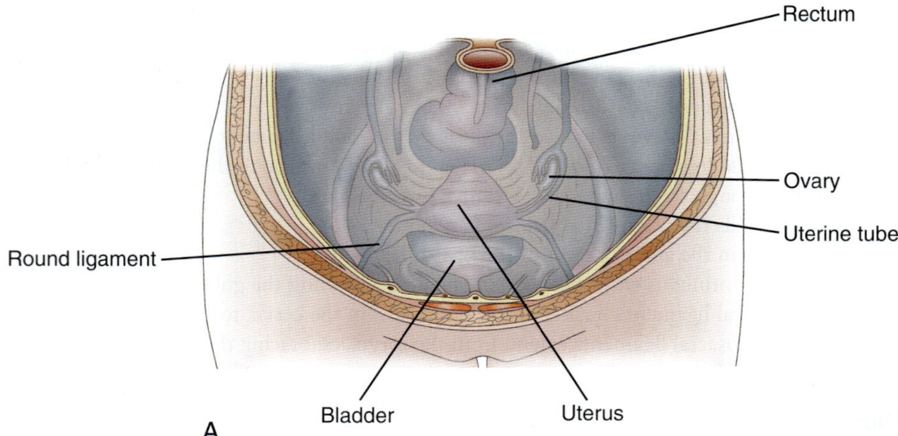

Fig. 4.29 (A) Relations of the peritoneum with internal genital organs viewed anteriorly (female).

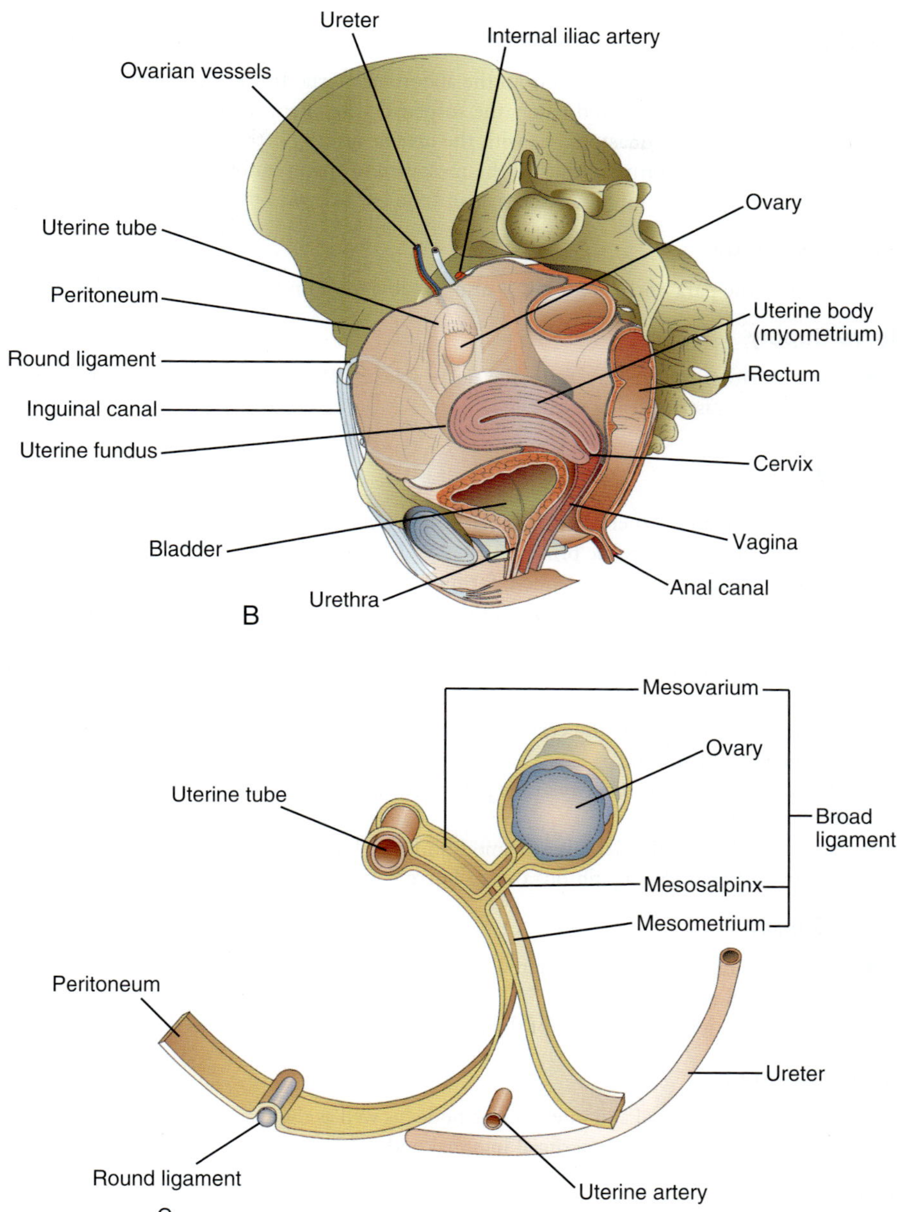

Fig. 4.29, cont'd **(B)** Relations of the peritoneum with internal genital organs, sagittal section (female). **(C)** Relations of the peritoneum to the ovary and related structures.

- The ovary lies in the side wall of the pelvis in the angle between the external and the internal iliac arteries on the obturator nerve (hence the referred pain)
- The ovary normally lies obliquely, with the tubal extremity being uppermost and medial. It is attached to the upper angle of the uterus by the ligament of the ovary

Blood Supply

- Via the ovarian artery, a branch from the abdominal aorta. It runs down behind the peritoneum, crosses the ureter and enters the suspensory ligament. It then gives off a branch to the uterine tube and anastomoses with the uterine artery
- The ovarian veins form a plexus in the mesovarium (pampiniform plexus). The right side drains directly to the inferior vena cava and the left side into the left renal vein

Lymph Drainage

- Drains to the para-aortic nodes (it is also possible to drain to the inguinal nodes)

Nerve Supply

- The sympathetic fibres are from the aortic plexus. Parasympathetic fibres are from the inferior hypogastric plexus

VAGINA

- It is approximately 10 cm long and has a transverse lumen. It runs in approximately the same direction as the pelvic brim
- The upper end is slightly expanded, forming the vaginal fornix (consisting of the anterior, posterior and lateral fornices) around the margin of the cervix. The posterior fornix is covered by peritoneum
- The ureter is initially adjacent to the lateral fornix and then passes to the anterior fornix to enter the bladder
- The anterior wall (below the cervix) is in contact with the base of the bladder and has the urethra embedded in it
- The vagina passes down between the pubovaginalis parts of the levator ani and through the urogenital diaphragm
- The vagina has a muscular layer of smooth muscle lined internally by a mucous membrane and covered externally by fibrous tissue. There is no muscularis mucosa and no glands

Blood Supply

- Via the vaginal branch of the internal iliac artery, as well as the uterine, inferior vesical and middle rectal arteries
- Veins initially join the plexuses of the pelvic floor and then drain into the internal iliac vein

Lymph Drainage

- Drains via the external and internal iliac nodes as well as the sacral lymph nodes, with lower portions draining to the superficial inguinal nodes

Nerve Supply

- The lower end receives sensory fibres from the perineal nerve and posterior labial branches of the pudendal nerve and the ilioinguinal nerve
  - Sympathetic nerves derived from the hypogastric plexuses supply the blood vessels and smooth muscle of the vaginal wall

FEMALE URETHRA (see Fig 4.26A)

- It is 4 cm in length, with all except the uppermost part being embedded within the anterior wall of the vagina

- It contains no internal sphincter
- It exits 2.5 cm behind the clitoris

Blood Supply

- Its superior aspect is supplied through the inferior vesical and uterine arteries, while its inferior aspect is supplied through the perineal branch of the internal pudendal artery

Lymph Drainage

- Primarily drains to the internal but also to the external iliac lymph nodes

Nerve Supply

- From the inferior hypogastric plexuses and the perineal branch/nerve of the perineal nerve

Part 16 Pelvic Peritoneum, Vessels and Nerves

PELVIC PERITONEUM

Pelvic Peritoneum in the Male (Fig 4.30A)

- It is draped over the pelvic viscera and extends from the pelvic brim across the pelvic walls and lines the pelvic cavity
- Anteriorly it is reflected to the upper surface of the bladder and forms the roof of the retropubic space
- Behind the bladder it forms the rectovesical pouch, with the retroperitoneal tissue forming the rectovesical fascia (of Denonvilliers)
- Laterally it has a continuous sheet melding with the parietal peritoneum at the pelvic brim

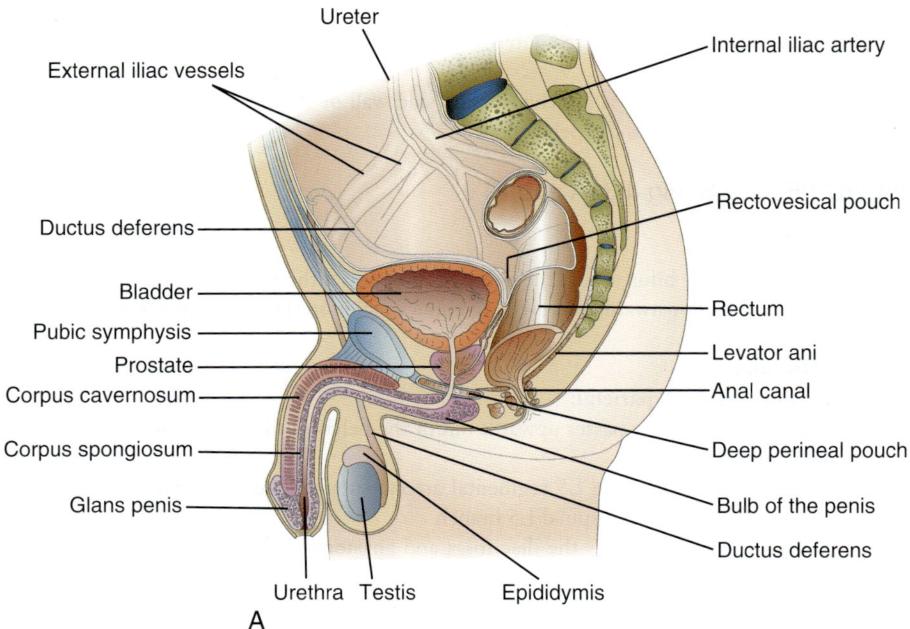

Fig. 4.30 **(A)** Relations of the pelvic peritoneum in males, sagittal section.

Continued on following page

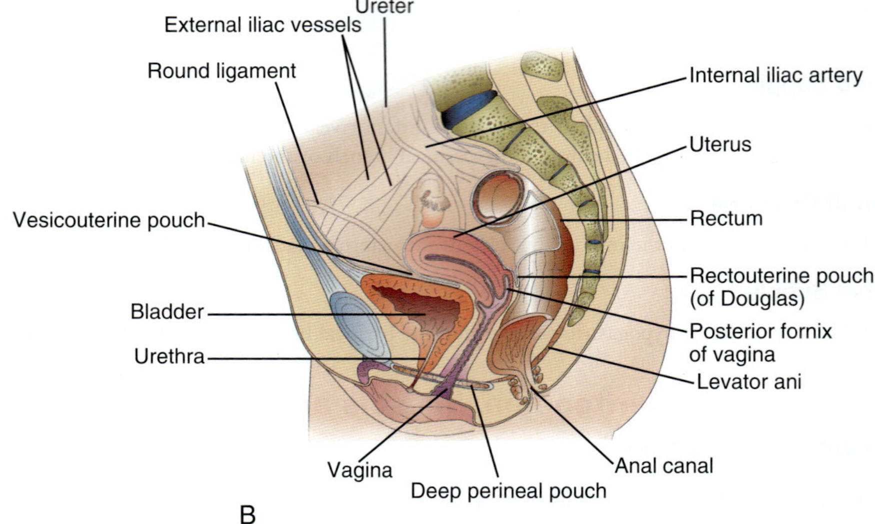

Fig. 4.30, cont'd (B) Relations of the pelvic peritoneum in females, sagittal section.

Pelvic Peritoneum in the Female (Fig 4.30B)

- It is largely the same as above, but altered owing to the presence of the uterus and the broad ligament
- From the back of the bladder, the peritoneum ascends over the front of the uterus to form the vesicouterine pouch
- From the back of the uterus, it is firmly attached to the posterior fornix of the vagina; it then dips down to form the rectouterine pouch (of Douglas) and then runs back up over the rectum and sacrum
- On each side the uterus is attached to the side wall of the pelvis by the broad ligament extending down towards the pelvic floor

PELVIC VESSELS (Fig 4.31A and B)

Internal Iliac Artery

The common iliac artery bifurcates at the pelvic brim opposite the sacroiliac joint, with the internal iliac artery passing downwards and dividing into a small posterior and a large anterior division.

Posterior Division

- **Three branches – all parietal:**
  - The iliolumbar artery passes upwards out of the pelvis in front of the lumbosacral trunk and deep to the psoas
    - Its lumbar branch (the L5 segmental artery) supplies the psoas and quadratus lumborum and gives off a spinal L5 branch
    - Its iliac branch supplies the iliac fossa and anastomoses around the anterior superior iliac spine
  - The lateral sacral artery runs down lateral to the anterior sacral foramina, supplying the roots of the sacral plexus and piriformis

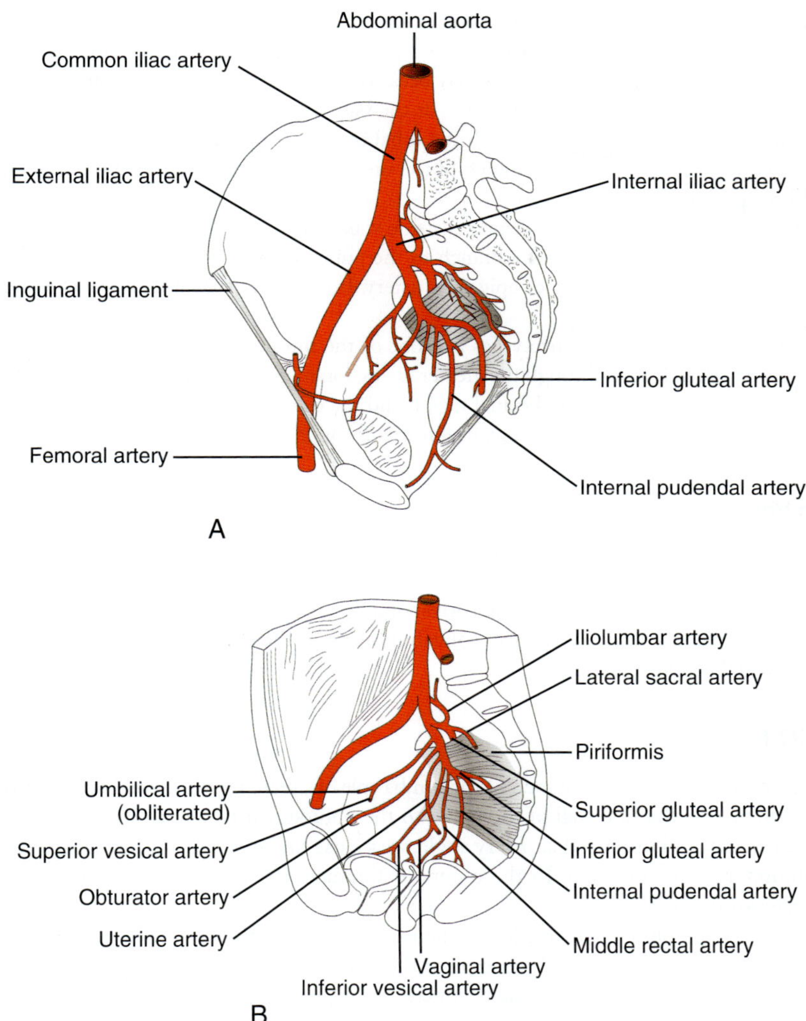

Fig. 4.31 **(A)** Branches of the internal iliac artery (male). **(B)** Branches of the internal iliac artery (female).

- The superior gluteal artery is the largest branch of the internal iliac artery and it exits through the greater sciatic foramen to enter the buttock

Anterior Division

- **Three arteries associated with the bladder:**
  - The superior vesical artery is the highest branch and is from the persistent, patent, proximal part of the fetal umbilical artery. The distal part becomes obliterated and forms the medial umbilical fold. It runs along the side wall of the pelvis and then turns medially to reach the upper part of the bladder. It supplies the bladder, adjacent ureter and ductus deferens
  - The inferior vesical artery supplies the trigone and lower bladder as well as the ureter, ductus deferens and seminal vesicle. It also usually gives rise to the prostatic artery
  - The obliterated umbilical artery

- **Three arteries to other viscera:**
  - The middle rectal artery, when present, runs towards and divides before entering the lower rectal wall. In the male, it may occasionally give off the prostatic artery
  - The uterine artery crosses the pelvis at the base of the broad ligament, turning upwards at the cervix. It anastomoses with the tubal branch of the ovarian artery
  - The vaginal artery, often a branch of the uterine artery, supplies the upper vaginal wall
- **Three parietal branches:**
  - The obturator artery passes along the side wall of the pelvis below the nerve to enter the obturator canal. It gives off a branch to the pubis periosteum and anastomoses with the pubic branch of the inferior epigastric artery. It may be at risk of damage when releasing a strangulated hernia
  - The internal pudendal artery lies in front of the inferior gluteal and pierces the parietal pelvic fascia. It exits through the greater sciatic foramen then passes back through the lesser sciatic foramen to supply the anal region and the external genitalia
  - The inferior gluteal artery runs backwards through the greater sciatic foramen into the buttock

Pelvic Veins

- There is a significant network of veins. The internal iliac vein is about 3 cm long and begins at the confluence of the gluteal veins and other vessels that accompany the internal iliacs. It then runs above and behind the corresponding artery
- The internal iliac vein also receives contributions from the uterine (vesicoprostatic in males) and rectal venous plexuses

PELVIC NERVES

- The obturator nerve is a branch of the lumbar plexus, piercing the medial wall of psoas and passing along the side wall of the pelvis to the obturator foramen. In its course, it runs in the external and internal iliac artery angle, very close to the ovary. The nerve runs above the obturator artery and vein. In the obturator foramen, the nerve divides into anterior and posterior divisions
- The accessory obturator nerve leaves the medial aspect of the psoas, but is otherwise similar to the femoral nerve and passes over the pubic ramus; it is derived from the posterior divisions of L3–4. It supplies the pectineus but is present in only one-third of individuals

SACRAL PLEXUS (Fig 4.32A–C)

- Much of L4 and all of L5 nerves enter the sacral plexus through the lumbosacral trunk, joining the anterior rami of the upper four sacral nerves
- The sacral plexus is a broad triangular structure resting on the piriformis beneath the fascial layer
- The sacral nerves give off branches and then divide into anterior and posterior divisions that branch. Two of these then reunite to form the sciatic nerve that supplies the lower limb

Branches from the Sacral Nerves (Six Starting with 'P')

- The piriformis is supplied by twigs from S1 and 2
- The perforating cutaneous nerve arises from S2 and 3 and supplies the skin over the buttock
- The posterior femoral cutaneous nerve arises from S2 and 3
- The parasympathetic pelvic splanchnic nerves arise from rootlets S2 and 3 (or S3 and 4)
- The pudendal nerve arises from the anterior surfaces of S2–4
- The perineal branch of S4 supplies the coccygeus and levator ani as well as the perianal skin

Branches from the Anterior Divisions (Three - Destined for the Flexor Compartment)

- The tibial part of the sciatic nerve originates from L4, 5, S1–3
- The nerve to the obturator internus supplies this muscle and the superior gemellus, and leaves the pelvis below the piriformis
- The nerve to the quadratus femoris originates from L4, 5, S1 and also supplies this muscle, the inferior gemellus and the hip joint

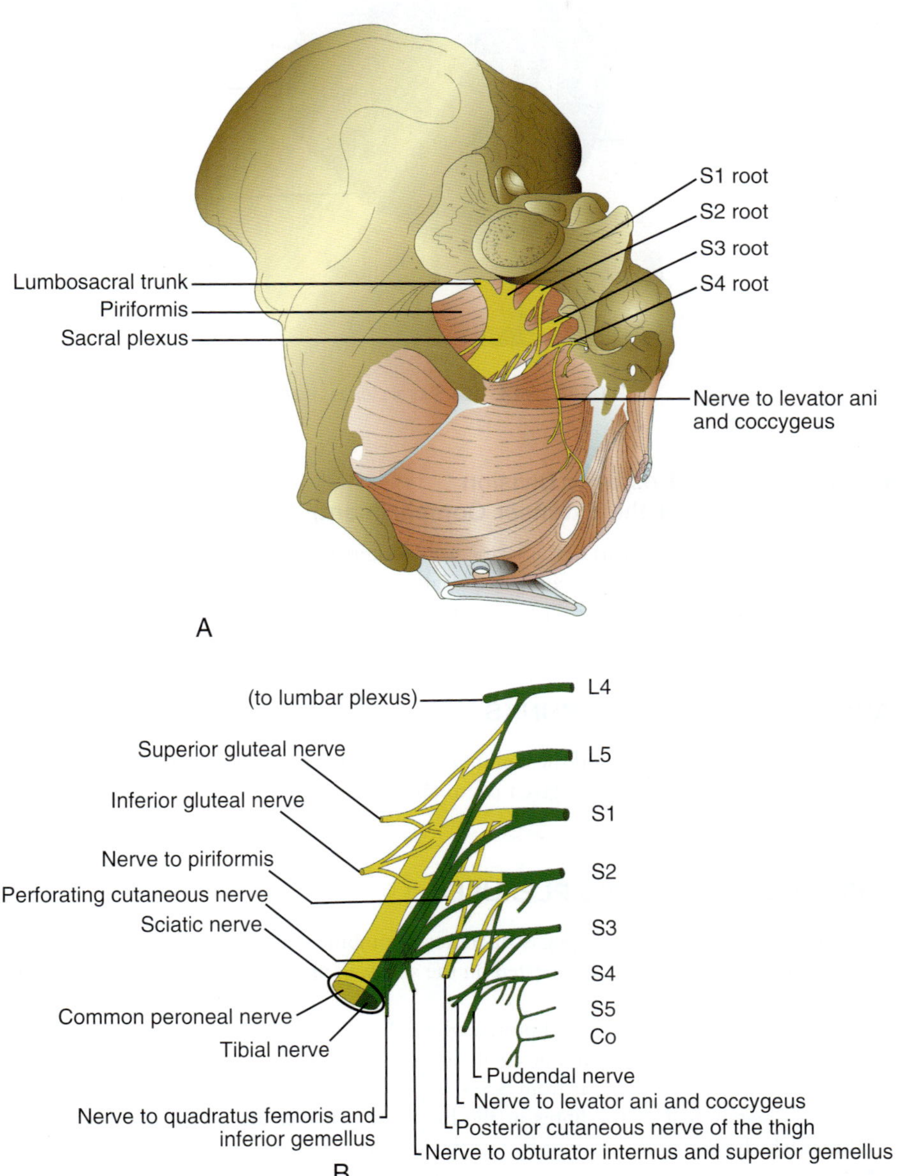

Fig. 4.32 **(A)** Sacral plexus. **(B)** Spinal branches.

Continued on following page

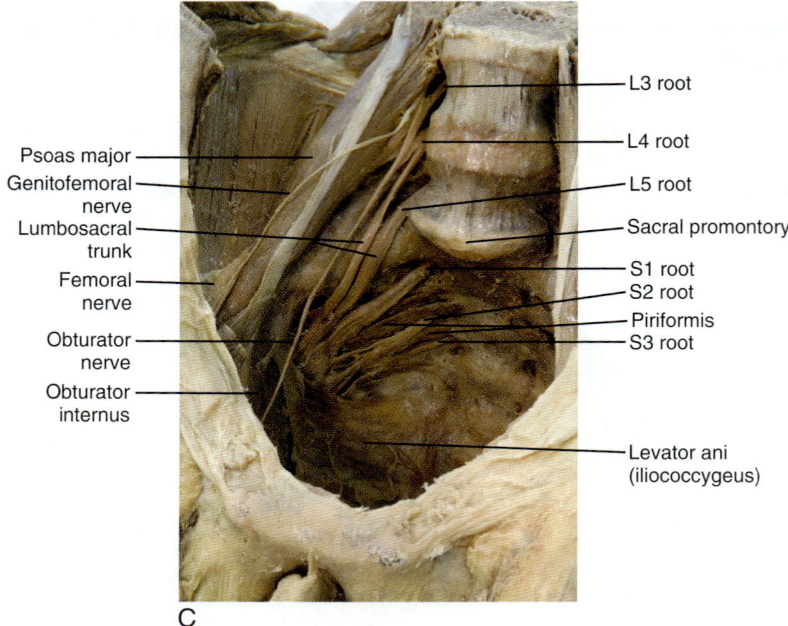

Fig. 4.32, cont'd **(C)** Sacral plexus, *in situ*.

Branches from the Posterior Division (Three – Destined for the Extensor Compartment)

- The common peroneal part of the sciatic nerve originates from L4, 5, S1, 2 and usually joins with the tibial part to form a combined sciatic nerve
- The superior gluteal nerve from L4, 5, S1 passes out above the piriformis
- The inferior gluteal nerve from L5, S1, 2 passes out below the piriformis

SACRAL SYMPATHETIC TRUNKS

These cross the pelvic brim behind the common iliac vessels, and each has the characteristic four ganglia. Somatic branches are then given off to all the sacral nerves and also to the lateral and median sacral vessels.

INFERIOR HYPOGASTRIC PLEXUSES

- The right and left inferior hypogastric plexuses combine to form a single pelvic plexus. This is an autonomic plexus and is located on the side wall of the pelvis, lateral to the rectum
- The sympathetic input is from:
  - The lumbar ganglia (pre- and postganglionic)
  - The sacral ganglia (pre- and postganglionic)
- The parasympathetic input is from S2–4
- Approximately half of the fibres in the hypogastric nerves are myelinated preganglionic fibres which relay to the inferior hypogastric plexus
- The remaining fibres (including all of the parasympathetic) pass through without relay
- The sympathetic vasoconstrictor fibres accompany all vessels and are also motor to the:
  - Bladder sphincter
  - Anal canal sphincter

  - Ductus deferens
  - Seminal vesicles
  - Prostatic muscle
  - Uterine muscle
- The pelvic parasympathetic nerves are:
  - Motor to the detrusor muscle
  - Secretomotor to the gut from the splenic flexure downwards
- Sensory supply
  - To abdominal viscera and gonads via the sympathetic pathways
- The cloacal derivatives, namely the bladder, rectal ampulla and anal canal, also receive sensory fibres from the pelvic parasympathetic pathway, as does the lower cervix and upper vagina

Part 17 Perineum (Fig 4.33A and B)

- It is the part of the body caudal to the pelvic diaphragm and contains the urogenital and anal triangles
- The skin on the side of the anal region is supplied by the inferior rectal nerve and a perineal branch of S4

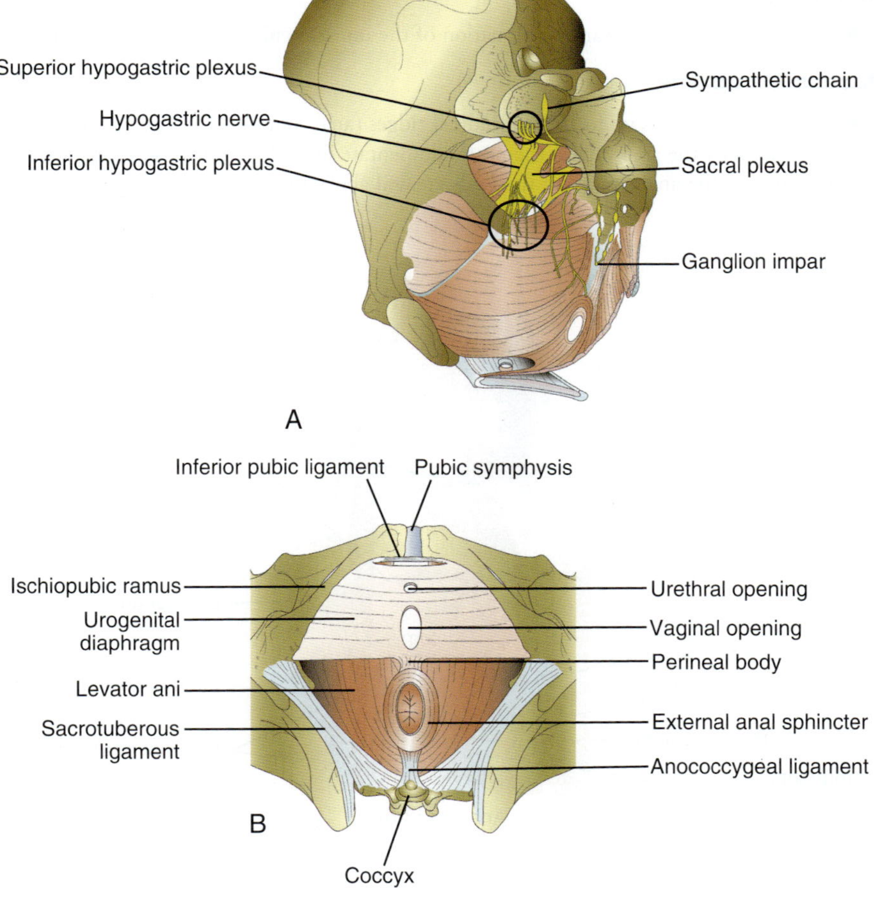

Fig. 4.33 **(A)** Perineum. **(B)** Urogenital and anal triangles of the perineum.

ANAL REGION (Fig 4.34)

Anal Canal

- The anal canal is the last 4 cm of the gastrointestinal tract and is developed from the anorectal canal and the proctodeum
- It consists of two muscle layers: internal (visceral) and external (skeletal), both of which are circular
- The junction between the rectum and the anal canal is at the pelvic floor and occurs at the level where the puborectalis part of the levator ani angles the gut forwards
- The anus can be considered as a tube within a funnel, with the levator ani down to the external sphincter being the funnel and the inner sphincter (a continuation of rectal muscle) as the inner tube

External Sphincter

- The rectal end of the anal canal blends with the puborectalis part of the levator ani (the line of fusion is the anorectal ring)
- The middle part is elliptical and is attached to the coccyx posteriorly and the perineal body anteriorly
- The lower subcutaneous part is the cuffing around the internal anal sphincter
- At the anorectal junction the outer longitudinal layer fuses with puborectalis

Internal Sphincter

- It is a thickened downward continuation of the inner circular muscle of the rectum

Mucous Membrane

- The upper third has up to 12 longitudinal ridges (anal columns) that are joined together at their bases by the anal valves (the pectinate/dentate line). The mucus-secreting anal glands secrete into the anal sinuses in the folds created above these valves.

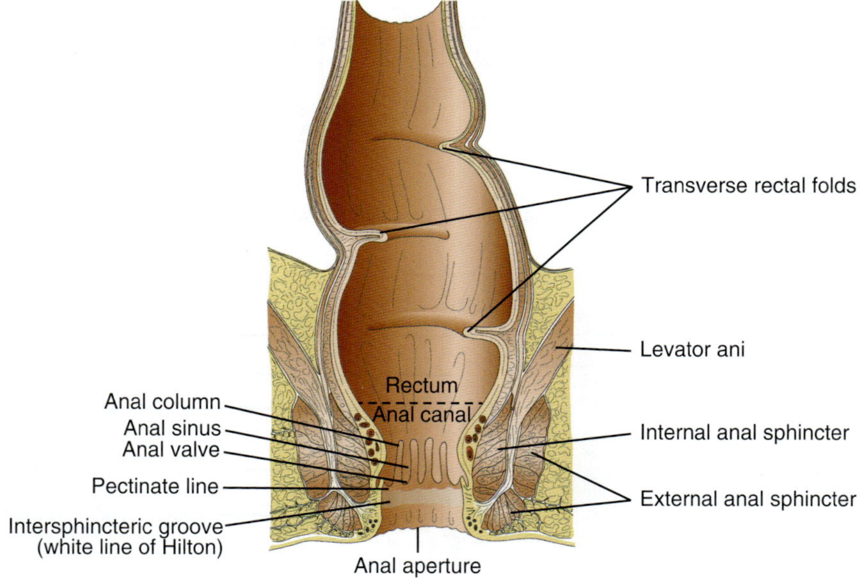

Fig. 4.34 Anal region, coronal section.

- Below this is a band of pecten which extends down to the intersphinteric groove (white line of Hilton). Below this is cutaneous skin and it is continuous with the anus
- The upper part develops from the cloaca and the lower part from the proctodeum

Blood Supply

- Blood supply to the muscular wall of the upper anal canal is from the superior rectal artery. The middle rectal and median sacral arteries contribute to a small section of the upper anal canal and the lower end also, including the mucous membrane, which is also supplied by the inferior rectal artery
- The veins correspond to the arterial supply and are continuous with the rectal venous plexus. The upper end drains via the portal system and the lower end via the internal iliac vein

Lymph Drainage

- Lymph drainage shows a watershed area corresponding with the vascular pattern

Nerve Supply

- The inferior rectal branches of the pudendal nerve supply the external sphincter
- The external sphincter has a high proportion of slow-twitch fibres that are almost always firing

ISCHIOANAL (ISCHIORECTAL) FOSSA (Fig 4.35)

- A wedge-shaped space positioned lateral to the anal canal and filled with fat
- The base is deep to the skin. Its medial wall is formed by the anal canal and levator ani. Its lateral wall is formed by the ischial tuberosity. The anterior apex is formed by the perineal body and the posterior boundary is the sacrotuberous ligament
- Each fossa has an anterior recess (above the urogenital diaphragm) and a much smaller posterior recess
- There is communication between the left and right sides
- Each fossa contains a fat pad (allows for dilation) and the pudendal canal, along with vessels and nerves
  - The pudendal canal contains the pudendal nerve and internal pudendal vessels. It can be considered as a splitting of the obturator fascia
  - The inferior rectal vessels run from the canal to the anus, arching upwards through the fat

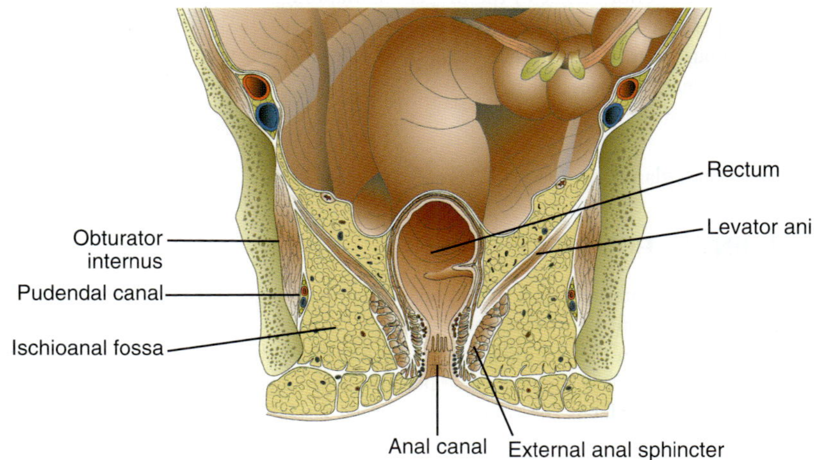

Fig. 4.35 Ischioanal fossa, coronal section.

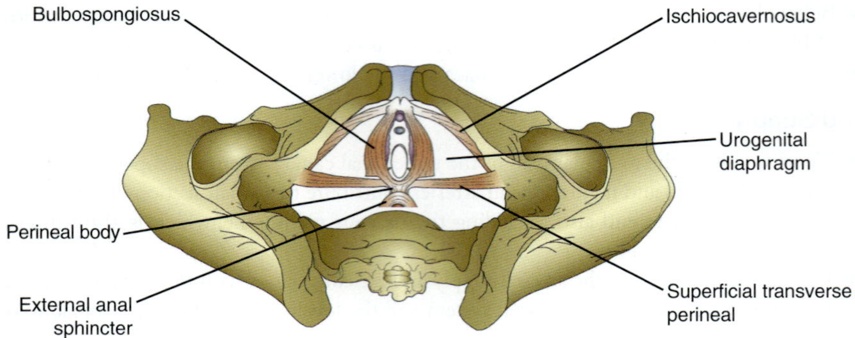

Fig. 4.36 Perineal body and its relations, inferior view (female).

CUTANEOUS NERVES

- The skin of the anal region is supplied by the inferior rectal nerve and the perineal branch of S4

PERINEAL BODY (CENTRAL PERINEAL TENDON) (Fig 4.36)

- A midline fibromuscular mass, in front of the anal canal and behind the posterior border of the perineal membrane
- The rectovesical/vaginal septum blends with it
- The external anal and external urethral sphincters blend with it, as do the levator prostatae, levator ani, bulbospongiosus and superficial/deep transverse perineal muscles

ANOCOCCYGEAL LIGAMENT

- A fibromuscular mass between the raphe and skin, separating the two ischioanal fossae

Part 18 Male Urogenital Region (Fig 4.37A and B)

The main constituents of the male urogenital region are the:

1. Urogenital diaphragm
2. Superior and inferior fasciae of the urogenital diaphragm
3. Superior perineal fasciae
4. Membranous parts of the urethra
5. Internal pudendal nerves
6. Dorsal nerve of the penis
7. Perineal nerves
8. Bulbourethral glands

DEEP PERINEAL POUCH

- The lower layer (inferior fascia of the urogenital diaphragm) or perineal membrane is an unyielding sheet of fibrous tissue and it anchors the penis
    - It is attached from the ischiopubic rami back to the ischial tuberosities
    - The anterior border is the transverse perineal ligament
    - The posterior border is the superficial perineal fascia (of Colles), which fuses with the perineal body
    - The membrane is pierced by the urethra and the bulbourethral ducts

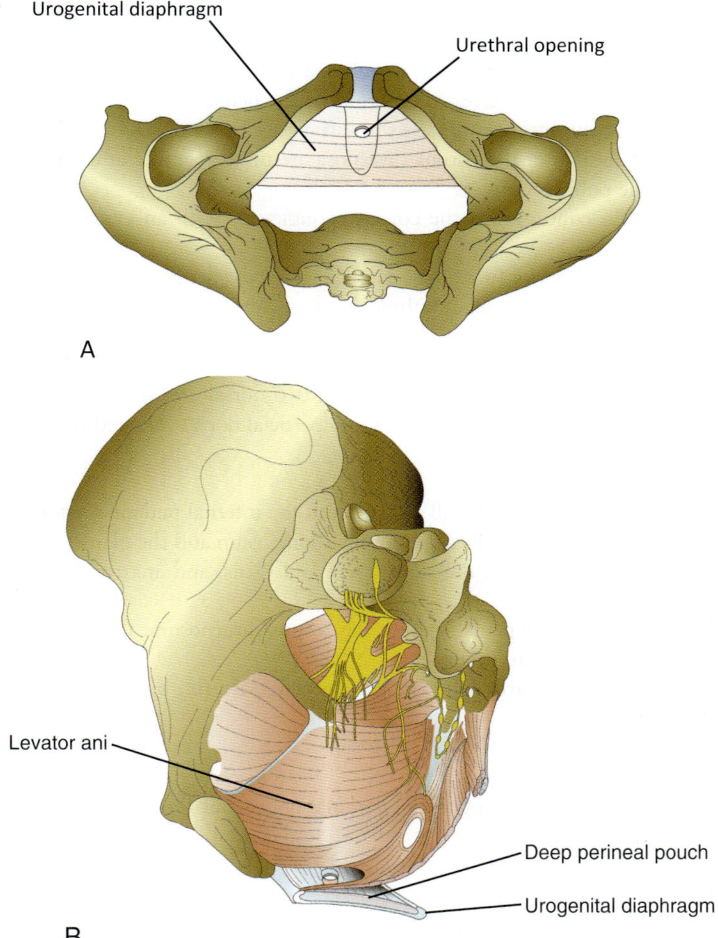

Fig. 4.37 **(A)** Male urogenital region, inferior view. **(B)** Male urogenital region, lateral view.

- The urogenital diaphragm lies above the perineal membrane and consists of the external urethral sphincter and the deep transverse perineal muscles
  - The bulbourethral glands lie one on each side of the membranous urethra (1 cm in diameter)
  - Their ducts run parallel to the urethra and pierce the perineal membrane. They make a small contribution to the seminal fluid
- The upper layer (superior fascia of the urogenital diaphragm) is poorly defined and forms part of the loose pelvic fascia

SUPERFICIAL PERINEAL POUCH

- The area between the superficial perineal fascia and the perineal membrane
- Colles' fascia is attached to the front of the pubic bone and is projected into the scrotal and penile expansions
- This will theoretically extend up into the anterior abdominal wall, but ends at the mid-axillary line
- It contains the root of the penis, the superficial perineal muscles and associated nerves and vessels

PENIS

- The root is attached to the perineal membrane and consists of the central bulb and two lateral crura, which each receive a deep artery of the penis
- The lateral crus continues forwards as the corpus cavernosum
  - The fibrous sheaths of the corpus cavernosa are fused together at a septum and are attached to the pubic symphysis
- The central bulb continues as the corpus spongiosum with an expanded terminus (the glans)
  - The bulb is the posterior (proximal) end of the corpus spongiosum; it accepts the urethra, arteries and ducts of the bulbourethral glands
- The two corpus cavernosa and corpus spongiosum are surrounded by the tunica albuginea and also loosely by the fascia of the penis (Buck's), a continuation of Scarpa's fascia
- Within Buck's fascia lie the deep dorsal vein, two dorsal arteries and two dorsal nerves. Outside the fascia, beneath the skin, lie the superficial dorsal vein and lymphatics

Blood Supply

- There are three pairs of arteries, all arising from the internal pudendal arteries
  - The artery to the bulb supplies the corpus spongiosum and the glans
  - The dorsal artery supplies the skin, fascia and glans, and anastomoses with the bulb artery
  - The deep artery of the penis supplies the corpus cavernosum. It forms a closed system and allows an erection to occur
- Venous drainage is primarily through the deep dorsal vein, but also parallels the above arterial supply

Lymph Drainage

- Skin lymphatics pass to the superficial inguinal nodes, but the glans and corpora drain to the deep inguinal nodes

Nerve Supply

- The skin is supplied by the pudendal nerves
- The bulbocavernosus and ischiocavernosus muscles are supplied by the perineal nerve (parasympathetic from the pelvic splanchnic nerves for erection and sympathetic from L1 for ejaculation)

SUPERFICIAL PERINEAL MUSCLES

- The bulb is overlaid with the bulbospongiosus muscles and each crura with its own ischiocavernosus. In addition there are the superficial transverse perineal muscles
- The bulbospongiosus arises from the perineal body and midline raphe, and inserts into the perineal membrane
- The ischiocavernosus arises from the posterior perineal membrane and the ischiopubic ramus, and inserts into the upper surface of corpus cavernosum
- The superficial transverse perineal muscle arises from the perineal membrane, and inserts into the perineal body to stabilise it

MALE URETHRA (see Fig 4.30A)

- It is 20 cm in length; 3.5 cm is prostatic, 1.5 cm is membranous and 15 cm is the penile urethra (bulbous and pendulous)

- When moving from the perineal membrane to the bulb, it makes a 90° turn
- The navicular fossa (containing the lacunae and urethral glands) lies at the distal tip of the urethra and is lined with stratified squamous rather than transitional epithelium
- The urethra is narrowest at the bladder neck, in the membranous part and at the proximal navicular fossa
- It has dilations at the prostatic part, bulb and navicular fossa
- The blood supply is from multiple sources: any adjacent vessels which pass through the prostate, urogenital diaphragm and corpus spongiosum
- The nerve supply is from the perineal nerve and inferior hypogastric plexus

SCROTUM

The subcutaneous tissue has no fat and contains part of the panniculus carnosus (dartos muscle), which sends a sheet into the midline septum. The dartos muscle is smooth muscle and is supplied by the sympathetic nerves from the genital branch of the genitofemoral nerve. The dartos overlies Colles' fascia.

- The blood supply is from the superficial and deep external pudendal arteries
- The anterior third is supplied by the ilioinguinal, and the posterior two-thirds is supplied by scrotal branches of the perineal nerve contributed laterally by the branches of the posterior femoral cutaneous nerve
- Lymph drainage is to the medial group of the superficial inguinal nodes

PERINEAL VESSELS AND NERVES

- The internal pudendal artery enters the deep perineal pouch from the anterior end of the canal, passing along the ischiopubic ramus. It gives off sets of arteries: the inferior rectal arteries, the perineal arteries and the dorsal and deep arteries of the penis
- The deep dorsal vein drains most of the blood from the corpora
- The pudendal nerve gives off an inferior rectal branch and then divides into the dorsal nerve of the penis and the perineal nerve

Part 19 Female Urogenital Region

The female external genitalia (collectively the vulva) include the:

1. Mons pubis
2. Labia majora/minora
3. Clitoris
4. Vaginal vestibule
5. Greater vestibular glands

These structures are analogous to male structures, but are functionally modified and don't undergo midline fusion.

- The mons pubis is the mound of skin containing pubic hair / hair follicles and subcutaneous fat which extends from the labia majora up to the pubi
- The labia majora are fatty cutaneous folds, with the round ligament of the uterus ending in the front of each labium
- The labia minora are cutaneous folds without fat. They enclose the vestibule and divide around the clitoris
- The body of the clitoris is formed by the corpora but the glans is from the bulb
- The vestibule contains the external urethral meatus, vaginal orifice and ducts of the greater vestibular glands

- The perineal membrane is wider than the male, but is weaker and is pierced transversely by the vagina. It provides the ischiocavernosus muscle to the clitoris and supports the bulbospongiosus and superficial transverse perineal muscles
- Muscles in the superficial perineal pouch comprise the ischiocavernosus muscle, the bulbospongiosus muscle and superficial transverse perineal muscle
- The greater vestibular glands lie at 4 o'clock and 8 o'clock, each with a 2 cm duct entering into the posterolateral vaginal orifice
- The lesser vestibular glands are minute openings between the urethra and the vagina
- The deep perineal pouch is traversed by the urethra and vagina, and contains urethral sphincters and transverse muscles along with nerves and vessels
- The perineal body is much more mobile in the female

Part 20 Pelvic Joints and Ligaments (Fig 4.38A and B)

The joints of the pelvis are the sacroiliac joint, sacrococcygeal joint and pubic symphysis, and the ligaments of the pelvis are the sacrotuberous, sacrospinous and iliolumbar ligaments.

SACROILIAC JOINT

- A synovial joint between the ilium and the sacrum
- It is an unusual joint because it has fibrocartilage (not hyaline) and jagged edges, and provides little movement
- This joint is supported by very strong bands posteriorly and weaker ones anteriorly
  - The anterior sacroiliac ligament is much stronger in the female
  - Dorsally there is a mass of ligaments, mainly the strong interosseous sacroiliac ligament
  - Stability is insured entirely by ligaments as the planes of the bony structure tend to diverge and push down the sacrum bones

SACROCOCCYGEAL JOINT

- A symphysis between the apex of the sacrum and the base of the coccyx. It contains a disc of fibrocartilage
  - The short ventral sacrococcygeal ligament unites the bones at the front
  - Two dorsal sacrococcygeal ligaments posteriorly, a short deep one and a superficial one, enclose the sacral hiatus
  - Laterally there are sacrococcygeal ligaments from the transverse process of the coccyx to the sacrum
  - Reasonable flexion and extension is possible at this joint (no side-to-side movement)

PUBIC SYMPHYSIS

- A secondary cartilaginous joint. Each pube is covered with hyaline cartilage and then both sides are joined by a mass of transversely running fibres

LIGAMENTS

Sacrotuberous Ligament

- A flat band along the posterior ilium from between the posterior superior and the posterior inferior iliac spines to the transverse tubercles of the sacrum and the ischial tuberosity

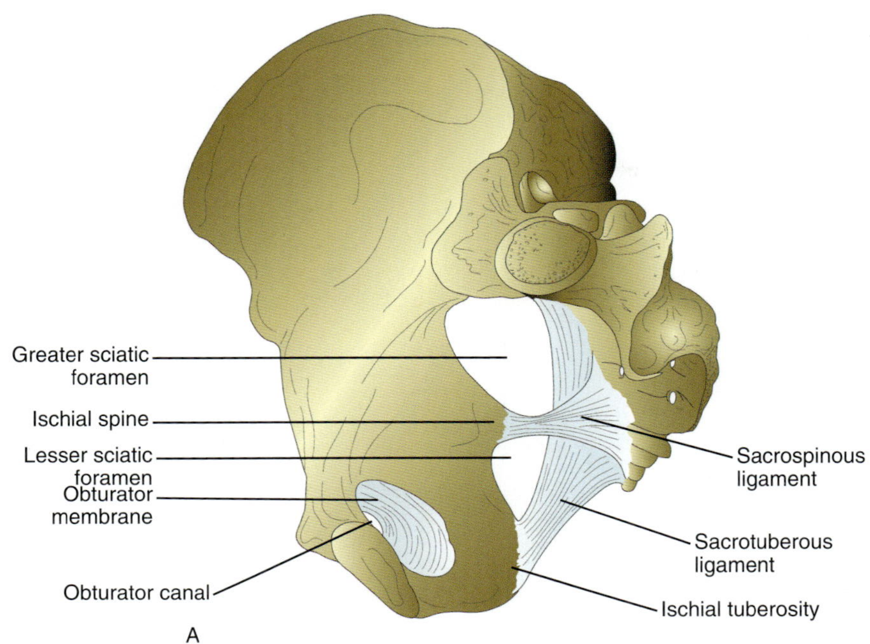

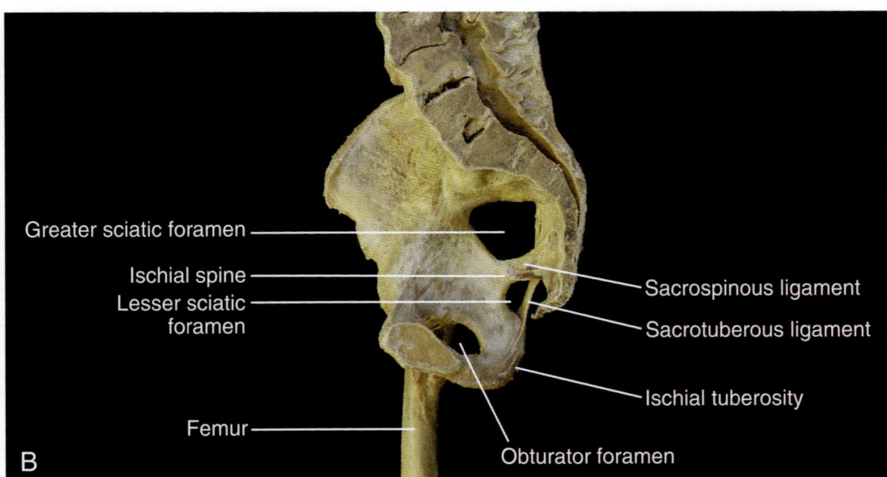

Fig. 4.38 **(A)** Joints and ligaments of the pelvis. **(B)** Joints and ligaments of the pelvis, cadaveric specimen; sagittal section.

Sacrospinous Ligament

- Lies on the pelvic aspect of the sacrotuberous ligament and runs from the coccyx and sacrum to the spine of the ischium

Iliolumbar Ligament

- Is shaped like a 'V' lying sideways, with its apex attached to the transverse process of L5. Its upper bands pass to the iliac crest, and its lower bands run laterally to blend with the sacroiliac ligament

Sacrospinous
ligament
Sacrotuberous
ligament
Ischial tuberosity

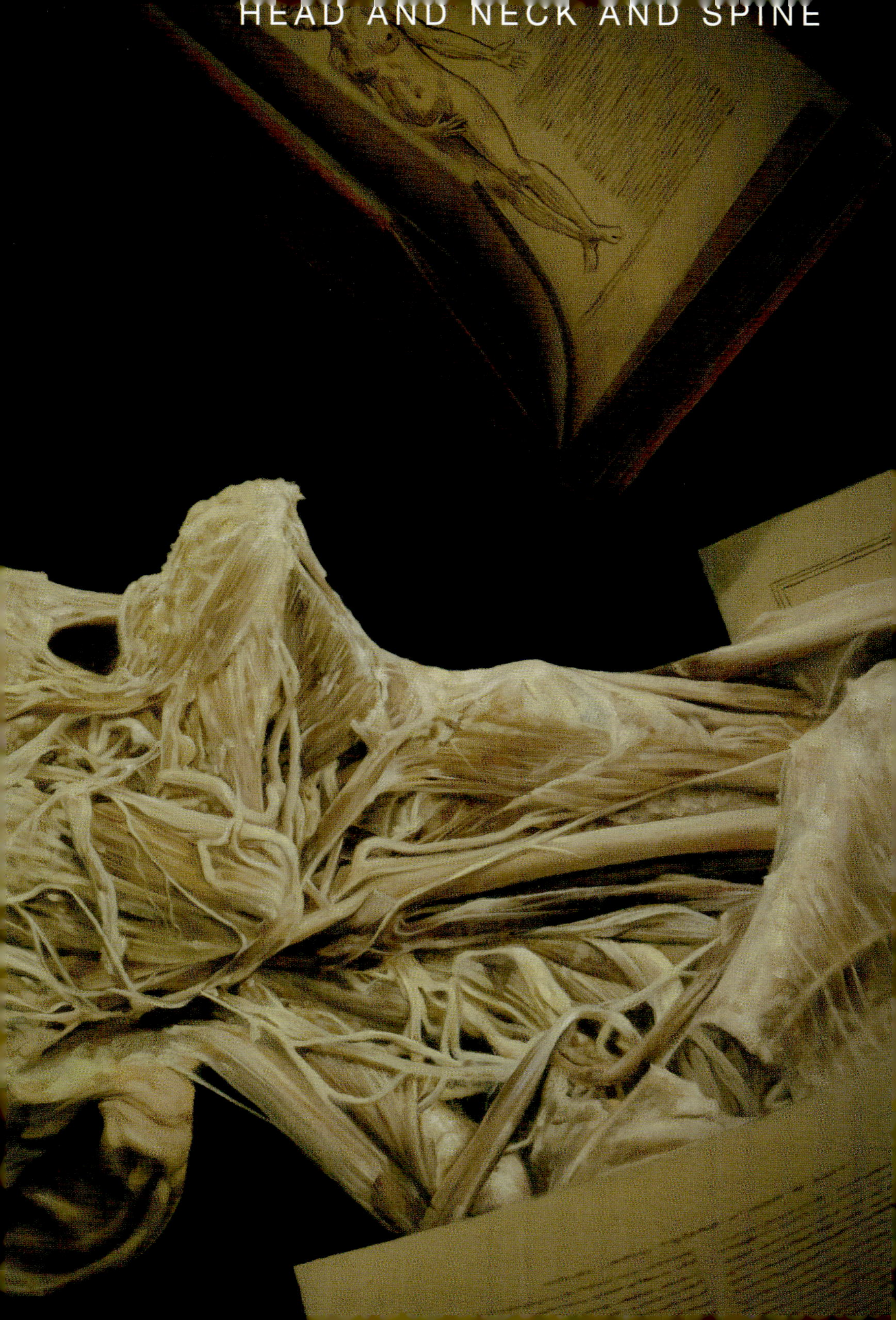

CHAPTER 5

Head and Neck and Spine

CHAPTER OUTLINE

Part 1 General Topography of the Neck

Deep to the skin, the cervical fascia divides into the superficial and deep fascia of the neck. The superficial fascia, or subcutaneous fascia, in the neck contains a thin sheet of muscle (the platysma), which begins in the superficial fascia of the thorax. The platysma muscle runs upwards to attach to the mandible and blends with the muscles of the face. The superficial fascia also contains cutaneous nerves (e.g. the terminal part of the cervical plexus) and superficial veins (e.g. the external and anterior jugular veins).

DEEP CERVICAL FASCIA

The deep fascia lies deep to the superficial fascia and is organised into several distinct layers: the investing layer, the pretracheal fascia, the prevertebral fascia and the carotid sheath.

Investing Layer

- Comparable to the deep fascia underlying subcutaneous fat elsewhere in the body
- Surrounds the neck like a collar and splits around: (1) the sternocleidomastoid, (2) the trapezius and (3) the parotid gland
- Meets the ligamentum nuchae posteriorly
- Extends superiorly from the external occipital protuberance along the superior nuchal line to the tip of the mastoid process
- Attached inferiorly to the pectoral girdle, the spine of scapula and the flat part of the clavicle

- Forms the suprasternal space by attaching its layers to the anterior and posterior borders of the jugular notch
- The external and anterior jugular veins, and all branches of the cervical plexus, pierce the investing fascia

Pretracheal Fascia

- Begins superiorly from the hyoid bone and the oblique line of the thyroid cartilage, and ends inferiorly in the upper thoracic cavity
- Fuses laterally with the front of the carotid sheath
- Encloses the thyroid gland (not adherent except at the isthmus and the second to fourth tracheal rings), trachea and oesophagus
- Lies deep to the infrahyoid muscles (sternohyoid, sternothyroid, omohyoid and thyrohyoid)
- Thymus and the parathyroid glands lie behind it
- Posterior to the pharynx, the pretracheal fascia is later referred to as the buccopharyngeal fascia and it separates the pharynx from the prevertebral fascia

Prevertebral Fascia

- A tough membrane surrounding the vertebral column and the muscles associated with it: prevertebral muscles, the anterior, middle and posterior scalene muscles and the deep muscles of the back
- Begins at the base of the skull in front of the longus capitis and rectus capitis, and extends sideways across the anterior, middle and posterior scalene muscles and the levator scapulae muscle
- Fades out laterally
- Covers the muscles comprising the floor of the posterior triangle
- All the cervical nerve roots lie deep to it, as does the third part of the subclavian artery
- The lymph nodes of the posterior triangle of the neck and the accessory nerve lie superficial to it
- It is prolonged as the axillary sheath
- Pierced by the four cutaneous branches of the cervical plexus (the great auricular, lesser occipital, transverse cervical and supraclavicular nerves)
- Provides a fixed base which the pharynx, oesophagus and carotid sheaths can glide against during any movement in the neck (e.g. swallowing)

Carotid Sheath

- This is not a fascia in the sense of a demonstrable membranous layer
- Surrounds the carotid artery (common and internal carotid artery), internal jugular vein and vagus nerve
- Internal jugular vein is located lateral to the common carotid artery, with the vagus nerve lying in between
- Is attached to the base of the skull and continues down to the aortic arch
- Cervical sympathetic trunk lies between the prevertebral fascia and the carotid sheath

TISSUE SPACES OF THE NECK

Between the fascial layers in the neck are spaces that may provide a conduit for the spread of the infection from the neck to the mediastinum. The most clinically important spaces are the prevertebral, retropharyngeal and pretracheal spaces.

- **Prevertebral space** is within the prevertebral fascia lying anterior to the bodies and the transverse processes of the cervical vertebrae. It extends from the base of the skull to the upper part of the posterior mediastinum

- **Pretracheal space** lies between the investing layer and the pretracheal layer (covering the anterior surface of the trachea and the thyroid gland). It extends between the neck and the anterior part of the superior mediastinum
- **Retropharyngeal space** is a space between the buccopharyngeal fascia (anteriorly) and the prevertebral fascia (posteriorly). It extends from the base of the skull to the diaphragm:
  - Superiorly, the retropharyngeal space is situated between the prevertebral fascia and the buccopharyngeal fascia
  - Continuous laterally with the parapharyngeal space
  - Continues anteriorly into the submandibular space (infection here causes Ludwig's angina)

Part 2 Triangles of the Neck

POSTERIOR TRIANGLE (Fig 5.1A and B)

The posterior triangle of the neck is on the lateral aspect of the neck in direct continuity with the upper limb.

Boundaries

- Posterior border of the sternocleidomastoid, the anterior border of the trapezius and the superior border of the clavicle (middle third)
- The apex of the triangle is at the superior nuchal line and the base lies on the clavicle (middle third)
- Roof is formed by the investing layer
- Floor consists of the prevertebral fascia and beneath the fascia are the splenius, levator scapulae, scalenus posterior, scalenus medius and scalenus anterior (from superior to inferior)

Contents

- At the apex is the occipital artery and greater occipital nerve
- Lymph nodes of the posterior triangle: the occipital nodes are at the apex and the supraclavicular nodes are at the base
- Accessory nerve emerges about halfway down the posterior border of the sternocleidomastoid and runs obliquely downwards to exit the posterior triangle by penetrating the anterior border of the trapezius

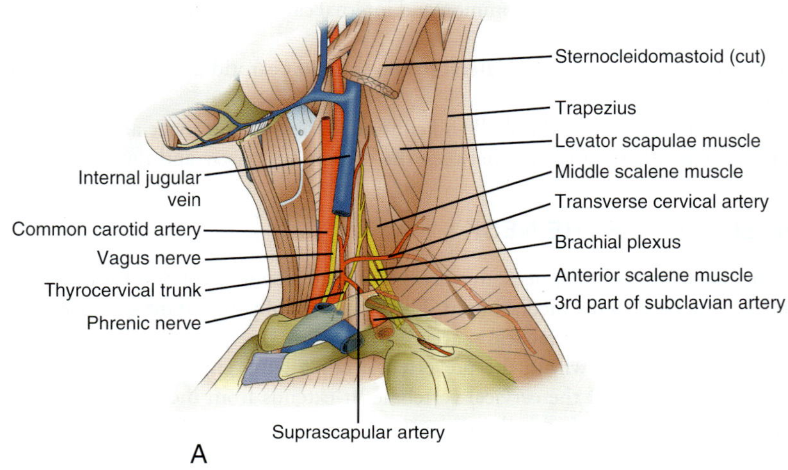

Fig. 5.1 **(A)** Boundaries and contents of the posterior triangle.

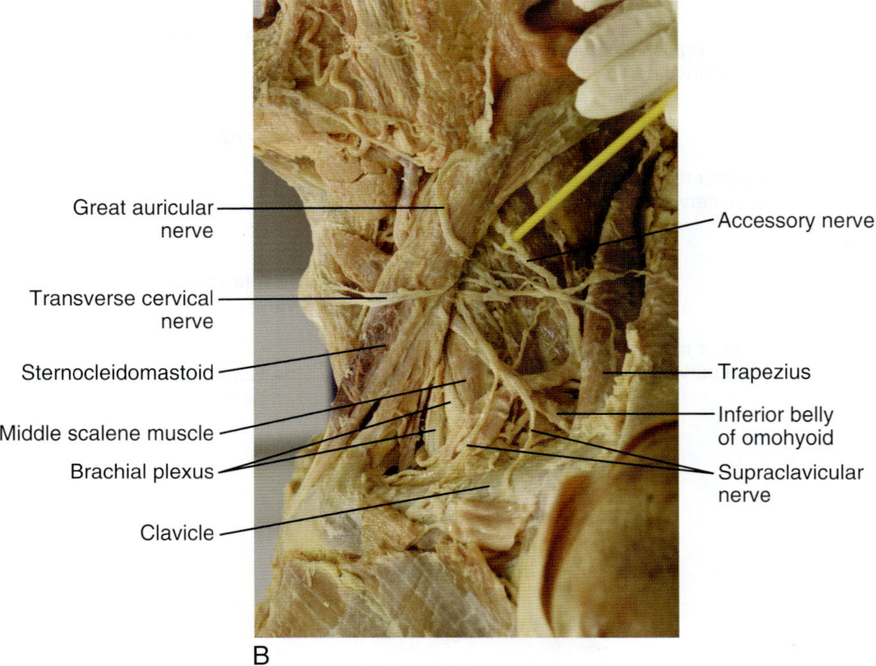

Fig. 5.1, cont'd **(B)** Posterior triangle (cadaveric dissection).

- Cutaneous branches of the cervical plexus pierce the fascia at the posterior border of the sternocleidomastoid
- Inferior belly of omohyoid crosses the lower medial part of the triangle
- Transverse cervical and suprascapular vessels are in the lower part of the triangle
- The third part of the subclavian artery
- Brachial plexus (at the base of the triangle)
- External jugular vein briefly appears in the anterior corner of the triangle

Cervical Plexus (Fig 5.2A and B)

Formed by simple roots between the anterior rami of the upper four cervical nerves. It consists of muscular (C1–3) and cutaneous (C2–4) branches.

Muscular Branches. Supplying the prevertebral and lateral vertebral muscles (e.g. the rectus capitis anterior, rectus capitis lateralis, longus colli, longus capitis). Other muscular branches are:

- Ansa cervicalis (having travelled via the hypoglossal nerve) – receives contributions from the anterior rami of the upper three cervical nerves (C1–3). It has two roots: superior (C1) and inferior (C2–3)
- From C1/superior root of the ansa cervicalis (hitch-hiked along the hypoglossal nerve) – innervates the thyrohyoid and geniohyoid musles
- From C2 and C3 to the sternocleidomastoid and C3 and C4 to the trapezius (proprioception)
- The inferior root of the ansa cervicalis (C2–3) – innervates the infrahyoid muscles

Cutaneous Branches

- C2 – supplies most of the posterior part of the neck extending up to the scalp, and forwards to the auricle and the face over the angle of the mandible
- C3 – supplies the cylindrical part of the neck

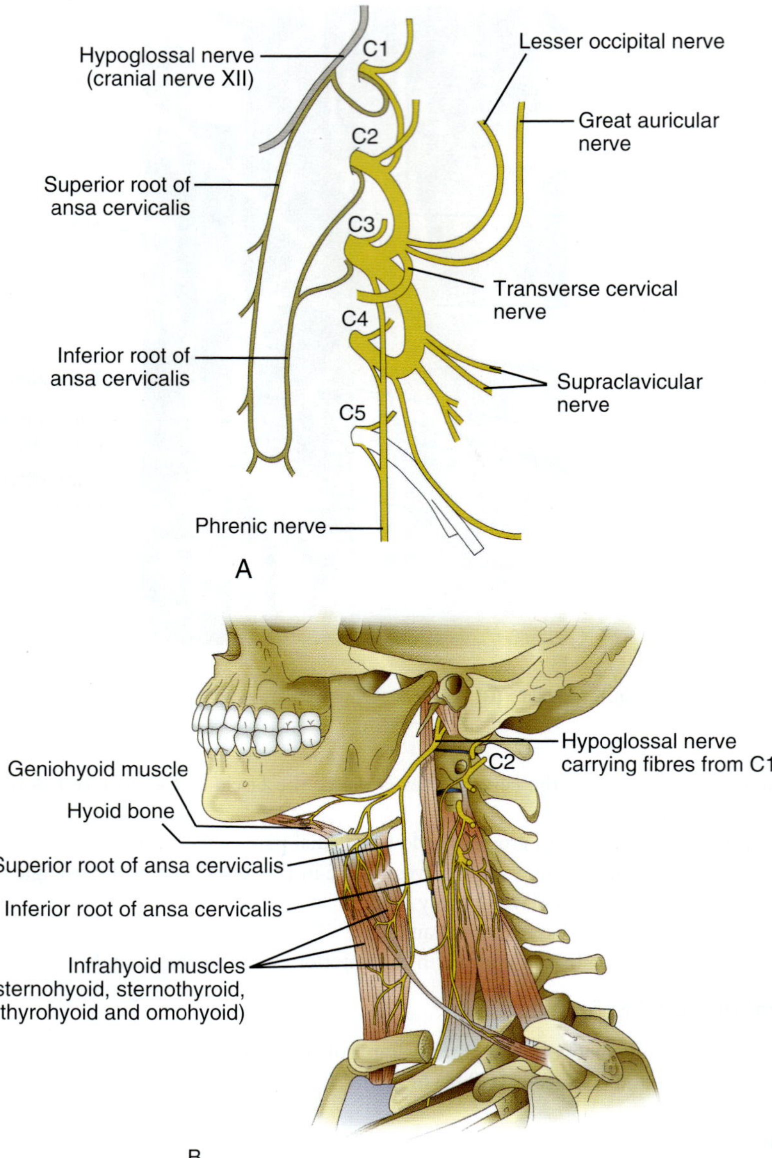

Fig. 5.2 (A) Cervical plexus. **(B)** Motor innervation of cervical plexus.

- C4 – extends over the clavicular region across the top of the shoulder and down to the scapular spine

ANTERIOR TRIANGLE (Fig 5.3)

The anterior triangle of the neck is outlined by the anterior border of the sternocleidomastoid muscle laterally, the inferior border of the mandible superiorly and the midline of the neck medially.

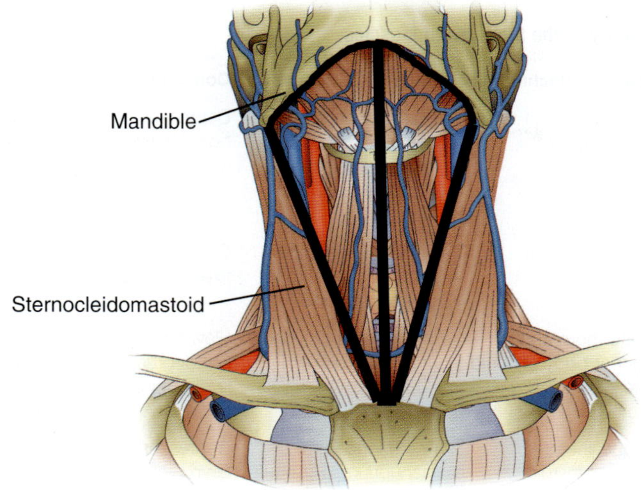

Fig. 5.3 Boundaries and contents of the anterior triangle of the neck.

It is further subdivided into several smaller anatomical triangles: the submandibular triangle, the submental triangle, the muscular triangle and the carotid triangle.

- Contains muscles which can be grouped according to their location relative to the hyoid bone: the suprahyoid and infrahyoid muscles:
  - Suprahyoid muscles: digastric, stylohyoid, mylohyoid and geniohyoid muscles
  - Infrahyoid muscles: sternohyoid, omohyoid, thyrohyoid and sternothyroid muscles
  - All of these are in the same plane as the rectus abdominis
- Contains the neck viscera: the thyroid gland, parathyroid glands, trachea, oesophagus and carotid sheath
- Contains numerous cranial nerves: the facial nerve, glossopharyngeal nerve, vagus nerve, accessory nerve and hypoglossal nerve
- Contains numerous peripheral nerves: the transverse cervical nerves from the cervical plexus and the upper and lower roots of the ansa cervicalis

SUPRAHYOID MUSCLES (Fig 5.4)

The four pairs of suprahyoid muscles are related to the submandibular and submental triangles and are described in the table below.

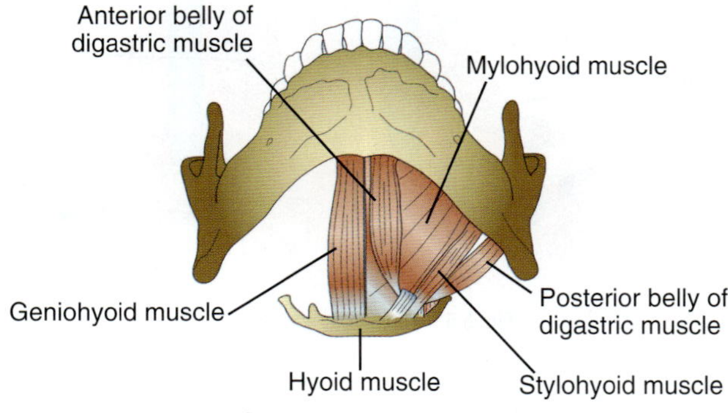

Fig. 5.4 Suprahyoid muscles, inferior view.

TABLE 5.1 ■ **Summary of the Suprahyoid Muscles**

Muscle	Superior Attachment	Inferior Attachment	Concentric Action	Innervation
Sternohyoid	Inferior border of body of hyoid bone	Posterior aspect of sternoclavicular joint and adjacent manubrium of sternum	Depresses hyoid bone after swallowing	Ansa cervicalis
Omohyoid	Inferior border of body of hyoid bone	Superior border of scapula medial to suprascapular notch	Depresses and fixes hyoid bone	Ansa cervicalis
Thyrohyoid	Greater horn and adjacent body of hyoid bone	Oblique line on lamina of thyroid cartilage	Elevates larynx but depresses hyoid bone	C1 fibres carried by the hypoglossal nerve (XII)
Sternothyroid	Oblique line of lamina of thyroid cartilage	Posterior aspect of manubrium	Depresses larynx	Ansa cervicalis

INFRAHYOID MUSCLES (Fig 5.5)

The four infrahyoid muscles are related to the muscular triangle and are described in the table below.

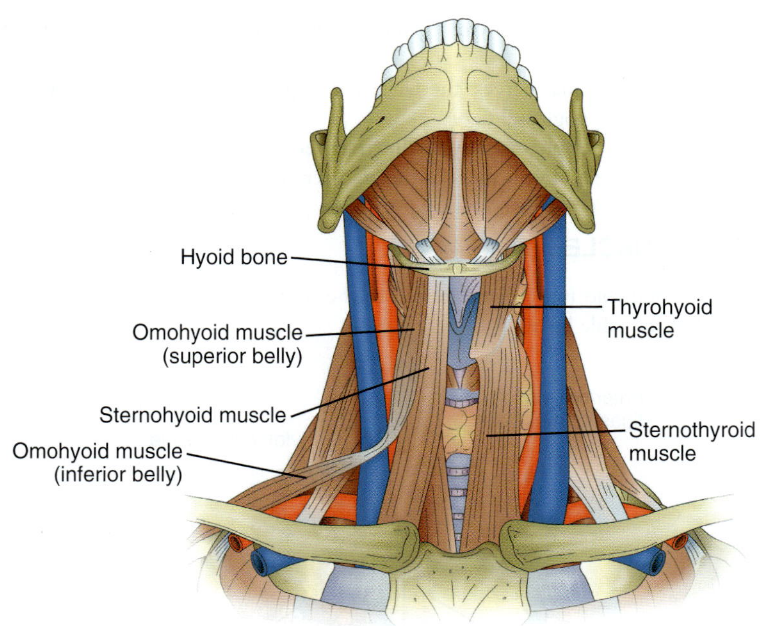

Fig. 5.5 Infrahyoid muscles.

TABLE 5.2 ■ **Summary of the Infrahyoid Muscles**

Muscles	Superior Attachment	Inferior Attachment	Concentric Action	Innervation
Digastric	Anterior belly: digastric fossa of mandible	Fibrous loop to lesser cornu of hyoid bone	Aids swallowing and depresses mandible	Anterior belly: mylohyoid
	Posterior belly: base of medial aspect of mastoid process		Aids swallowing and depresses mandible	Posterior belly: facial nerve (VII) before it enters parotid gland
Stylohyoid	Base of styloid process	Lateral area of body of hyoid bone	Elevates and retracts hyoid bone	Facial nerve (VII) before it enters parotid gland
			Aids swallowing and retracts hyoid bone	
Mylohyoid	Mylohyoid line on mandible	Body of hyoid bone and fibres from muscle on opposite side	Elevates hyoid bone and supports and raises the floor of the mouth	Mylohyoid nerve
			Aids in mastication and swallowing	
Geniohyoid	Inferior mental spine of mandible	Anterior surface of body of hyoid bone	Elevates and retracts hyoid bone Depresses mandible	C1 fibres carried by hypoglossal nerve (XII)

THYROID GLAND

- Consists of two lobes with an isthmus which connects the two lobes in front of the second, third and fourth tracheal rings
- Lies deep to the infrahyoid muscles
- Has its own capsule and is also enclosed by an envelope of pretracheal fascia

Thyroid Gland and Its Relations (Fig 5.6)

- Lateral lobe is pear-shaped, with a narrow upper pole and broader lower pole and it looks triangular in cross-section, with lateral, medial and posterior surfaces:
  - Lateral surface – lies deep to the sternothyroid and sternohyoid muscles
  - Medial surface – lies against the lateral side of the larynx and upper trachea, the lower pole extends as low as the sixth tracheal ring. The cricothyroid and inferior constrictor muscles are medial muscular relations of this surface, with the external laryngeal nerves approaching the thyroid from above and recurrent laryngeal nerves from below
  - Posterior surface – overlaps the medial part of the carotid sheath. The parathyroid glands usually lie in contact with this surface
- Recurrent laryngeal nerves
  - Approach the medial surface of the gland from below, just in front of the tracheo-oesophageal groove
  - The left recurrent laryngeal nerve is more likely to lie deep to the inferior thyroid artery than superficial to it, but on the right there is an equal chance of it lying deep or superficial to the artery
  - It always lies behind the pretracheal fascia and behind the cricothyroid joint
  - At the level of the upper border of the isthmus, it may divide into two: the anterior (motor) and posterior branches (purely sensory)

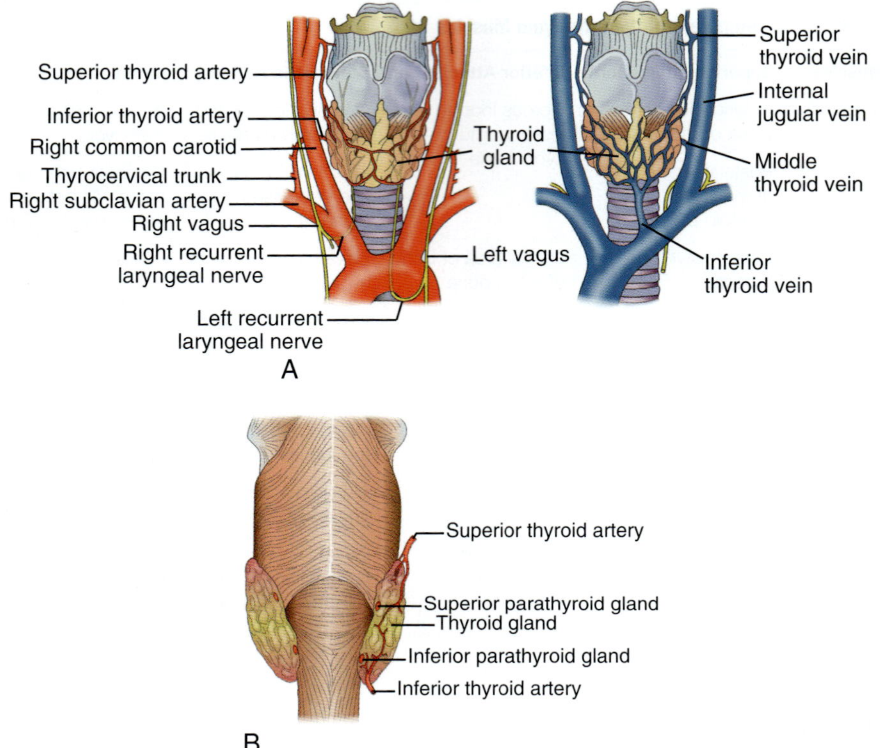

Fig. 5.6 **(A)** Thyroid gland and its relations. Left: Relations to arteries and nerves. Right: Relations to veins and lymphatics. **(B)** Posterior view of the thyroid gland showing the parathyroid glands and their blood supply.

- The smaller external laryngeal nerve runs downwards to supply the cricothyroid behind the superior thyroid artery
- The isthmus joins the anterior surfaces of the lobes and is firmly adherent to the second to fourth tracheal rings
  - An arterial anastomosis between the superior and inferior thyroid arteries runs across the upper part of the isthmus
  - The pyramidal lobe (+/−) may project forwards on the left, representing the caudal end of the thyroglossal duct

Blood Supply

- Superior thyroid artery (first branch from anterior aspect of external carotid) gives off its sternocleidomastoid and superior laryngeal branches before piercing the pretracheal fascia to reach the summit of the upper pole
  - The external laryngeal nerve lies immediately behind the artery
  - Divides into the anterior and posterior branches on the gland
  - Anastomoses with an ascending branch of the inferior thyroid artery from the lower lobe
- Inferior thyroid artery originates from the thyrocervical trunk and runs upwards behind the lower pole to divide outside the pretracheal fascia into four or five branches that pierce the fascia separately. It gives off the oesophageal and inferior laryngeal braches before its terminal branches to the gland

- Thyroid ima artery enters the lower part of the isthmus in less than 5% of individuals and originates from the brachiocephalic trunk or the right common carotid artery, or directly from the arch of the aorta

Venous Drainage

This is from three sources: (1) superior thyroid vein, which drains into either internal jugular vein or facial vein, (2) middle thyroid vein, which drains directly into internal jugular vein, and (3) inferior thyroid vein, which forms a plexus which drains into brachiocephalic veins (primarily into the left brachiocephalic vein).

Lymph Drainage

- Follows the arteries
- Upper pole to the anterosuperior group, and lower pole to the posteroinferior group of the deep cervical nodes

Nerve Supply

- Sympathetic supply is from the middle cervical ganglion, entering the gland via the inferior and superior thyroid arteries
- Parasympathetic supply is from the vagus nerve

Structure

- Consists of a mass of rounded follicles full of colloid (iodine-containing product of epithelial cells)
- Is the only endocrine gland to store its secretions outside of its cells
- Development – develops as a proliferation of cells from the caudal end of the thyroglossal duct

PARATHYROID GLANDS (see Fig 5.6B)

- Lie behind the lateral lobe of the thyroid gland (but may be within or outside of the thyroid's capsule of pretracheal fascia)
  - Usually four brownish-yellow coloured glands with a total weight <200 mg – two on each side and not necessarily level with each other
  - Superior glands are more constant in position and usually lie at the back of the thyroid gland at the level of the first tracheal ring and above the inferior thyroid artery
  - Inferior glands are more variable and are usually behind the lower pole (below the inferior thyroid artery and lateral to the recurent laryngeal nerve)
- Blood supply is via the inferior thyroid artery
- Lymph drainage is the same as in the thyroid gland

TRACHEA

- Begins at the lower border of the cricoid cartilage at the level of C6 in continuity with the larynx
- C-shaped rings are closed posteriorly by the trachealis muscle
- Lies in the midline of the neck

OESOPHAGUS

- Extends from the cricopharyngeus at C6 (lower border of the cricoid cartilage)
- Initially outer fibres are attached to the cricoid cartilage and arytenoid cartilages, but the fibres then spiral downwards
- Lies slightly over to the left

CAROTID SHEATH

- Divides into upper and lower parts
- Upper part:
  - Extends from the level of the bifurcation of the common carotid artery (C3/4) to the base of the skull around the margins of the carotid canal
  - Contains the internal carotid artery, the internal jugular vein and the last four cranial nerves for some or all of its course (glossopharyngeal nerve, vagus nerve, accessory nerve and hypoglossal nerve)
  - Boundaries are:
    - Medially: the pharynx
    - Laterally: the deepest part of the parotid gland and superior to this is the styloid process and three muscles which originate from the process (the stylohyoid, stylopharyngeus and styloglossus)
    - Anteriorly: the infratemporal fossa
    - Posteriorly: the cervical sympathetic trunk
- Lower part:
  - Extends from the sternoclavicular joint vertically upwards to the level of the bifurcation of the common carotid artery (C3/4 or at the upper border of the thyroid cartilage)
  - Contains the common carotid artery, internal jugular vein, vagus nerve and ansa cervicalis
  - Posteriorly, it is free to slide over the prevertebral fascia, but anteriorly it is connected to the deep fascia of sternocleidomastoid
  - The sheath is very thin over the internal jugular vein so it can freely dilate to increase blood flow
  - Dead space around the internal jugular vein contains the inferior deep cervical lymph nodes

Part 3 Suprahyoid Region

SUBMANDIBULAR FOSSA AND GLAND

These are described in Part 12 Mouth and Hard Palate (the section on the oral cavity).

GREAT VESSELS OF THE NECK (Fig 5.7A and B)

Common Carotid Artery

- Left common carotid originates from the aortic arch
- Right common carotid originates from the brachiocephalic trunk
- Gives off no branches proximal to its bifurcation to the internal and external carotid arteries
- Lies in the medial part of the carotid sheath and lateral to the larynx and trachea
- Internal jugular vein lies further laterally, with the vagus nerve lying in between
- Sympathetic trunk lies behind the artery and is outside the carotid sheath
- Surface marking is drawn by a line from the sternoclavicular joint to the greater horn of the hyoid
- Carotid body is a small yellowish-grey structure lying behind the bifurcation and contains chemoreceptors

External Carotid Artery

- From the bifurcation it slopes upwards, initially medial and then anterior to the internal carotid artery

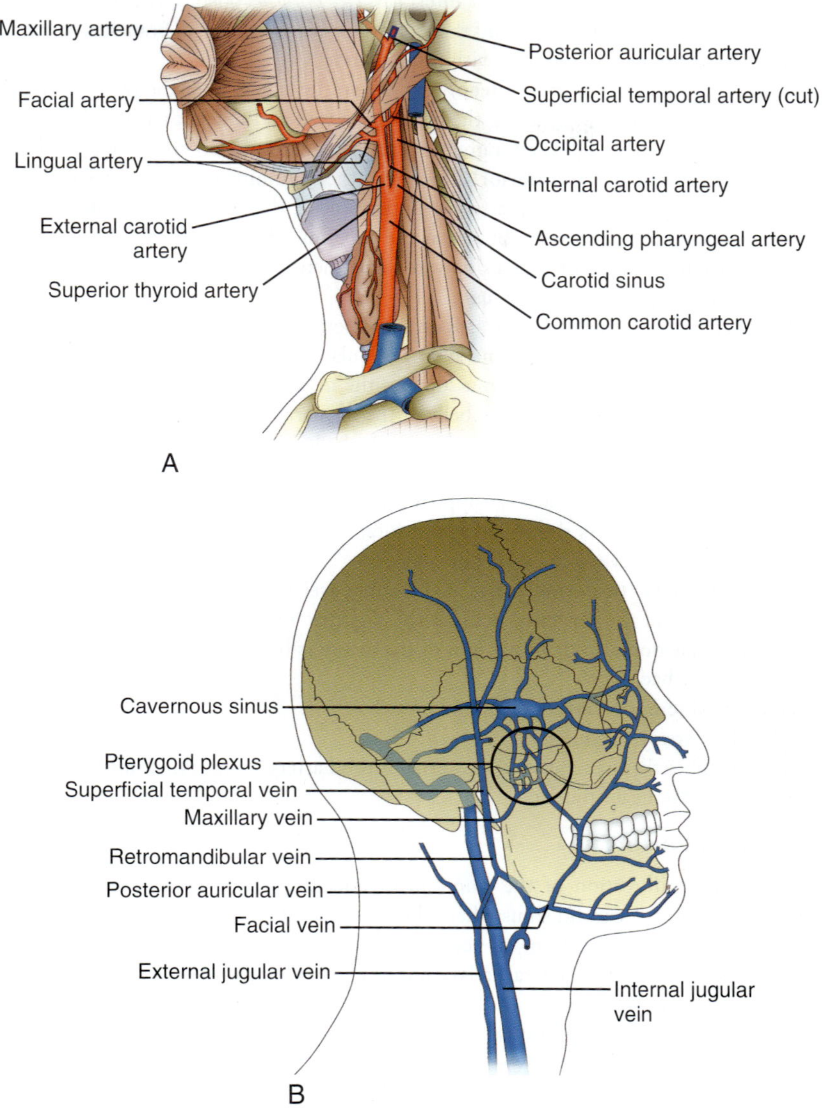

Fig. 5.7 (A) Great vessels of the neck and their relations. **(B)** Venous drainage of the head.

- Passes deep to the posterior belly of digastric and stylohyoid, then pierces the deep lamina of the parotid gland where it further divides into the maxillary and superficial temporal arteries
- Within the gland, it is separated from the internal carotid artery by the deep part of the gland and the pharyngeal structures (stylopharyngeus, glossopharyngeal nerve and pharyngeal branch of vagus nerve)
- The surface marking is drawn as a line from the greater horn of the hyoid to a point just in front of the tragus of the ear

- Gives off six branches: *three branches* anteriorly, *two branches* posteriorly, *one branch* medially (deep) before the parotid gland, and then it ends in its two terminal branches (the maxillary and superficial temporal arteries) within the gland:
  - **A**scending pharyngeal artery (**deep**) runs up on the side wall of the pharynx deep to the internal carotid artery supplying the pharyngeal wall and the soft palate (also sends meningeal branches through the foramen lacerum, jugular foramen and hypoglossal canal)
  - **S**uperior thyroid artery (**anterior**) arises from the beginning of the external carotid artery, and runs vertically downwards to the upper pole of the thyroid. The external laryngeal nerve lies behind it. Its main branch is the superior laryngeal artery
  - **L**ingual artery (**anterior**) passes upwards and then forwards along the upper border of the hyoid, deep to the hyoglossus
  - **F**acial artery (**anterior**) runs upwards on the superior constrictor muscle, deep to the digastric muscle, stylohyoid muscle and submandibular gland. It gives off a tonsillar branch (to the tonsil and soft palate). Later, it supplies the mandible, and then gives off a submental artery which supplies the anterior belly of the digastric and mylohyoid muscles
  - **P**osterior auricular artery (**posterior**) arises at the level of the digastric muscle, sometimes within the parotid gland. It runs up superficial to the styloid process and across the upper border of the digastric muscle, supplying the skin over the mastoid process. The stylomastoid branch enters the stylomastoid foramen, supplies the facial nerve and gives off the stapedial artery (to the stapedius muscle)
  - **O**ccipital artery (**posterior**) arises at the same level as the facial artery and passes on the lower border of the posterior belly of the digastric muscle. It gives off two branches to the sternocleidomastoid. The origin of the artery is hooked by the hypoglossal nerve. It supplies the back of the scalp
  - **S**uperficial temporal artery (terminal branch)
  - **M**axillary artery (terminal branch)
  - To remember the branches of the external carotid artery: **S**ome **A**natomists **L**ike **F**reaking **O**ut **P**oor **M**edical **S**tudents

Internal Carotid Artery

- Arises at the bifurcation of the common carotid artery and, at its beginning, it bulges slightly to form the carotid sinus where the arterial wall is thin and contains baroreceptors (supplied by the glossopharyngeal nerve)
- Originates as an external (lateral) relation to the external carotid artery, but quickly courses posteriorly and deep
- Has no branches in the carotid sheath
- Behind the internal carotid artery is the sympathetic trunk
- Superior laryngeal branch of the vagus nerve passes obliquely behind to reach its medial side and divide into the internal and external laryngeal nerves

Internal Jugular Vein

- Emerges from the jugular bulb at the posterior compartment of the jugular foramen
  - Receives the inferior petrosal sinus as its first tributary, and then passes down to lie on the lateral side of the internal carotid artery and later the common carotid artery
  - Other tributaries are the pharyngeal plexus and the facial, lingual, superior and middle thyroid veins
  - Deep cervical nodes lie close throughout
  - Inferior root of ansa cervicalis curls around the lateral border to unite with the superior root
  - Surface marking is drawn as a line from the lobe of the ear to the sternal end of the clavicle

Part 4 Prevertebral Region

PREVERTEBRAL MUSCLES OF THE NECK (Fig 5.8)

CERVICAL SYMPATHETIC TRUNK (Fig 5.9)

The cervical part of the sympathetic trunk lies anterior to the longus colli and longus capitis muscles, and posterior to the common carotid artery below and the internal carotid artery above.

- Superior cervical ganglia lie in the area around C1 and C2
- Gives off branches to the internal and external carotid arteries, pharynx, superior cardiac plexus and cervical spinal nerves C1–4

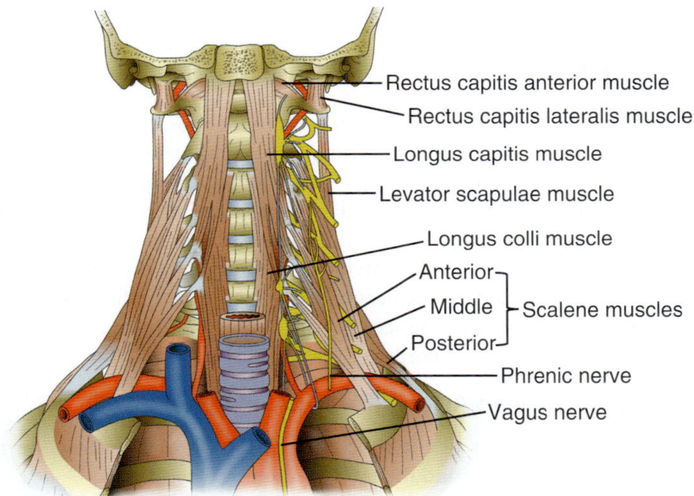

Fig. 5.8 Prevertebral muscles of the neck.

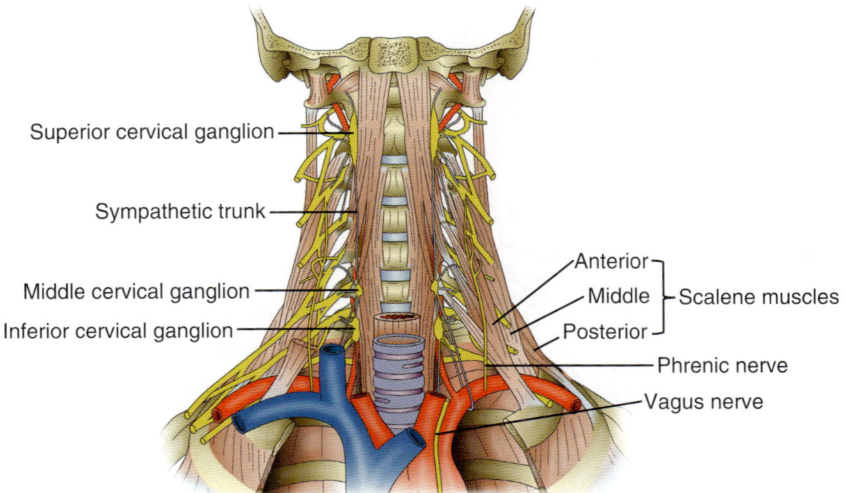

Fig. 5.9 Cervical sympathetic trunks.

Part 5 Root of the Neck

The root of the neck is the area immediately above the superior thoracic aperture and axillary inlets. It contains structures passing between the neck, the thorax and the upper limb: the vessels, nerves, lymphatics, upward extensions of the thoracic cavity and scalene muscles.

- Arteries: the subclavian arteries and its branches, and the common carotid arteries
- Nerves: the vagus nerve, recurrent laryngeal nerves, phrenic nerves and the cervical part of the sympathetic trunks
- Lymphatics
- The extension of the thoracic cavity: the pleural cavity, the cupula and the apical part of the superior lobe of the lung
- Scalene muscles: anterior, middle and posterior scalene muscles

SUBCLAVIAN ARTERY

The subclavian arteries on both sides arch upwards out of the thoracic cavity to enter the root of the neck and then the axilla. The right subclavian artery begins behind the sternoclavicular joint as one of two terminal branches of the brachiocephalic trunk. The left subclavian artery begins lower in the thorax than the right, originating directly from the arch of the aorta. Both the left and right subclavian arteries run posterior to the anterior scalene muscle, whereas the left and right subclavian veins run anterior to the anterior scalene muscle. Both subclavian arteries are divided into three parts by the anterior scalene muscles such that the first part extends from its origin to the anterior scalene muscle, the second part lies behind the muscle and the third part reaches from the muscle to the lateral border of the first rib.

Branches of the Subclavian Artery (Fig 5.10A and B)

- Branches from the first part of the subclavian artery (three branches) are the vertebral artery, the thyrocervical artery and the internal thoracic artery:
  - The vertebral artery arises from the upper convexity of the subclavian artery, runs upwards and disappears into the foramen of the transverse process of C6

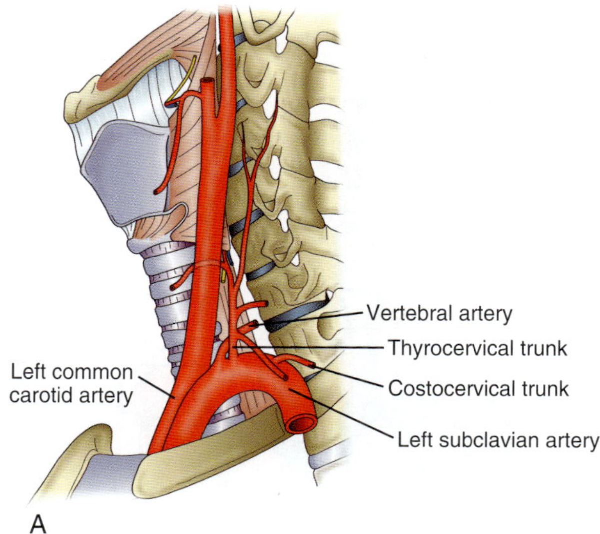

Fig. 5.10 **(A)** Branches of the subclavian artery.

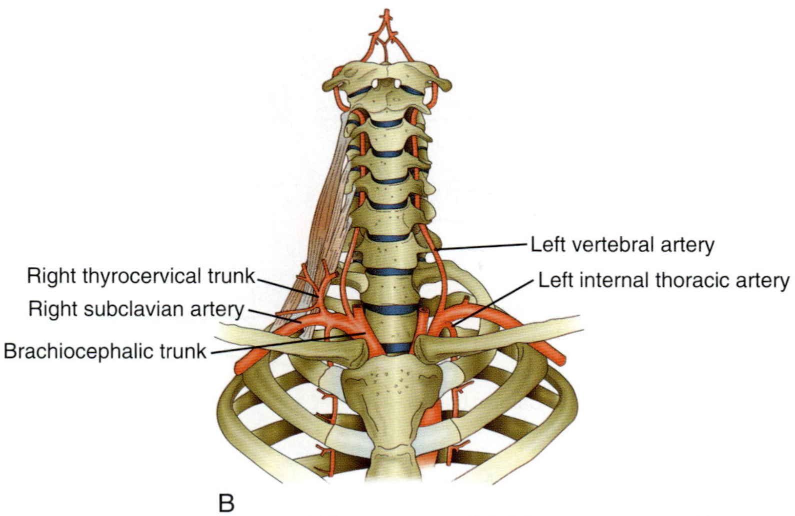

Fig. 5.10, cont'd (B) Vertebral arteries and their relations.

- The thyrocervical artery divides into the transverse cervical, suprascapular and inferior thyroid arteries
- The internal thoracic artery runs downwards over the apex of the lung, crossing the phrenic nerve

- The second part of the subclavian artery has only one branch: the costocervical artery
  - The costocervical artery divides into a descending branch (the superior intercostal artery) and an ascending branch (deep cervical artery)
- The third part of the subclavian artery has only one branch: the dorsal scapular artery
  - The dorsal scapular artery runs laterally in front of the middle scalene muscle and disappears deep towards the levator scapulae muscle, to contribute to the scapular anastomosis

VAGUS NERVE (Fig 5.11A and B)

It leaves the skull through the jugular foramen between CN IX and CN XI. It travels downwards in the carotid sheath, between the internal carotid artery and internal jugular vein. At the root of the neck, it passes in front of the subclavian artery and behind the subclavian vein to enter the mediastinum.

RECURRENT LARYNGEAL NERVES (see Fig 5.6)

Right Recurrent Laryngeal Nerve

- Branches off the right vagus nerve as it reaches the lower edge of the first part of the subclavian artery, passes around the subclavian artery and runs upwards in a groove between the trachea and the oesophagus

Left Recurrent Laryngeal Nerve

- Branches off the left vagus nerve as it crosses the arch of the aorta, passes below and behind the arch of the aorta and runs upwards along the trachea

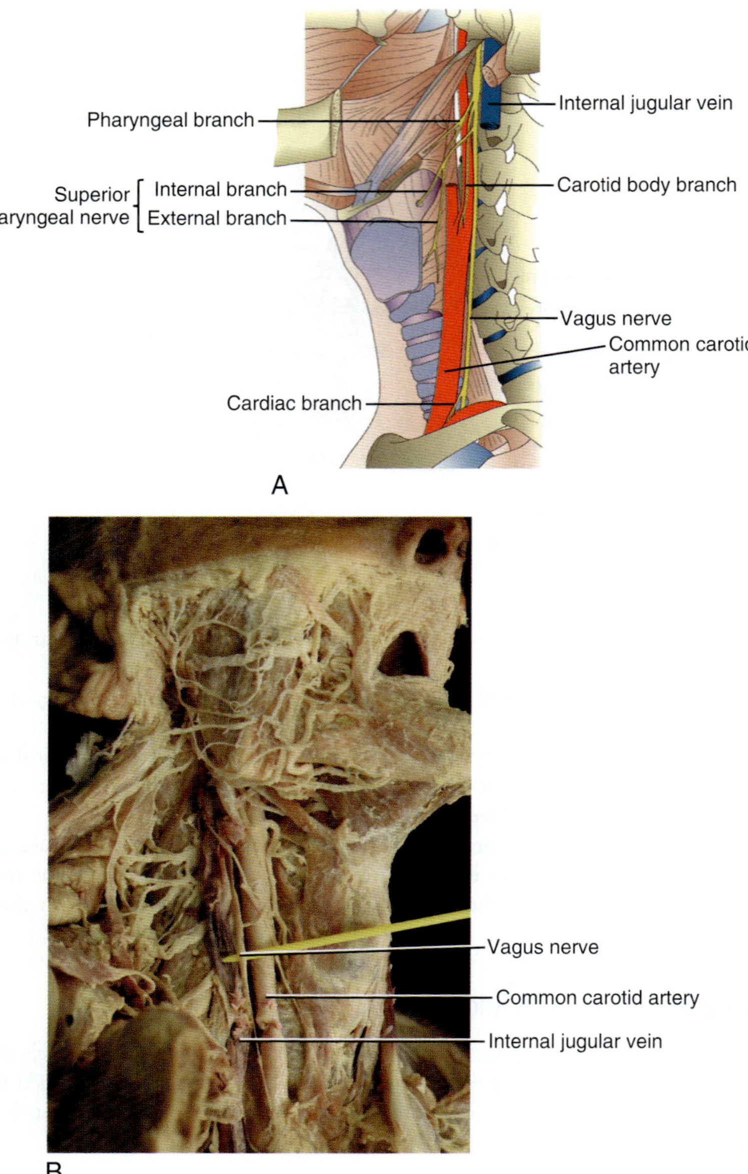

Fig. 5.11 **(A)** Vagus nerve and its relations. **(B)** Vagus nerve (cadaveric dissection).

PHRENIC NERVE (Fig 5.12)

The phrenic nerve (C3–5) runs downwards over the anterior scalene muscle, across the dome of the pleura, anterior to the subclavian artery and behind the subclavian vein.

ANTERIOR SCALENE MUSCLE

- A key muscle to understanding the structures at the root of the neck
- Arises from C3–6, with four slender tendons lying end to end with those of the longus capitis

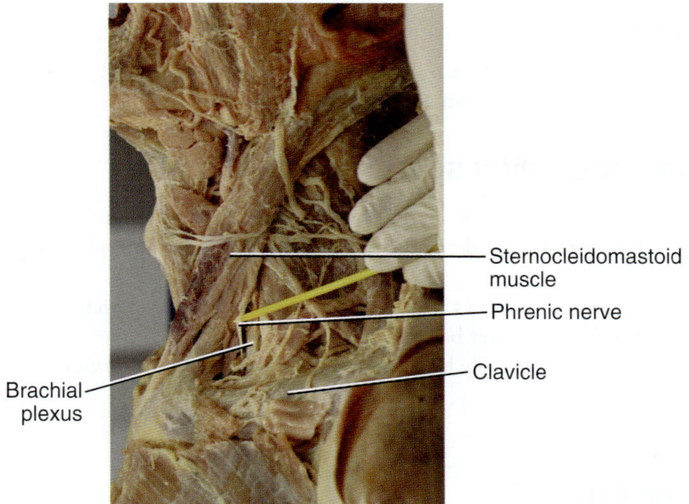

Fig. 5.12 Phrenic nerve (at the root of the neck: cadaveric dissection).

- Ends in a narrow tendon attached to the scalene tubercle and the ridge of the inner border of the upper surface of the first rib
- Is covered with a prolongation of the prevertebral fascia
- Is innervated segmentally (C4–6)

Anterior Relations

- Phrenic nerve passes vertically downwards plastered by the prevertebral fascia. The nerve then crosses the subclavian artery. From the suprapleural membrane, it passes medially towards the apex of the lung, anterior to the vagus
- The ascending cervical artery (from the inferior thyroid artery or thyrocervical artery) runs up medial to the phrenic nerve on the prevertebral fascia
- Transverse cervical and suprascapular arteries lie between the scalenus anterior and the carotid sheath
- Vagus nerve
- Internal jugular vein (surrounded by the inferior deep cervical lymph nodes)
- Subclavian vein lies in a groove on the first rib, lying lower than the insertion of the scalenus anterior

Medial Relations

- Pyramidal space
  - Formed by the longus colli muscle, medial edge of the scalenus anterior muscle, (lateral) and the subclavian artery and the neck of the first rib (base). The carotid tubercle (Chassaignac'c tubercle) is at the apex of the pyramid and it is called the carotid tubercle because the common carotid artery lies on it
  - Common carotid artery lies immediately in front of the pyramidal space
  - Space contains the stellate ganglion, vertebral artery and veins, inferior thyroid artery and thoracic duct and the first part of the subclavian artery with its three branches

Posterior Relations

- Anterior scalene muscle is separated from the middle scalene muscle by the subclavian artery and anterior rami of C7/T1
- Second part of the subclavian artery and its branch

Lateral Relations

- The trunks of the brachial plexus
- The third part of the subclavian artery and its branch

MIDDLE AND POSTERIOR SCALENE MUSCLES

- Middle scalene muscle arises from the posterior tubercles and intertubercular laminae of all cervical vertebrae to the quadrangular area between the neck and subclavian groove of the first rib
- Posterior scalene muscle arises from posterior tubercles of the lower cervical vertebrae to the second rib along its outer border
- Both are supplied segmentally by the anterior rami of the lower cervical nerves (C3–8)

Part 6 Face

SKIN OF THE FACE

Tension lines run in an onion-skin-like pattern from mouth to ear and wrinkles run at right angles to the muscle pull.

TABLE 5.3 ■ **Summary of the Muscles of the Face**

Muscle			Relative Attachment	Innervation	Concentric Action
ORBITAL GROUP	Orbicularis oculi	Palpebral part	Medial palpebral ligament	Lateral palpebral raphe	Closes the eyelids gently
		Orbital part	Nasal part of frontal bone	Fibres form an uninterrupted ellipse around orbit	Closes the eyelids forcefully
			Frontal process of maxilla		
			Medial palpebral ligament		
NASAL GROUP	Nasalis	Transverse part	Maxilla just lateral to nose	Aponeurosis across dorsum of nose with muscle fibres from the other side	Compresses nasal aperture
		Alar part	Maxilla over lateral incisor	Alar cartilage of nose	Draws cartilage downwards and laterally, opening nostril
	Others	Procerus	Nasal bone and upper part of lateral nasal cartilage	Skin of lower forehead between eyebrows	Draws down medial angle of eyebrows, producing transverse wrinkles over bridge of nose
		Depressor septi	Maxilla above medial incisor	Mobile part of the nasal septum	Pulls nose inferiorly

TABLE 5.3 ■ **Summary of the Muscles of the Face** (Continued)

Muscle			Relative Attachment	Innervation	Concentric Action
ORAL GROUP	Depressors	Depressor anguli oris	Oblique line of mandible below canine, premolar, and first molar teeth	Skin at the corner of mouth Blends with orbicularis oris	Draws corner of mouth downwards and laterally
		Depressor labii inferioris	Anterior part of oblique line of mandible	Lower lip at midline Blends with muscle from opposite side	Draws lower lip downwards and laterally
	Elevators	Levator labii superioris	Infraorbital margin of maxilla	Skin of upper lateral half of upper lip	Raises upper lip Helps form nasolabial furrow
		Levator labii superioris alaeque nasi	Frontal process of maxilla	Alar cartilage of nose and upper lip	Raises upper lip and opens nostril
		Levator anguli oris	Maxilla below infraorbital foramen	Skin at the corner of the mouth	Raises corner of mouth Helps form nasolabial furrow
	Others	Mentalis	Mandible inferior to incisors	Skin of chin	Raises and protrudes lower lip as it wrinkles skin on chin
		Zygomaticus major	Posterior part of lateral surface of zygomatic bone	Skin at the corner of the mouth	Draws the corner of the mouth upwards and laterally
		Zygomaticus minor	Anterior part of lateral surface of zygomatic bone	Upper lip just medial to corner of mouth	Draws the upper lip upwards
		Orbicularis oris	From muscles in area Maxilla and mandible in midline	Forms ellipse around mouth	Presses the cheek against teeth Compresses distended cheeks
OTHER MUSCLES OR GROUPS	Occipitofrontalis	Frontal belly	Skin of eyebrow	Into galea aponeurotica	Wrinkles forehead Raises eyebrows
		Occipital belly	Lateral part of superior nuchal line of occipital bone and mastoid process of temporal bone	Into galea aponeurotica	Draws scalp backwards
	Others	Anterior auricular	Anterior part of temporal fascia	Into helix of ear	Draws ear upwards and forwards
		Superior auricular	Epicranial aponeurosis on side of head	Upper part of auricle	Elevates ear
		Posterior auricular	Mastoid process of temporal bone	Convexity of concha of ear	Draws ear upwards and backwards

MUSCLES OF THE FACE (Fig 5.13)

Functionally differentiated to form groups around the orifices as sphincters and dilators. They are all innervated by the facial nerve (CN VII).

Motor Supply of the Face (see 5.13A)

The facial nerve is the major motor supply of the face.

- Temporal branches emerge from the upper border of the parotid gland and cross the zygomatic arch up to the frontalis and the anterior and posterior auricularis
  - Action: wrinkling the forehead
- Zygomatic branches have two parts: upper and lower. The upper part innervates the frontalis and upper orbicularis oculi and the lower part innervates the lower orbicularis oculi and muscles below the orbit
  - Action: paralysis prevents blinking
- Buccal branches supply the buccinator and the upper lip muscles (e.g. the upper part of the orbicularis oris)
  - Action: paralysis prevents emptying of the cheek pouches
- A marginal mandibular branch emerges from the lower border of the parotid gland and supplies muscles of the lower lip (e.g. the lower part of the orbicularis oris)
  - Injury to this nerve may result in permanent paralysis of the lower lip
  - It is at risk when making incisions along the lower border of the jaw
- A cervical branch passes vertically downwards and supplies the platysma

In summary, the facial nerve exits the skull through the stylomastoid foramen and immediately gives off the posterior auricular nerve, which passes back and up to supply the occipital part of the occipitofrontalis. The next branch, which comes off the facial nerve, innervates the posterior belly of the digastric and stylohyoid muscles. The facial nerve then enters the posteromedial surface of the parotid gland and divides into an upper temporozygomatic and a lower cervicofacial branch.

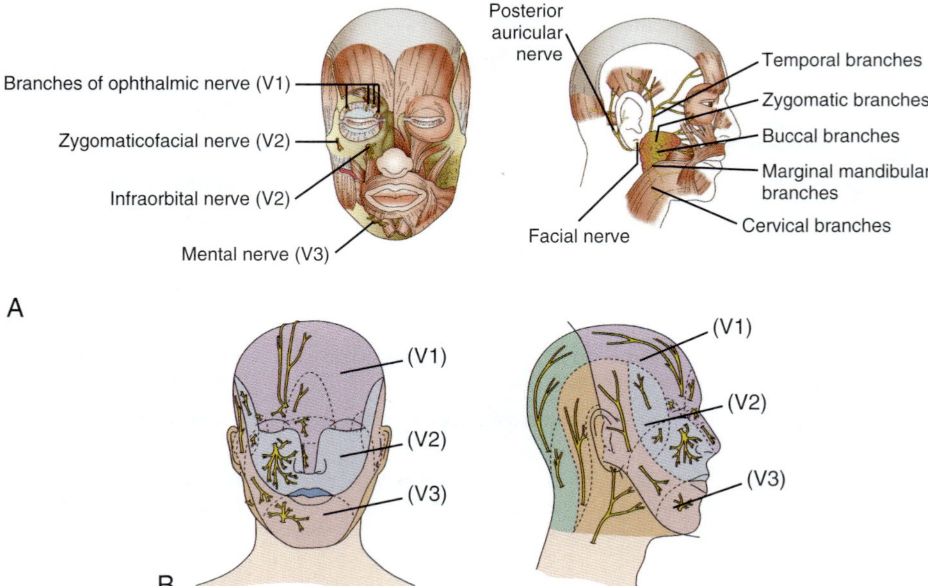

Fig. 5.13 **(A)** Motor supply of the face. Left: Muscles and foramina of the face. Right: Branches of the facial nerve. **(B)** Sensory supply of the face. Left: Anterior view. Right: Lateral view.

The branching pattern of the facial nerve is variable as it runs through the superficial part of the parotid gland. Five branches eventually emerge from the anterior border of the parotid gland: the temporal, zygomatic, buccal, marginal mandibular and cervical branches.

SENSORY SUPPLY OF THE FACE (see Fig 5.13B)

The trigeminal nerve (CN V) is the major sensory supply of the face. It has three branches: the ophthalmic nerve (CN V1), the maxillary nerve (CN V2) and the mandibular nerve (CN V3), and they give off five, three and three cutaneous branches respectively.

- **Ophthalmic nerve**
  - Lacrimal nerve supplies a small area of the skin over the lateral part of the upper eyelid
  - Supraorbital nerve passes up through a notch/foramen to supply the forehead and scalp
  - Supratrochlear nerve passes up on the medial side through the frontal notch and supplies the middle of the forehead
  - Infratrochlear nerve supplies the skin on the medial part of the upper eyelid and the bridge of the nose
    - The above four branches also supply the upper eyelid conjunctiva
  - External nasal nerve supplies the middle external nose down to the tip, and the ciliary branches supply the cornea
- **Maxillary nerve**
  - Infraorbital nerve emerges through its foramen, immediately breaking up into three branches: the palpebral, labial and nasal branches
  - Zygomaticofacial nerve emerges from a foramen on the zygomatic bone and supplies the overlying skin
  - Zygomaticotemporal nerve emerges in the temporal fossa through a foramen in the temporal surface of the zygomatic bone, supplying the hairless part of the temple
- **Mandibular nerve**
  - Auriculotemporal nerve passes around the neck of the mandible and ascends over the posterior root of the zygomatic arch
    - Auricular part supplies the external acoustic meatus, tympanic membrane and the skin of the auricle below
    - Temporal part supplies the hairy skin over the temple
  - Buccal nerve supplies a thumbprint-sized area over the cheek, below the zygomatic bone
  - Mental nerve is a cutaneous branch of the inferior alveolar nerve. It supplies the skin and mucous membrane of the lower lip and labial gum

BLOOD SUPPLY OF THE FACE (Fig 5.14)

- Facial artery is the highest of the three branches from the anterior aspect of the external carotid artery

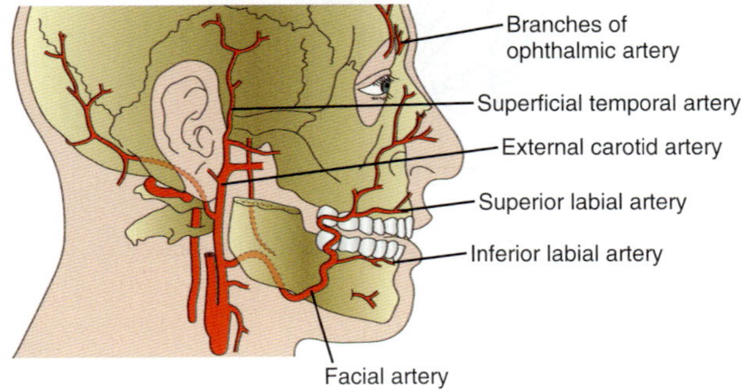

Fig. 5.14 Arterial supply of the face.

  - Gives off the superior and inferior labial artery
- Superficial temporal artery (a terminal branch of the external carotid artery) supplies the temple
  - Gives off the transverse facial artery
- Ophthalmic artery (from internal carotid artery) gives off the supraorbital and supratrochlear branches, which freely anastomose with the superficial temporal artery branches

VENOUS RETURN OF THE FACE (see Fig 5.7B)

The superficial veins are normally the main venous return of the face.

- The facial vein follows the facial artery to the lower border of the mandible, where it pierces the investing layer of the neck and is joined by the retromandibular vein
- The facial vein communicates with the cavernous sinus via the ophthalmic veins
  - Blood from the forehead will normally flow via the facial vein, but if there is any blockage then retrograde flow can occur
  - A 'danger triangle' extends to the upper lip and nearby cheek
  - Further communication is via the deep facial vein, which receives a vein from the cavernous sinus through foramen ovale

LYMPH DRAINAGE OF THE FACE (Fig 5.15)

- Lymph drains into three superficial groups of nodes from three wedge-shaped blocks:
  - Submental nodes receive lymph from the chin and tip of tongue
  - Submandibular nodes receive lymph from an area which extends from the central forehead and frontal sinuses through the anterior half of the nose and maxillary sinuses
  - Preauricular group receives lymph from the forehead, temple, orbital contents and cheek
- Eventually all drain to the deep cervical nodes

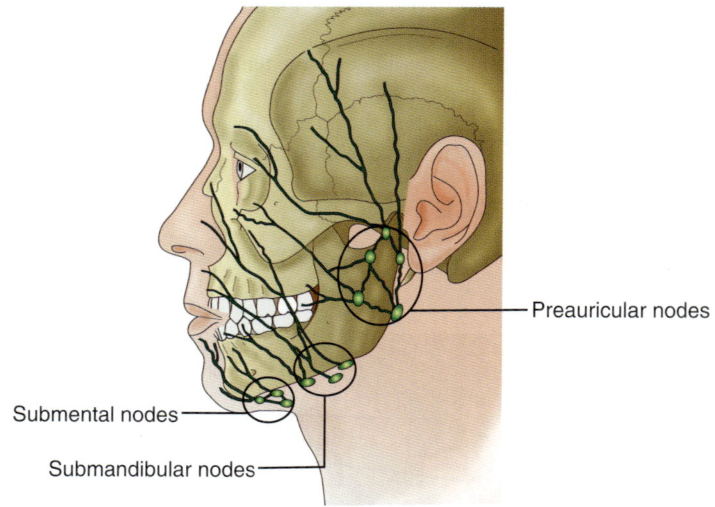

Fig. 5.15 Lymph drainage of the face.

Part 7 Scalp (Fig 5.16A and B)

The scalp is a multilayered structure that extends anteriorly from the superciliary arches to the external occipital protuberance and the superior nuchal lines posteriorly. It continues laterally down to the zygomatic arch. It consist of five layers: **S**kin, **C**onnective tissue (dense), **A**poneurotic layer, **L**oose connective tissue and **P**ericranium (**SCALP**). The first three layers are anchored

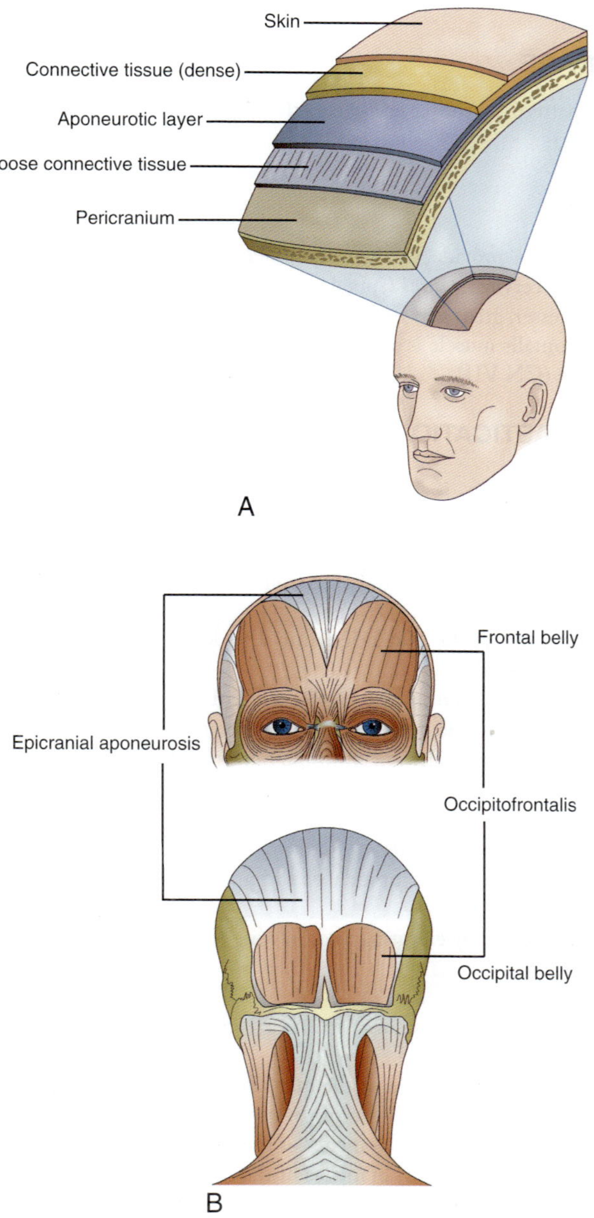

Fig. 5.16 (A) Layers of the scalp. **(B)** Occipitofrontalis and the epicranial aponeurosis. Top: Anterior view, showing frontalis muscular part. Bottom: Posterior view, showing occipitalis muscular part.

tightly together. The dense connective tissue layer contains the neurovascular structures. The loose connective tissue facilitates movement of the scalp over the calvaria. Infection tends to localise and spread through this layer because of its consistency.

BLOOD SUPPLY

- Branches of the external carotid artery and ophthalmic artery (a branch of the internal carotid artery)
- Venous return is similar to the pattern of the arteries

LYMPH DRAINAGE

- Follows the pattern of the arteries (e.g. the lymphatics in the occipital region drain to occipital nodes)

NERVE SUPPLY

- Two major sources provide the sensory innervation of the scalp: the trigeminal nerve (CN V) and the cervical nerves (spinal cord level C2 and C3, including the great auricular nerve and the lesser, great and third occipital nerves)
- The occipitofrontalis muscle is a muscle of facial expression and is therefore innervated by the facial nerve (CN VII)

MUSCLES OF MASTICATION

Masseter Muscle

- Arises from the zygomatic arch and consists of three parts: the superficial, intermediate and deep parts
- Superficial part – the largest part arising from the anterior two-thirds of the lower border of the zygomatic arch
  - Fibres slope down at 45° and insert into a wide area from the angle of the mandible upwards and forwards
- Intermediate part – arises from the middle third of the zygomatic arch
- Deep part – arises from the deep surface of the zygomatic arch
  - Fibres pass vertically downwards into the ramus of the mandible
- Masseteric nerve passes down between the deep and intermediate parts
- Branch of the superficial temporal or transverse facial artery runs forwards between the superficial and intermediate parts
- Innervated by the masseteric branch of the anterior division of the mandibular nerve (CN V3)
- Action: closing the jaw by elevating and drawing forwards the angle of the mandible

Temporalis Muscle

- Arises over the temporal fossa over the area between the inferior temporal line and the infratemporal crest
- Inserts into the coronoid process of the mandible and the anterior margin of the ramus of the mandible
- Blood suppy is via the temporal branches of the maxillary artery
- Innervated by the two temporal branches of the mandibular nerve (CN V3)

Medial and Lateral Pterygoid Muscles (Fig 5.17)

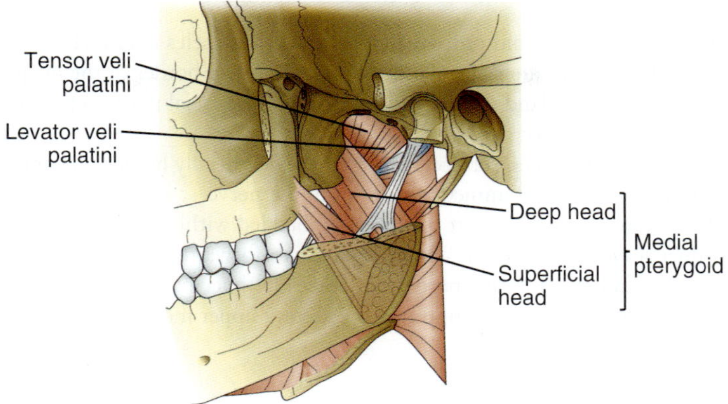

Fig. 5.17 Medial pterygoid muscle.

Part 8 Parotid Region

PAROTID GLAND (Fig 5.18)

The parotid gland is predominantly a serous salivary gland with an irregular shape. It fills a gap between the mastoid process, the ramus of the mandible and the styloid process. It has an upper and a lower pole and three surfaces: lateral, anterior and deep.

- Upper pole is a small concave surface adhering to the external acoustic meatus near the temporomandibular joint
- Lower pole is rounded, lying below and behind the angle of the mandible
- Lateral surface is subcutaneous and almost flat
- Anterior surface is U-shaped, adhering to the ramus of the mandible. The masseter muscle lies on the outer surface and the medial pterygoid on the inner surface
    - Parotid duct and the branches of the facial nerve emerge from the anterior border
    - Deep to the parotid duct and the branches of the facial nerve, the terminal branches of the external carotid artery (superficial temporal and maxillary arteries) lie within the gland

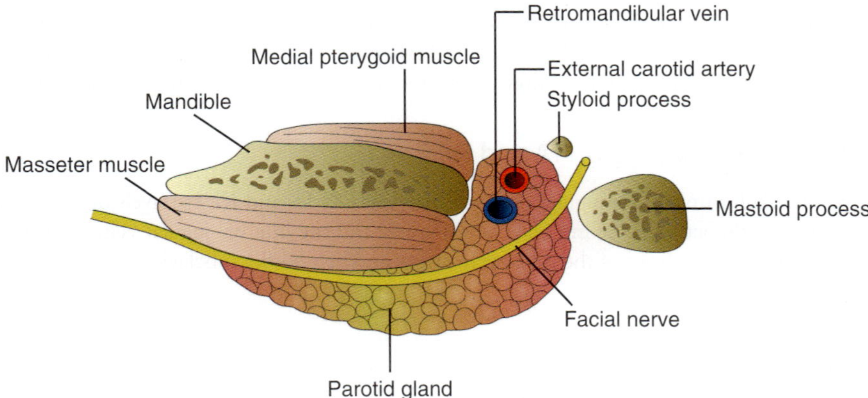

Fig. 5.18 Parotid gland and its neurovascular relations (transverse section of the left gland viewed superiorly).

- Deep surface (posteromedial):
  - Lies behind the ramus of the mandible, against the styloid process and its three attached muscles and ligaments
  - Is indented by the mastoid process and its attached muscles (sternocleidomastoid)
- External carotid artery enters the gland through the lower border of the deep surface
- Embedded within the gland are (superficial to deep) the facial nerve, retromandibular vein and external carotid artery
- Facial nerve enters the deep surface, but emerges superficially behind the anterior border
- Retromandibular vein runs immediately deep to the nerve
- Arterial structures are the deepest structures embedded within the gland
- Parotid duct leaves the anterior surface and passes forwards across the masseter muscle, then turns around the anterior border to pierce the buccinator muscle. It opens on the mucous membrane of the cheek opposite the second upper molar

Blood Supply

- External carotid artery
- Venous return via the retromandibular vein

Lymph Drainage

- Follows the external carotid artery and drains to the upper group of the deep cervical nodes

Nerve Supply

- Parotid gland receives its sensory innervation from the auriculotemporal nerve (a branch of the mandibular nerve (CN V3))
- Parotid fascia receives its sensory innervation from the great auricular nerve (C2)
- Secretomotor fibres arise from the cell bodies in the otic ganglion and reach the parotid gland by hitch-hiking via the auriculotemporal nerve
- Sympathetic fibres reach the gland from the superior cervical ganglion via the external carotid artery and middle meningeal arteries

Part 9 Infratemporal Region

Some contents have been explained in previous sections (e.g. the carotid sheath, mandibular nerve).

GLOSSOPHARYNGEAL NERVE (Fig 5.19)

It leaves the skull through the jugular foramen and lies deep to the styloid apparatus. It then runs down wards and forwards between the internal and external carotid arteries, curves around the lateral border of the stylopharyngeus and continues in an anterior direction to reach the base of the tongue.

VAGUS NERVE (see Fig 5.11A and B)

It leaves the skull through the jugular foramen between CN IX and XI. It travels downwards in the carotid sheath, between the internal carotid artery and the internal jugular vein. At the root of the neck, it passes in front of the subclavian artery and behind the subclavian vein to enter the mediastinum.

ACCESSORY NERVE

It leaves the skull through the middle part of the jugular foramen posterior to CN X, runs posterolaterally, either medial or lateral to the internal jugular vein, crosses the transverse process of

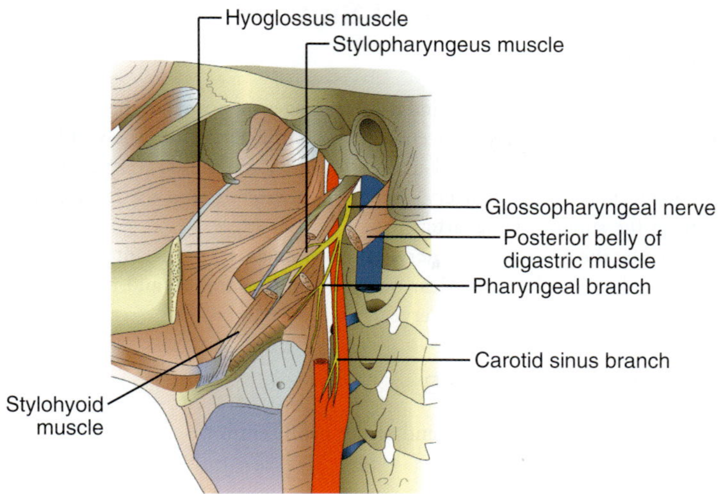

Fig. 5.19 Glossopharyngeal nerve and its relations.

the atlas and passes medial to the styloid process and posterior belly of the digastric muscle to perforate the sternocleidomastoid muscle and reach the posterior triangle of the neck.

HYPOGLOSSAL NERVE (Fig 5.20)

It leaves the skull through the hypoglossal foramen, passes between the internal carotid artery and the internal jugular vein and crosses three arteries (the occipital, external carotid and lingual arteries) deep to the posterior belly of digastric to reach the tongue. A branch from the anterior ramus of C1 hitchhikes with it. This branch innervates some of the suprahyoid muscles (thyrohyoid and geniohyoid).

Part 10 Pterygopalatine Fossa

Some contents have been explained in other sections (e.g. maxillary nerve, maxillary vessels).

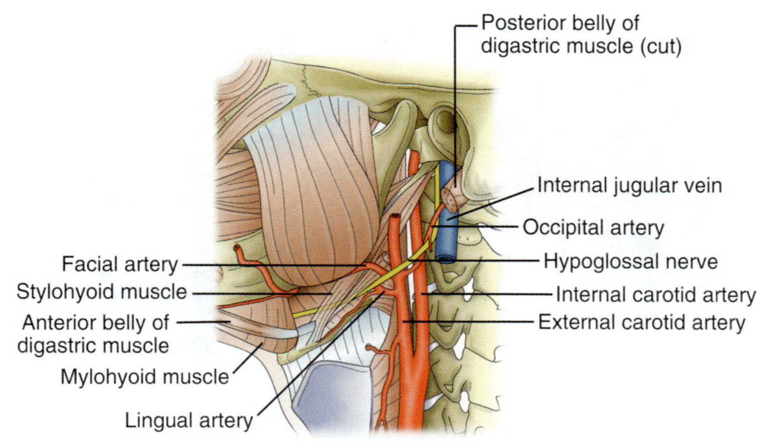

Fig. 5.20 Hypoglossal nerve and its relations.

Part 11 Nose and Paranasal Sinuses

EXTERNAL NOSE

- Consists of the nasal bone (bridge) and nasal cartilages supported in the midline by the septum
- Covering skin contains many sebaceous glands and extends into the vestibule
- Blood supply is via the dorsal nasal artery (from the ophthalmic atery), external nasal artery (from the anterior ethmoidal artery), lateral nasal artery (from the facial artery) and septal artery (from the superior labial artery)
- Is innervated by the external nasal nerve (the terminal part of the anterior ethmoidal nerve), the supratrochlear and infratrochlear nerves (from the frontal and nasociliary nerves) and nasal branches of the infraorbital nerve

NASAL CAVITY (Fig 5.21A and B)

- From the nostrils to the posterior end of the nasal septum

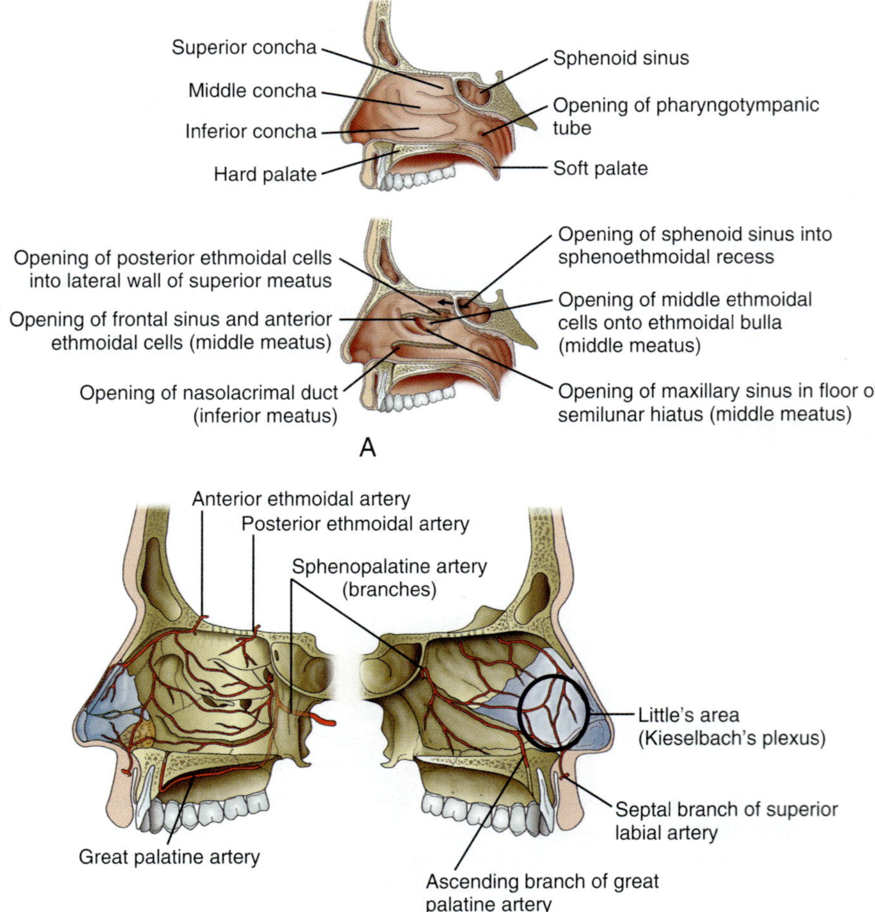

Fig. 5.21 **(A)** Nasal cavity, midline sagittal section. Top: Turbinates intact. Bottom: Turbinates cut, revealing the ostia of the paranasal sinuses. **(B)** Arterial supply of the nasal cavity. Left: Arteries of the lateral wall. Right: Arteries of the medial wall.

- Most of the cavity is the respiratory area, which is lined with respiratory mucus and pseudostratified ciliated columnar epithelium
  - Vestibular area is the area just inside the nostril
  - Olfactory area contains the receptors for smell
- Floor is the roof of the mouth (hard palate)
- Lateral wall is the medial wall of the orbit superiorly and the medial wall of the maxillary sinus inferiorly
- Roof is very narrow, with the medial and lateral walls very close together
- Nasal conchae:
  - Lowest is the longest
  - Middle and upper are joined anteriorly
  - Each has a space beneath it: the superior, middle and inferior meatuses, with the sphenoethmoidal recess uppermost
  - Sphenoidal sinus opens into the sphenoethmoidal recess
  - Posterior ethmoidal air cells enter into the superior meatus
  - Nasolacrimal ducts enter into the inferior meatus (2 cm behind the nostril)
  - Middle meatus receives all other openings: the frontal sinuses, anterior and middle ethmoidal aircells and maxillary sinuses

Blood Supply

- Main artery is the sphenopalatine (the end of the maxillary artery passing through the sphenopalatine foramen)
  - Anastomoses with the septal branch of the superior labial and ascending branch of the greater palatine over the lower anterior part of the septum (Little's area), where it forms Kieselbach's plexus
  - Kieselbach's plexus is a common site for anterior epistaxis
- Anterior and posterior ethmoidal arteries supply the roof and the anterior part of the lateral wall
- Veins drain to the pterygoid plexus: the facial vein, ophthalmic vein and inferior cerebral vein

Lymph Drainage

- Runs with the veins rather than the arteries, and drains to the submandibular, deep cervical and retropharyngeal nodes

Nerve Supply

- Olfactory area is supplied via the olfactory receptors, which are extensions of the olfactory nerve
- Vestibular area is supplied via the infraorbital nerve
- Respiratory area is supplied anteriorly via the anterior ethmoidal nerve and the anterior superior alveolar nerve, and posteriorly via branches from the pterygopalatine ganglion and the greater palatine nerve

PARANASAL SINUSES

- Frontal sinus – is absent at birth; others are rudimentary, expanding between 6 and 7 years and again after puberty
- Maxillary sinus – is a pyramid-shaped space within the body of the maxilla
  - Base is at the lateral wall of the nose
  - Apex is in the zygomatic process of the maxilla
  - Roof is the floor of the orbit

  - Floor is the alveolar part of the maxilla
  - Ostium is high up and well back on the nasal wall, and opens into the middle meatus
  - Blood supply: branches from the facial, maxillary, infraorbital and greater palatine arteries
  - Nerve supply: branches of the maxillary nerve (CN V2)
  - Lymph drainage: submandibular nodes
- Ethmoidal sinus – lies between the orbit and the nose. It is not a single cavity and it is divided up into numerous cells: anterior, middle and posterior ethmoidal air cells
  - Blood supply: branches of the external and internal carotid arteries (supraorbital, anterior and posterior ethmoidal and sphenopalatine arteries)
  - Nerve supply: branches of the ophthalmic nerve (CN V1) and maxillary nerve (CN V2)
  - Lymph drainage: submandibular and retropharyngeal nodes
- Sphenoidal sinus – occupies the body of the sphenoid bone
  - Initially lies in the pituitary fossa, but as it enlarges it extends backwards into the basiocciput
  - Bounded superiorly by the pituitary fossa and middle cranial fossa, laterally by the cavernous sinus and internal carotid artery and posteriorly by the posterior cranial fossa and pons
  - Ostium is in the anterior wall of the sinus and opens into the sphenoethmoidal recess
  - Blood supply: branches of the external and internal carotid arteries (posterior ethmoidal and sphenopalatine arteries)
  - Nerve supply: branches of the maxillary nerve (CN V2)
  - Lymph drainage: retropharyngeal nodes
- Frontal sinus – is not present at birth and usually appears in the second year of life
  - Extends from the medial end of the eyebrow into the squamous part of the frontal bone and backwards into the orbital part
  - Ostium is in the lower medial corner
  - Blood supply: branches of the internal carotid artery (supratrochlear, supraorbital and anterior ethmoidal arteries)
  - Nerve supply: branches of the ophthalmic nerve (CN V1)
  - Lymph drainage: submandibular nodes

Part 12 Mouth and Hard Palate

The oral cavity consists of the roof (the hard and soft palate), floor (the muscular diaphragm and tongue) and lateral walls (fascia and a layer of skeletal muscle). It opens anteriorly to the oral fissure and posteriorly to the oropharyngeal isthmus.

ROOF OF THE ORAL CAVITY

- The roof of the oral cavity, or palate, consists of an anterior hard palate and a posterior soft palate:
  - The hard palate is covered by mucosa and is formed by the palatine process of the maxilla (anterior three-quarters) and the horizontal plates of the palatine bones (posterior quarter)
  - The soft palate hangs off the posterior edge of the hard palate. Much of its bulk is made of mucous and serous glands within the mucous membrane of its oral surface. It consists of an aponeurosis and five pairs of muscles, and acts as a valve during the co-ordinated process of swallowing to prevent reflux of material into the nasopharynx
    - Tensor veli palatini
    - Levator veli palatini
    - Palatopharyngeus
    - Palatoglossus
    - Musculus uvulae

  - All muscles of the soft palate are innervated by the pharyngeal plexus (CN X) except for tensor veli palatini (CN V3).

FLOOR OF THE ORAL CAVITY

- The floor of the oral cavity is formed by:
  - Paired mylohyoid muscles connected in the midline by a raphe
  - Paired geniohyoid muscles
  - Tongue
  - Submandibular glands (deep portion)

Tongue

The tongue is a muscular structure covered with a mucous membrane that forms part of the floor of the oral cavity and the anterior wall of the oropharynx. It is divided into the dorsum, tip, inferior surface and root.

- The dorsum faces in two directions:
  - Anterior two-thirds (oral part) is covered by mucous membrane, into which the underlying muscles are inserted
    - Stratified squamous keratinising variety
    - Roughened with papillae
    - There are no glands on the dorsum of the anterior two-thirds of the tongue
  - Posterior third (pharyngeal part) extends from the sulcus terminalis to the epiglottis
    - Foramen caecum (apex of the sulcus) is the remains of the thyroglossal duct
    - No papillae behind the sulcus
    - Nodular appearance from the presence of underlying mucous and serous glands

Muscles of the Tongue

- Intrinsic muscles (origins and insertions are within the tongue)
  - Superior and inferior longitudinal, transverse and vertical muscles
- Extrinsic muscles
  - Genioglossus, hyoglossus, styloglossus and palatoglossus

Blood Supply

- Lingual artery

Lymph Drainage

- The tip drains to the submental nodes, the anterior part drains to the submandibular nodes and then to the deep cervical nodes, and the posterior part drains directly to the deep cervical nodes

Nerve Supply

- All muscles are supplied by the hypoglossal nerve (except the palatoglossus, which is supplied by the pharyngeal plexus). The sensory innervation is by three nerves:
  - Oral part (anterior two-thirds): the lingual nerve, which is a major branch of the mandibular nerve (CN V3), provides the general sensory supply and the chorda tympani, which is a branch of the facial nerve, provides the special sensory supply (taste)
  - Posterior third: the glossopharyngeal nerve provides the general sensory and the special sensory supply (taste)
  - Vallecula: the internal laryngeal nerve

Submandibular Gland (Fig 5.22A)

The submandibular gland is hook-shaped with two arms: a larger arm (superficial part) and a smaller arm (deep part). To reach the gland, the layers that need to be dissected are: the skin, the subcutaneous fat, the platysma and the investing layer of deep cervical fascia.

- There are three muscles closely related to the submandibular gland: the mylohyoid, the hyoglossus and the posterior belly of the diagastric muscle
- There are a number of structures running across the gland: the facial vein, the facial artery and the lymph nodes
- There are three nerves at risk during submandibular excision: the marginal mandibular branch of the facial nerve, the lingual nerve and the hypoglossal nerve
- The **lingual nerve** (Fig 5.22B) lies above the deep portion of the submandibular gland and loops under its duct from lateral to medial, deep to the mylohyoid and on the surface of the hyoglossus

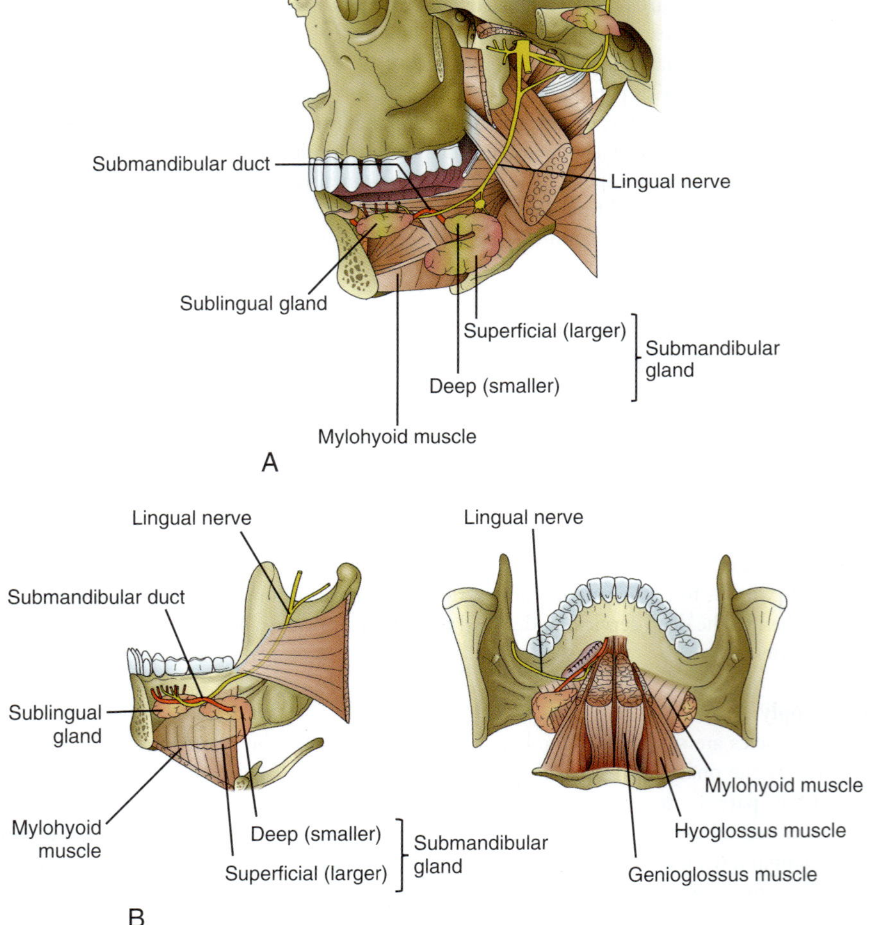

Fig. 5.22 **(A)** Submandibular gland and its relations. **(B)** Lingual nerve and its relations. Left: Lateral view. Right: Posterior view.

- The submandibular duct (or Wharton's duct) originates from the superficial part, although it emerges from the deep part. It terminates at the sublingual papilla next to the base of the frenulum of the tongue

LATERAL WALLS OF THE ORAL CAVITY

- The lateral walls of the oral cavity are formed by the cheeks. Each one consists of fascia and a thin layer of skeletal muscle (buccinator) sandwiched between the skin and the oral mucosa
  - The buccinator muscle is one of the muscles of facial expression and it is in the same plane as the superior constrictor muscle of the pharynx. These two muscles provide continuity between the walls of the oral and the pharyngeal cavities
  - The buccinator muscle holds the cheeks against the alveolar arches and keeps food between the teeth when chewing
  - As with other muscles of facial expression, it is innervated by the facial nerve (CN VII)

Part 13 Pharynx and Soft Palate (Fig 5.23A–C)

PHARYNX

The pharynx is formed by skeletal muscles and fascia. This musculofascial half-cylinder extends from the base of the skull to the upper border of the oesophagus (C6 vertebral level). It can be divided into three regions: the nasopharynx, the oropharynx and the laryngopharynx.

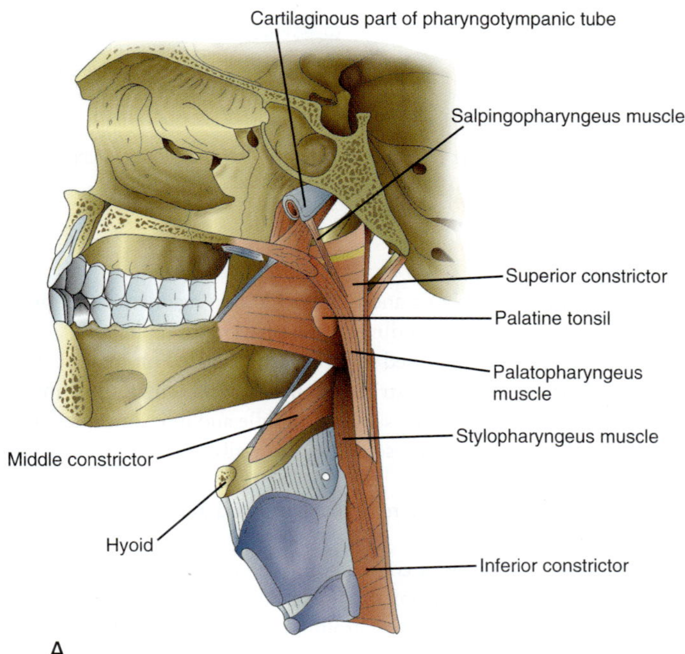

Fig. 5.23 **(A)** Musculature of the pharynx (longitudinal and constrictor muscles), sagittal section.

Continued on following page

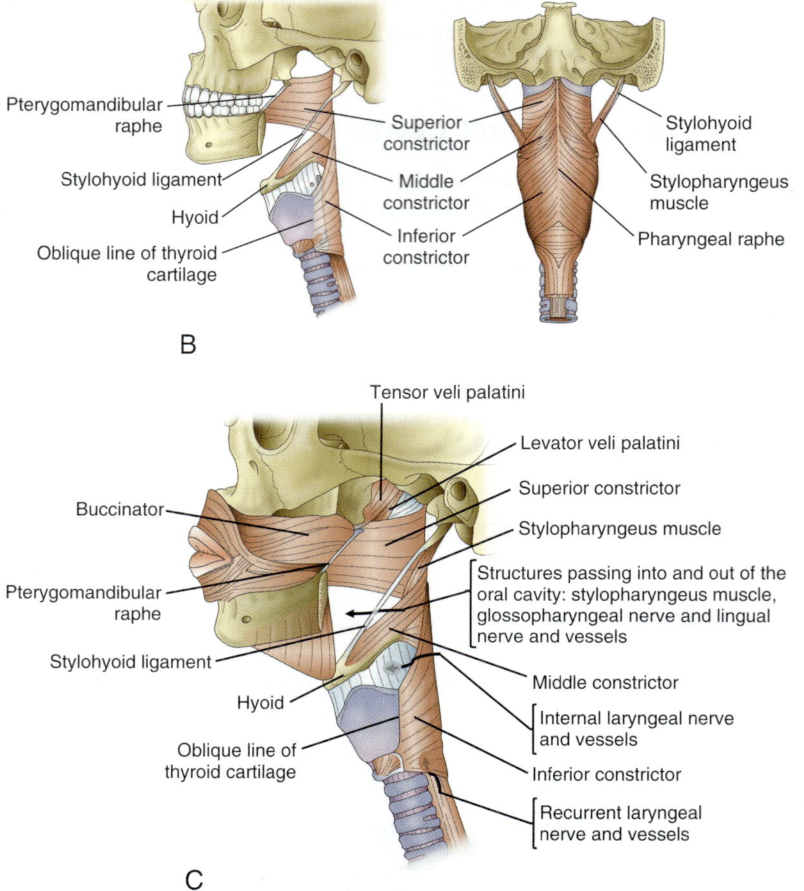

Fig. 5.23, cont'd **(B)** Musculature of the pharynx (longitudinal and constrictor muscles). Left: Lateral view. Right: Posterior view. **(C)** Gaps between muscles in the pharyngeal wall.

Pharyngeal Wall

The pharyngeal wall is attached to bone and cartilage, and to ligament superiorly and anteriorly. The two sides meet posteriorly in the midline at the pharyngeal raphe.

- Muscles of the pharynx are organised into two groups based on the direction of their fibres relative to the pharyngeal wall: constrictors (circular) and longitudinal muscles (vertical)
  - Constrictor muscles comprise the superior, middle and inferior constrictor muscles. They overlap each other in a fashion resembling the walls of three flowerpots stacked one on another
    - Gaps between the muscles are reinforced by fascia and provide routes for structures to pass through the wall
    - Muscle fibres of the superior constrictor arise outside the pharyngobasilar fascia
    - Middle constrictor arises from the angle between the stylohyoid ligament and the greater horn of the hyoid, arching around to the median raphe
    - Inferior constrictor arises from the oblique line of the thyroid cartilage and the cricoid
  - Longitudinal muscles include the salpingopharyngeus, palatopharyngeus and stylopharyngeus muscles. From their sites of origin, they run downwards and attach to the

pharyngeal wall. Their function is to elevate the wall and/or assist swallowing, pulling up and over a bolus of food and pushing it through the pharynx to the oesophagus
- All muscles are innervated by the vagus nerve (CN X) *except* the stylopharyngeus, which is supplied by the glossopharyngeal nerve (CN IX).

Structures Passing Through the Gaps

- Above the superior constrictor: tensor and levator veli palatini muscles
- Between the superior and middle constrictors (oropharyngeal triangle): muscles, nerves and vessels passing into and out of the oral cavity (e.g. the stylopharyngeus muscle, the glossopharyngeal nerve (CN IX) and the lingual nerve and vessels)
- Between the middle and inferior constrictors: the internal laryngeal vessels and nerve (the branch of the superior laryngeal nerve)
- Below the inferior constrictor: the recurrent laryngeal nerve and inferior laryngeal vessels

Blood Supply

- Via many different sources: the ascending pharyngeal, ascending palatine, lingual, tonsillar, greater palatine, pterygoid canal, and superior and inferior laryngeal arteries
- The upper part of the pharynx is supplied by the branches of the external carotid artery (e.g. the lingual, maxillary and facial arteries) and the lower part by branches of the subclavian artery (e.g. the inferior thyroid artery of the thyrocervical trunk)
- Importantly, the major blood supply to the palatine tonsil is from the facial artery (tonsillar branch)
- Venous return is by the pharyngeal plexus: veins drain superiorly into the pterygoid plexus and inferiorly to the facial and internal jugular veins

Lymph Drainage

- Lymphatic vessels drain into the deep cervical lymph nodes (paratracheal, infrahyoid and retropharyngeal nodes)
- Importantly, the palatine tonsils drain into superior jugulodigastric nodes

Nerve Supply

- Motor and sensory innervation is mainly by the pharyngeal plexus (branches of the vagus nerve (CN X) and glossopharyngeal nerve (CN IX))
- All muscles are innervated by the vagus nerve (CN X) *except* for the stylopharyngeus (CN IX)
- Sensory innervation is subdivided: nasopharynx (maxillary nerve (CN V2)), oropharynx (glossopharyngeal nerve (CN IX)) and laryngopharynx (vagus nerve (CN X))

SOFT PALATE

- Continues posteriorly from the hard palate as a mobile fold and acts as a valve: closing the oropharynx isthmus and nasopharynx during swallowing
- Is acted upon by five different muscles, supplied by the pharyngeal plexus (CN X), except for the tensor veli palatini (CN V3)
- Tensor veli palatini has two components: a vertically oriented part, originating from the base of the skull and the cartilage of the pharyngotympanic tube, and a horizontal fibrous palatine aponeurosis, which fans out to meet its opposite number. The two parts are connected by a narrow tendon at the pterygoid hamulus. Its function is to tense the soft palate and open the pharyngotympanic tube
- Levator veli palatini arises from the apex of the petrous temporal bone and the pharyngotympanic tube. It passes down to insert into the palatine aponeurosis. It pulls the soft palate up and back to shut off the nasopharynx

- Palatopharyngeus originates from the superior surface of the palatine aponeurosis and adjacent hard palate, and arches down posteriorly on the inner aspect of the pharynx to the thyroid cartilage. The palatine tonsil sits just anterior it. The part of the muscle fixed to the hard palate elevates the larynx and pharynx during swallowing. The part attached to the palatine aponeurosis helps to narrow the oropharyngeal isthmus
- Palatoglossus arises from the inferior surface of the palatine aponeurosis and passes down in front of the palatine tonsil to insert into the side of the tongue. It helps to narrow the oropharyngeal isthmus and elevate the tongue
- The musculus uvula passes back from the hard palate and fuses with its counterpart in the uvula. Together they elevate and retract the uvula, helping the levator veli palatini close the pharyngeal isthmus

Part 14 Larynx (Fig 5.24A and B)

The larynx is a musculoligamentous structure with a cartilaginous framework, located above the lower respiratory tract. It has important functions in protecting the airway and for phonation. It continues inferiorly with the trachea and opens superiorly into the laryngopharynx. It is composed of:

- Cartilages, joints, ligaments, membranes and muscles
- Three singular cartilages: the epiglottis, thyroid and cricoid
- Three pairs of cartilages: the arytenoids, corniculates and cuneiforms
- Three pairs of joints: the cricothyroid, cricoarytenoid and arytenocorniculate
- Ligaments and fibroelastic membranes: the thyrohyoid membrane with its ligaments, the hyoepiglottic and cricotracheal ligaments, the cricothyroid membrane with its ligament and the quadrangular membrane with its ligament

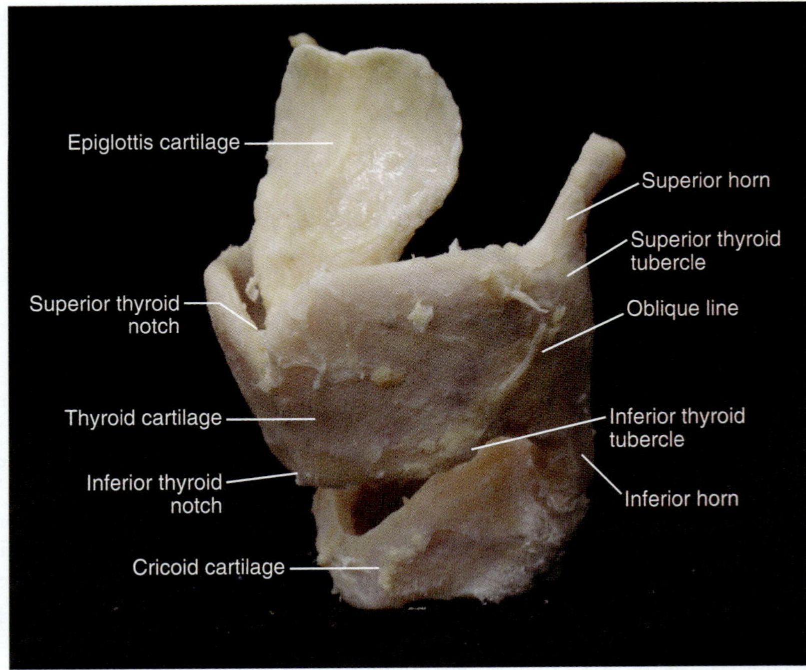

Fig. 5.24 (A) Larynx, cartilaginous framework.

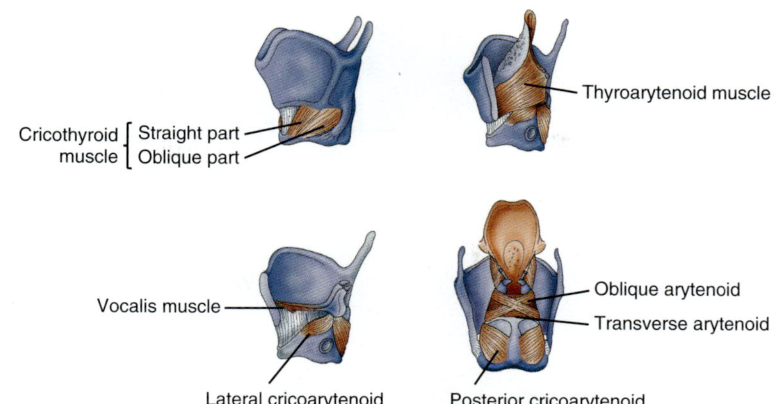

Fig. 5.24, cont'd **(B)** Larynx, musculoligamentous structure. Top left: Lateral view. Top right: Lateral view, parasagittal section, revealing structure of the epiglottis. Bottom left: Lateral view, sagittal section, epiglottis removed. Bottom right: Posterior view.

- Muscles: the intrinsic and extrinsic muscles, and specifically the posterior cricoarytenoid and cricothyroid (intrinsic muscles), are important
  - *Posterior cricoarytenoid* muscles are the most important as they are the only ones that abduct the vocal cords
  - Cricothyroid contraction lengthens the vocal cords
  - The recurrent laryngeal nerve supplies motor to all intrinsic muscles (*except the cricothyroid, which is innervated by the superior laryngeal branches of CN X*)

DIVISIONS OF THE LARYNX (Fig 5.25)

The larynx is divided into three areas by pairs of mucosal folds: the vestibular and vocal folds. These divisions are: the vestibule, the laryngeal ventricle or middle part (very thin and between folds) and the infraglottic space.

- The piriform recess lies on either side of the laryngeal inlet. It is bounded medially by the aryepiglottic fold and laterally by thyroid cartilage. It is a common place for food or foreign bodies (e.g. a fish bone) to become trapped
- Vocal folds or true vocal cords produce sounds when they are adducted and air is forced between them. The rima glottidis is the space between the two adjacent true vocal cords
- During forced closure (heavy lifting or straining), the rima glottidis, rima vestibuli and lower part of the vestibule are completely closed. The rima vestibuli is the space between the two adjacent vestibular folds (false vocal cords)
- During swallowing, the rima glottidis, rima vestibuli and vestibule are closed. The larynx moves upwards and forwards and this action causes the epiglottis to swing downwards to narrow the laryngeal inlet as well as open the oesophagus. All these actions prevent food from entering the respiratory tract

BLOOD SUPPLY

- The superior and inferior laryngeal arteries are the two major blood supplies of the larynx. They originate from the superior and inferior thyroid arteries, respectively
- The superior laryngeal veins drain into the superior thyroid veins, which in turn drain into the internal jugular vein. The inferior laryngeal veins drain into the left brachiocephalic veins via the inferior thyroid veins

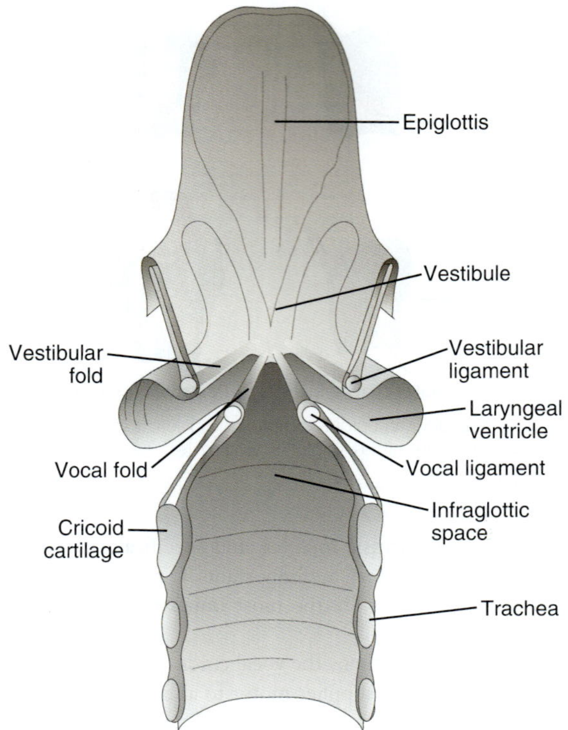

Fig. 5.25 Divisions of the larynx, coronal section, posterior view.

LYMPH DRAINAGE

- Lymphatics above the vocal folds drain into the deep cervical nodes associated with the bifurcation of the common carotid artery, while those below drain into the deep nodes associated with the upper trachea

NERVE SUPPLY

- Sensory and motor innervation of the larynx is by two branches of the vagus: the superior and the recurrent laryngeal nerves
- The recurrent laryngeal nerve supplies motor innervation to all intrinsic muscles (*except the cricothyroid*), as well as sensory innervation below the vocal folds
- The superior laryngeal nerve divides into internal and external branches. The external laryngeal nerve innervates the cricothyroid, and the internal laryngeal nerve is mainly sensory and supplies the laryngeal cavity above the vocal folds

ANATOMY OF CRICOTHYROIDOTOMY AND TRACHEOSTOMY

Tracheostomy is performed to relieve airway obstruction or to protect the airways, and can be employed in an emergency or planned. Cricothyroidotomy is a safer alternative in an emergency situation. These procedures may be technically challenging owing to patient factors (e.g. obese patients or those with a short neck).

Cricothyroidotomy

Surgical cricothyroidotomy and needle cricothyroidotomy are important emergency procedures in advanced life support. In surgical cricothyroidotomy, the patient is suitably positioned with the neck extended. After palpating the gap between the inferior thyroid notch and cricoid cartilage in the midline, the medic makes a transverse incision down to and then through the cricothyroid membrane in order to insert a tube. Needle cricothyroidotomy is a temporising measure. Once the patient has been stabilised, a formal tracheostomy can be performed for definitive airway management. Some structures may be at risk of injury – such as a branch of the superior thyroid artery, which runs over the cricothyroid membrane. Other complications include injury to the trachea or oesophagus, etc.

Tracheostomy

The patient is suitably prepared and positioned. Palpable midline structures are used as reference points. These points are (from inferior to superior): the suprasternal notch, the cricoid cartilage and the superior thyroid notch. A horizontal incision (in relation to the midline) is made midway between the suprasternal notch and the cricoid cartilage. The skin, platysma and superficial veins (communicating veins between the anterior jugular vein) are divided, together with the investing layer of the deep fascia of the neck. The strap muscles are retracted laterally to expose the thyroid isthmus. Pretracheal fascia encloses the thyroid isthmus, which usually overlies the second and third tracheal rings. The thyroid isthmus with its fascia is divided and oversewn before incising the second and third tracheal rings; the first tracheal ring must be avoided. It is important to stick to the midline in order to avoid injuring the recurrent nerves, carotid sheath and inferior thyroid veins. In an emergency, a vertical midline incision may be used rather than a transverse cervical incision.

Part 15 Orbit and Eye

ORBIT

- The orbit is a pyramid-shaped cavity (base is anterior); the bones which contribute to its framework are:
  - Medial wall – consisting of four bones, which are the maxilla, lacrimal, ethmoid and sphenoid bones
  - Lateral wall – consisting of the zygomatic bone and the greater wing of the sphenoid bone
  - Floor – mainly consisting of the maxilla, with small contributions from the zygomatic and palatine bones
  - Roof – mainly consisting of the frontal bone, with a small contribution from the sphenoid bone

EYELIDS

The layers that constitute the eyelid from superficial to deep are:

- Skin and subcutaneous tissue
- Orbicularis oculi muscle (includes the orbital and palpebral parts)
- Orbital septum
- Tarsus
- Conjunctiva

Orbicularis Oculi Muscle

The voluntary muscle of the eyelid (orbicularis oculi) is innervated by the facial nerve (temporal branch). Any damage to the nerve results in the inability to close or blink the ipsilateral upper eyelid, and the lower eyelid droops away. This is associated with corneal ulcers and spillage of tears.

To minimise the risk of nerve injury and such sequelae, surgical landmarks can be used to estimate the course of the zygomatic branch of the facial nerve.

Orbital Septum

Deep to the palpebral part of the orbicularis oculi, it is an extension of periosteum into both the upper and the lower eyelids from the margin of the orbit.

Tarsus

Two muscles associated with the tarsus raise the eyelid – namely the levator palpebrae superioris muscle and the superior tarsal muscle.

- Levator palpebrae superioris muscle is innervated by the occulomotor nerve
- Superior tarsal muscle is innervated by postganglionic sympathetic fibres from the superior cervical ganglion
- Loss of function of either of these muscles results in falling of the upper eyelid – namely complete ptosis (levator palpebrae superioris muscle impaired) or partial ptosis (superior tarsal muscle impaired)

Conjunctiva

- The structure of the eyelid is completed by the conjunctiva, which extends from the posterior surface of the eyelid to the eyeball at the junction between the sclera and the cornea

LACRIMAL APPARATUS

The lacrimal apparatus is involved in the production, movement and drainage of fluid from the surface of the eyeball. It is made of the lacrimal gland and its ducts, the lacrimal canaliculi, the lacrimal sac and the nasolacrimal duct.

- The lacrimal gland is a serous gland with a large orbital part (the lacrimal fossa) and a small palpebral part and has approximately 12 ducts which lead to the superior fornix
  - Sensory innervation: ophthalmic nerve (CN V1)
  - Secretomotor: parasympathetic and sympathetic
    - Parasympathetic fibres leave the superior salivatory nucleus (the facial nerve/CN VII), enter the greater petrosal nerve and continue with this nerve until it becomes the nerve of the pterygoid canal. The nerve of the pterygoid canal joins the pterygopalatine ganglion. From the pterygopalatine ganglion, the fibres join the maxillary nerve (CN V2) and continue with it until the zygomatic nerve branches off from it. They travel with the zygomatic nerve until it gives off the zygomaticotemporal nerve, which eventually distributes fibres in a small branch that joins the lacrimal nerve (V1)
    - Sympathetic fibres follow a similar pathway to parasympathetic fibres. Sympathetic fibres (from the superior cervical ganglion) travel along the plexus surrounding the internal carotid artery. They then leave the plexus as the deep petrosal nerve and join the parasympathetic fibres in the nerve of the pterygoid canal. From here, they follow the same path as the parasympathetic fibres

MUSCLES OF THE EYEBALL (Fig 5.26)

The muscles of the eyeball can be conceptualised as two groups: **intrinsic muscles** and **extrinsic (extraocular) muscles**. The intrinsic muscles control the shape of the lens and the size of the pupil. The extrinsic muscles are involved in movement of the eyeball (six muscles) and raising the upper eyelid (one muscle). A detailed knowledge of their attachments, function and innervation is essential for examining both the eye and the nervous system.

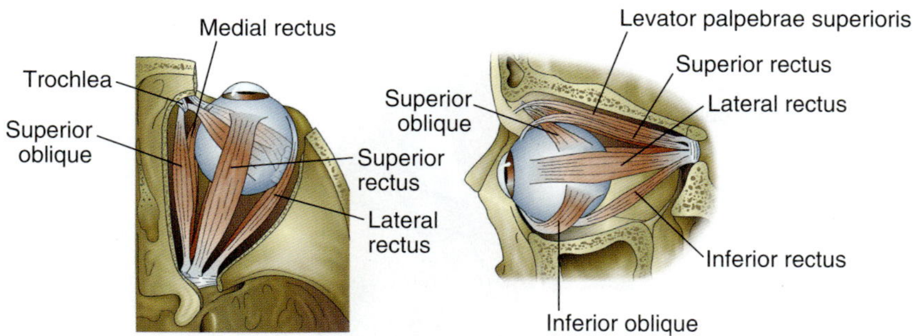

Fig. 5.26 Muscles of the orbit. Left: Superior view. Right: Lateral view.

- Intrinsic muscles: the ciliary, sphincter pupillae and dilator pupillae muscles
- Extrinsic muscles: the superior, inferior, medial and lateral recti, superior and inferior oblique and levator palpebrae superioris muscles
- The common tendinous ring is a thickening of the periosteum (periorbita) in the posterior part of the orbit around the optic canal and the central part of the superior orbital fissure. The ring is also the point of origin of the extraocular muscles (superior, inferior, lateral and medial rectus)

Blood Supply (Fig 5.27)

- An anastomosis between the internal carotid artery (ophthalmic artery) and the external carotid artery (maxillary, facial and superficial temporal arteries)
- The ophthalmic artery supplies the posterior two-thirds of the orbital part of the optic nerve
- Venous return is via the superior and inferior ophthalmic veins

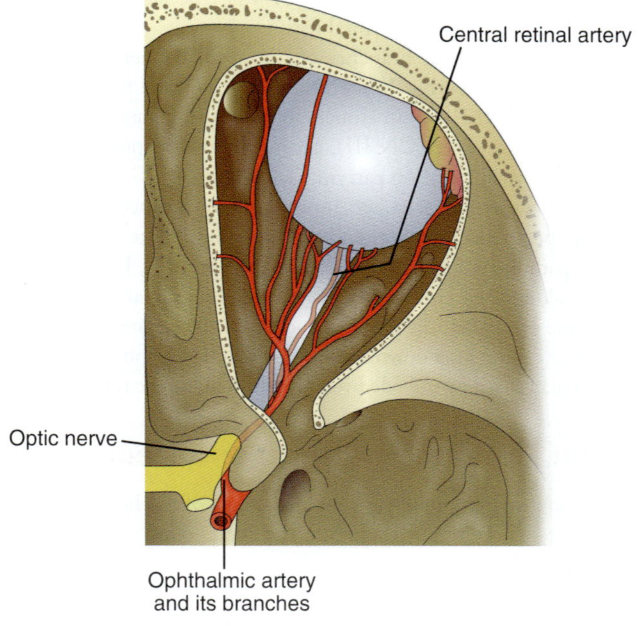

Fig. 5.27 Blood supply of the orbit.

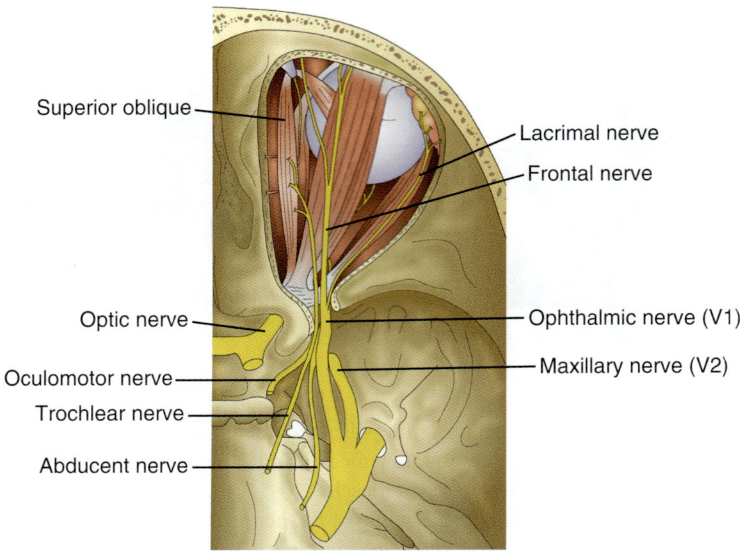

Fig. 5.28 Nerves of the orbit.

Lymph Drainage

- Via the preauricular and parotid nodes and then to the deep cervical lymph nodes

Nerve Supply (Fig 5.28)

- Numerous nerves travel into and/or through the orbit and innervate structures within the orbital cavity: the optic nerve, oculomotor nerve, trochlear nerve, abducent nerve, ophthalmic nerve (CN V1) and maxillary nerve (CN V2)
- Optic nerve is the nerve of vision (CN II) and enters the orbit through the optic canal
- Three branches of the ophthalmic nerve (CN V1) (the lacrimal, frontal and nasociliary nerves) enter through the superior orbital fissure
- The infraorbital and zygomatic branches of the maxillary nerve (CN V2) pass from the pterygopalatine fossa to the orbit through the inferior orbital fissure
- All intrinsic musles of the eye are innervated by the parasympathetic nervous system through the oculomotor nerve (CN III), except the dilator pupillae (by the sympathetics from the superior cervical ganglion carrying T1 fibres)
- All extrinsic (extraocular) muscles are innervated by the oculomotor nerve, except the lateral rectus (by the abducent nerve) and the superior oblique (by the trochlear nerve)
- Any intracranial pathology (e.g. increased intracranial pressure, head trauma, infections) may affect the nerves along their course. An increase in intracranial pressure will first affect the abducent nerve (the eye is medially deviated and cannot move laterally from midline), then the trochlear nerve (eye cannot look down and in) and finally the optic nerve (oedema of the optic disc or papilloedema caused by impeded venous return along the retinal veins)

Part 16 Lymph Drainage of Head and Neck

An overall picture of the distribution of the lymph drainage of the head and neck is summarised below and outlying nodes all eventually drain into the deep nodes.

- Named according to their positions:
  - Submental nodes lie below the chin near the midline
  - Submandibular nodes are further lateral and are below the mandible

  - Anterior cervical nodes lie along the anterior jugular vein
  - Superficial cervical nodes lie along the external jugular vein
  - Nodes may lie in the infrahyoid, prelaryngeal or pretracheal position
  - Occipital nodes lie over the upper attachment of the trapezius
  - Posterior auricular nodes lie over the upper part of the sternocleidomastoid
  - Preauricular nodes lie outside and within the parotid gland

DEEP CERVICAL NODES

- Scattered along the carotid sheath (in front and behind), largely under the sternocleidomastoid, and divided into two groups:
- Upper group:
  - Includes the jugulodigastric and jugulo-omohyoid nodes
  - Collects lymph from the back of the tongue, tonsil, ear, nose, sinuses, upper pharynx and larynx
- Lower group:
  - Constitutes the supraclavicular group
  - Collects from the face, anterior scalp, anterior tongue, lower pharynx and larynx, thyroid gland and mediastinum (and on the left side may receive lymph from the stomach)
- Widespread intercommunication
- Lymph from the lower end of the deep cervical chain is collected in the jugular lymph trunk
  - Left jugular lymph trunk drains into the thoracic duct
  - Right jugular lymph trunk drains into the right lymphatic duct or the right brachiocephalic vein

Part 17 Temporomandibular Joint

A synovial joint between the head of the mandible and the auricular fossa and auricular tubercle of the temporal bone.

- Is divided into an upper and a lower joint by a fibrocartilaginous disc attached around its periphery to the inner aspect of the joint capsule
  - Is attached anteriorly near the head of the mandible (mobile) and posteriorly near the temporal bone (immobile)
  - There is no hyaline cartilage in this joint, so it is an atypical joint
  - Anterior margin of the disc receives the upper fibres of the lateral pterygoid
  - Three extracapsular ligaments are associated with the joint: the lateral, sphenomandibular and stylomandibular ligaments
  - Movements of the mandible include depression, elevation, protrusion and retraction

Part 18 Ear (Fig 5.29)

The ear is the organ of hearing and balance. It has three parts: the external ear, the middle ear and the inner ear.

EXTERNAL EAR

- It has two parts: the auricle and the external acoustic meatus
- The auricle is on the side of the head and assists in capturing sound
- The external acoustic meatus extends between the deepest part of the concha and the tympanic membrane (about 2.5 cm). Importantly, it does not follow a straight course. The lateral third is the cartilaginous part and the medial two-thirds is the bony tunnel

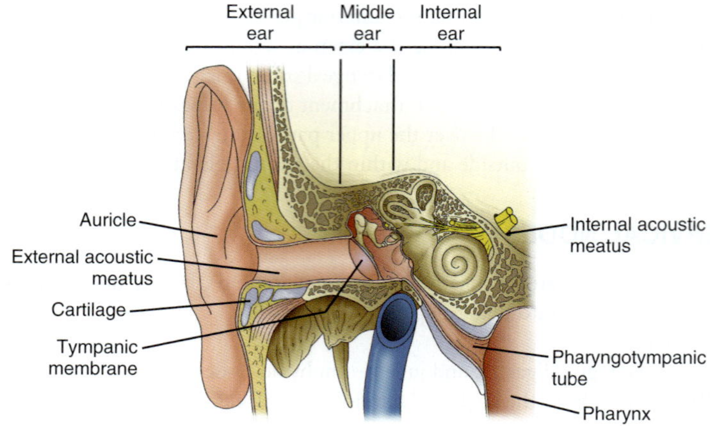

Fig. 5.29 External, middle and inner ear.

- The sensory innervation of the external ear is from different sources, and knowledge of this is clinically important (e.g. swimmer's ear):
  - Auricle: superficially by the cervical plexus, mandibular nerve (CN V3) and the deeper parts by vagus nerve (CN X) and facial nerve (CN VII)
  - External acoustic meatus: by CN V3, CN X and CN VII
  - Tympanic membrane: outer surface by CN V3, CN X, CN VII and CN IX (a small contribution) and the inner surface by CN IX

MIDDLE EAR

The middle ear is an air-filled space with two parts (the tympanic cavity and the epitympanic recess) within the temporal bone and lined by mucous membrane. Within its boundaries, it transmits structures (e.g. the chorda tympani nerve), contains structures (e.g. the ossicles) and communicates with other spaces (e.g. the nasopharynx).

BOUNDARIES AND RELATIONS

- Tegmental wall (roof): separates the middle ear from the middle cranial fossa
- Jugular wall (floor): separates the middle ear from the internal jugular vein. On its medial border, a branch of the glossopharyngeal nerve (CN IX) enters the middle ear to join the tympanic plexus
- Membranous wall (lateral wall): separates the middle ear from the epitympanic recess and almost entirely consists of the tympanic membrane, except the upper part
- Mastoid wall (posterior wall): separates the middle ear from the mastoid air cells inferiorly and continues superiorly to the mastoid antrum via the aditus. The posterior wall is partially complete. Importantly, the tendon of the stapedius muscle and a branch of the facial nerve (CN VII) (chorda tympani nerve) enter the middle ear through the posterior wall
- Carotid wall (anterior wall): separates the middle ear from the internal carotid artery inferiorly. The pharyngotympanic tube and tensor tympani muscle enter the middle ear superiorly. The anterior wall is also partially complete. Importantly, branches from the internal carotid plexus (caroticotympanic nerves) enter the middle ear, and the chorda tympani nerve exits through the inferior part of the anterior wall

- Labyrinthine wall (medial wall): separates the middle ear from the lateral wall of the inner ear and is associated with the promontory (bulging of wall due to cochlea) covered by the mucous membrane containing the tympanic plexus (formed by the glossopharyngeal nerve (CN IX) and the caroticotympanic nerves), the oval and round windows and the lesser petrosal nerve (a branch of the tympanic plexus). The lesser petrosal nerve leaves the middle ear, runs along the middle cranial fossa and exits it to reach the otic ganglion, carrying preganglionic parasympathetic fibres

Contents

- Auditory ossicles: the malleus, incus and stapes
- Muscles associated with the ossicles: the tensor tympani and stapedius
- Chorda tympani nerve
- Tympanic nerve plexus: the tympanic branch of the glossopharyngeal nerve and caroticotympanic nerves of the internal carotid plexus

Blood Supply

- Its major blood supply comes from two large branches: the tympanic branch of the maxillary artery and the mastoid branch of the occipital or posterior auricular arteries
- Its venous drainage is via the pterygoid plexus of veins and superior petrosal sinus

Lymph Drainage

- Drains to the parotid, retropharyngeal and deep cervical nodes

Nerve Supply

- Innervated by the tympanic plexus
- Understanding the contents and relations of the middle ear is important for clinical practice. For instance, the chorda tympani nerve is most often injured during middle-ear surgery (e.g. otosclerosis) and leaves 20% of patients with changes in taste and dryness of the mouth. Numerous factors influence whether injury to the chorda tympani causes symptoms, including anatomical variables

Parts 19 and 20 Vertebral Column and Osteology of Vertebrae

The vertebral column is made up of five parts: the cervical, thoracic, lumbar, sacral and coccygeal vertebrae.

- In the fetus, the column lies flexed along its whole length like the letter C. After birth, secondary curvatures (lordosis) develop in the cervical and lumbar regions

CHARACTERISTICS OF VERTEBRAE (Fig 5.30)

- Ventral body and dorsal (neural) arch enclosing the vertebral foramen
  - Arch gives off spinous process and transverse processes
  - At the back of the sides of the body are the superior and inferior articular facets
    - Between the body and the transverse processes are the pedicles, and between the transverse processes and the spinous process are the laminae
    - Pedicles are shorter than the body, to allow for transmission of the spinal nerves through the intervertebral foramen
    - At the root of the transverse processes are the superior and inferior articular processes

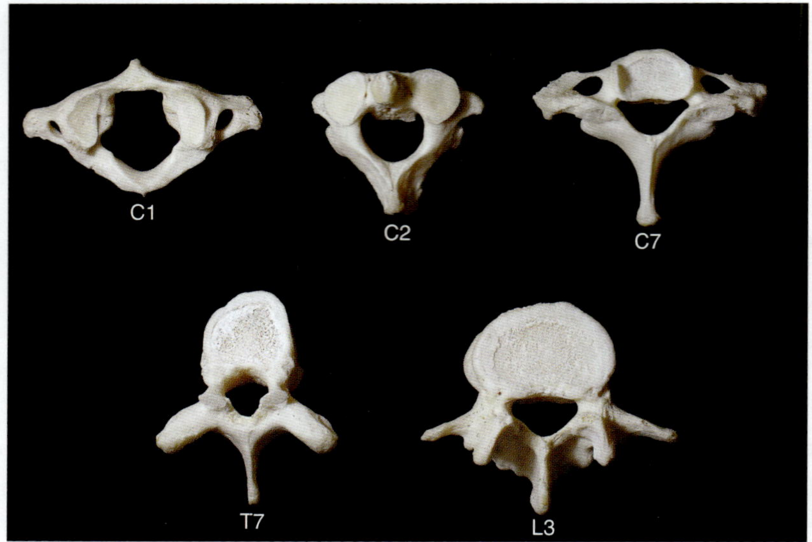

Fig. 5.30 Characteristics of vertebrae (upper row: C1, C2, C7; lower row: T7 and L3).

- **Typical cervical vertebrae** (Fig 5.31C)
  - Vertebral body is short in height, square-shaped when viewed from above and has a concave superior surface and a convex inferior surface
  - Each transverse process is trough-shaped and perforated by a round foramen transversarium
  - Spinous process is short and bifid
  - Vertebral canal is triangular

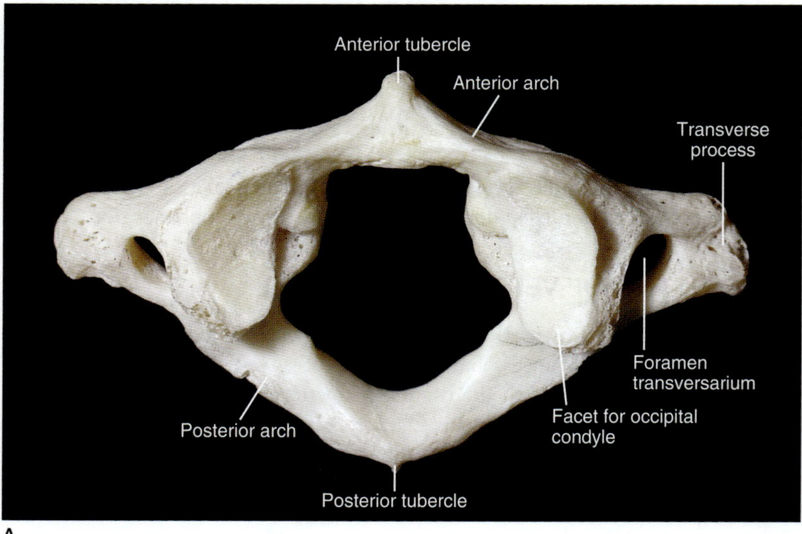

Fig. 5.31 **(A)** First cervical vertebra.

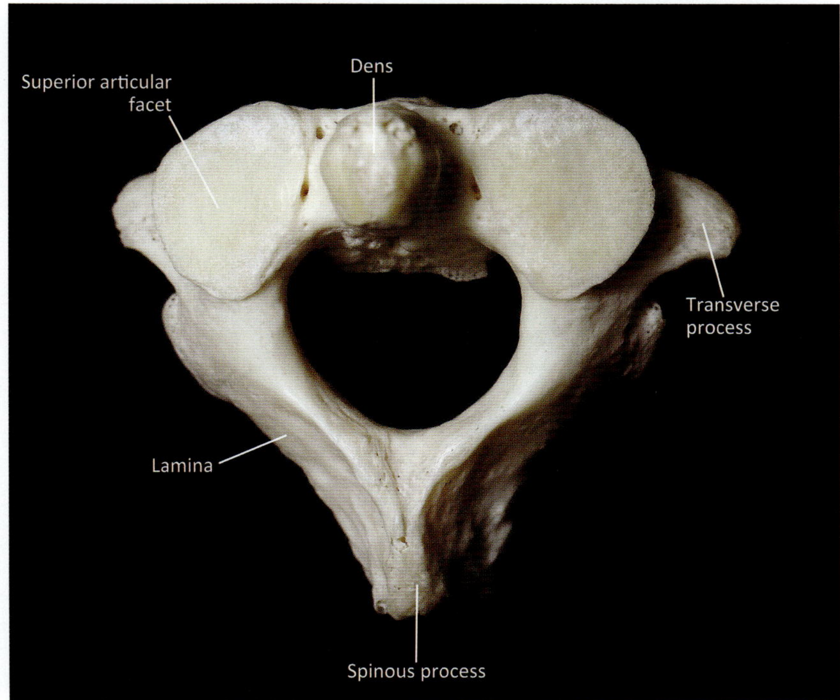

B

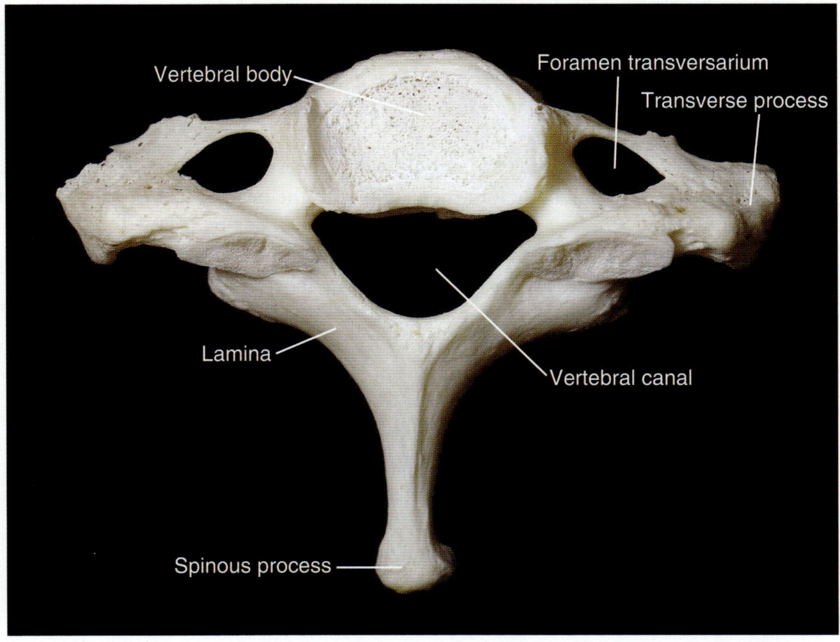

C

Fig. 5.31, cont'd **(B)** Second cervical vertebra. **(C)** Typical cervical vertebra (C7).

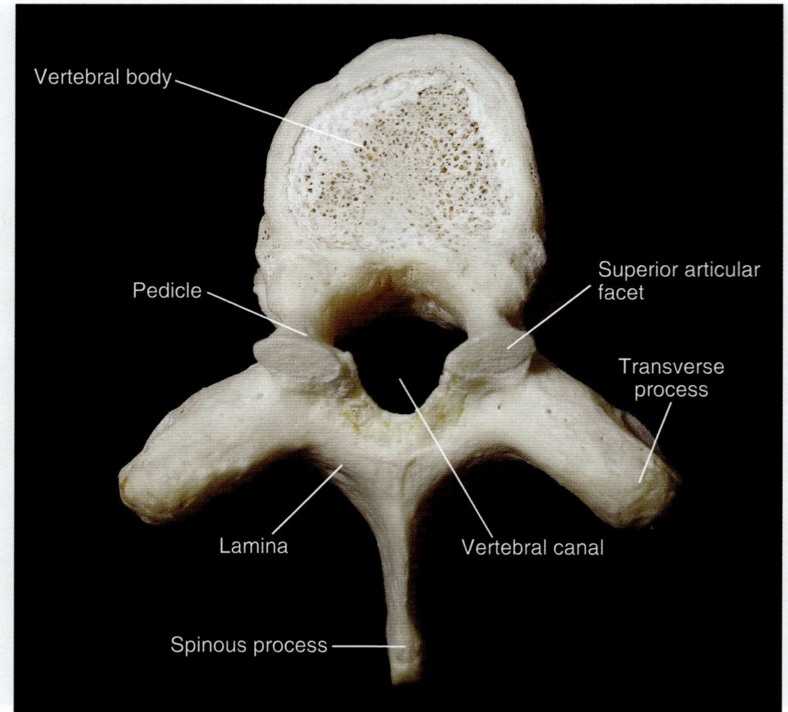

Fig. 5.32 Typical thoracic vertebra (T7).

  - First and second cervical vertebrae (the atlas and the axis) are specialised to ease movement of the head
  - Cervical rib is formed by elongation of the costal element of C7
- **Typical thoracic vertebrae** (Fig 5.32)
  - Typical thoracic vertebra has two partial facets (superior and inferior costal facets) on each side of the vertebral body for articulation with the head of its own rib and the head of the rib below
  - Each transverse process has a facet for articulation with the tubercle of its own rib
  - Vertebral body is heart-shaped when viewed from above
  - Vertebral canal is circular
- **Typical lumbar vertebrae** (Fig 5.33)
  - Characterised by their large size
  - No facets for articulation with ribs
  - Transverse processes are generally thin and long
  - Vertebral body is cylindrical
  - Vertebral canal is triangular in shape and larger than the thoracic vertebrae
- The **sacrum** is a single bone that represents the five fused sacral vertebrae
  - Two large L-shaped facets for articulation with the pelvis

VERTEBRAL JOINTS

- Joints between the bodies comprise the intervertebral discs with associated anterior and posterior longitudinal ligaments
  - Each intervertebral disc is a secondary cartilaginous joint or symphysis

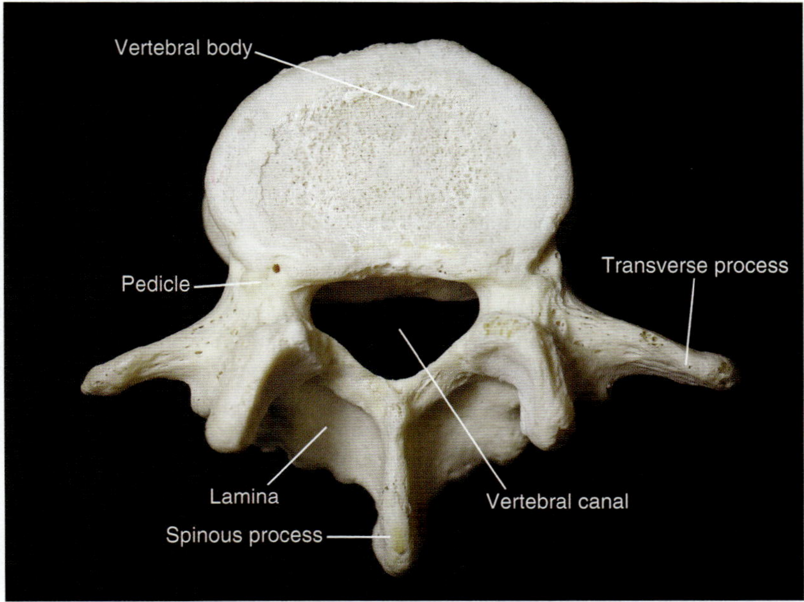

Fig. 5.33 Typical lumbar vertebra (L3).

- Upper and lower surfaces of the vertebral body are covered completely by a thin plate of hyaline cartilage
- Annulus fibrosus is a peripheral ring of concentric layers with alternating perpendicular fibres uniting discs
  - Inside is the nucleus pulposus (from the embryonic notochord)
- Paracentral or foraminal disc herniation typically affects the nerve emerging *below* the disc space
  - For example: a herniated L4/5 disc will press on the L5 nerve root
  - A central disc herniation is potentially more serious because the protrusion occurs directly posteriorly. In the lower lumbar region, this presses on the cauda equina nerve root and results in bladder and bowl dysfunction as well as nerve root pain
- Anterior longitudinal ligament extends from the anterior tubercle of the atlas to the front of the upper part of the sacrum
- Posterior longitudinal ligament extends from the back of the atlas to the sacral canal

- Joints between the arches (zygapophyseal joints)
  - Facet joints are synovial joints
    - Nerve supply: From the nerve of and the nerve above the segment
  - Ligamentum flava are yellow (elastic) and join the contiguous borders of adjacent laminae
    - Extend from the front of the upper laminae to the back of the lower lamina
  - Supraspinous ligament joins the tips of the adjacent spinous processes (e.g. ligamentum nuchae in the neck)
  - Interspinous ligaments unite the spinous processes in the lumbar region
  - Intertransverse ligaments are similar weak sheets joining the transverse processes
- Canal of the vertebral column narrows from above downwards and is closed on all sides apart from at the intervertebral foramina
  - Intervertebral foramina house the spinal nerves and posterior root ganglia, and give passage to arteries and veins

MOVEMENTS

- Flexion, extension and abduction (lateral flexion) are possible in the cervical, thoracic and lumbar regions
- The degree of movement varies between the three regions (cervical, thoracic and lumbar regions)
- Head movements occur at the atlanto-occipital and atlantoaxial joints
- Thoracic region – articular facets lie on the circumference of a circle allowing greater degree of rotation
- Cervical region – articular facets have a similar slope to thoracic vertebrae but are not on a circular arc; therefore, there is limited rotation and abduction occurs with some rotation
- Atlas lacks a vertebral body and, as a result, there is no intervertebral disc between C1 and C2. It is ring-shaped and composed of two lateral masses interconnected by an anterior arch and posterior arch
- Axis is characterised by the dens and a large spinous process
  - Dens carries no weight and weight is transmitted through the lateral masses
  - Bifid spinous process is very large (muscular attachments)
  - Rotation takes places at the atlantoaxial joint
- Lumbar region – articular facets lie in the anteroposterior direction and this limits rotation
- Vertebrae and longitudinal muscles are supplied by segmental arteries
- Venous drainage is via the internal venous plexus and external venous plexus

SPINAL CORD

The spinal cord extends from the foramen magnum to approximately the level of the disc between L1/L2 in adults (varies between T12 and L3) but is longer in neonates (L3/L4). The distal part of the spinal cord is cone-shaped (conus medullaris) and a fine filament of connective tissue (filum terminale) continues inferiorly from the tip of the conus medullaris. Also, the terminal cluster of the posterior and anterior roots of the lumbar, sacral and coccygeal nerves (cauda equina) runs inferiorly to reach their exit points from the vertebral canal.

- The spinal cord is not uniform in diameter and it has two enlargements associated with the origin of the spinal nerves, which innervate the upper (C5–T1) and lower limbs (L1–S3)
- Its external surface has a number of fissures (anterior and posterior median fissures) and sulci (posterolateral sulci)
- Blood supply comes from two sources: longitudinally oriented vessels (a single anterior spinal and two posterior spinal arteries originating from the vertebral arteries) and segmental spinal arteries (originating from the vertebral and deep cervical arteries in the neck, the posterior intercostal arteries in the thorax and the lumbar arteries in the abdomen)
  - The anterior and posterior spinal arteries are reinforced along their length by several segmental arteries, the largest of which is called '*the artery of Adamkiewicz*'. The artery of Adamkiewicz arises in the lower thoracic or upper lumbar region (usually on the left side)

Part 21 Cranial Cavity and Meninges (Figs 5.34–5.36)

CRANIUM

The cranium is formed by the articulation of 22 bones attached to each other by sutures (except the mandible). The cranium can be subdivided into the upper domed part (calvaria), the base of the skull and the facial skeleton (viscerocranium).

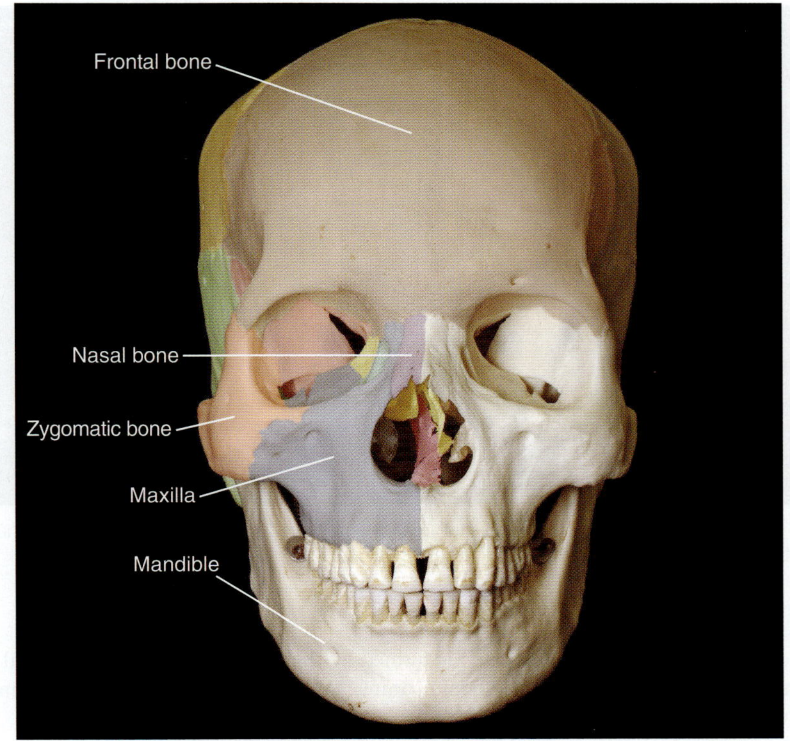

Fig. 5.34 Cranium, anterior view.

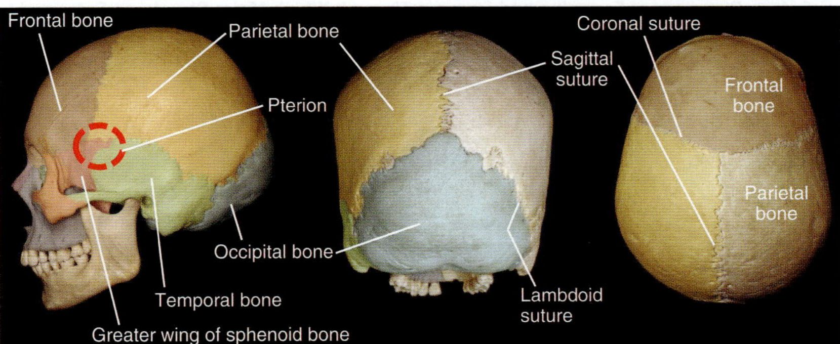

Fig. 5.35 Cranium. Left: Lateral view. Middle: Posterior view. Right: Superior view.

- Calvaria is formed by the paired temporal and parietal bones and the unpaired frontal, sphenoid and occipital bones
- Floor of the cranial cavity is divided into the anterior, middle and posterior cranial fossae and is formed by the frontal, ethmoid, sphenoid, temporal, parietal and occipital bones

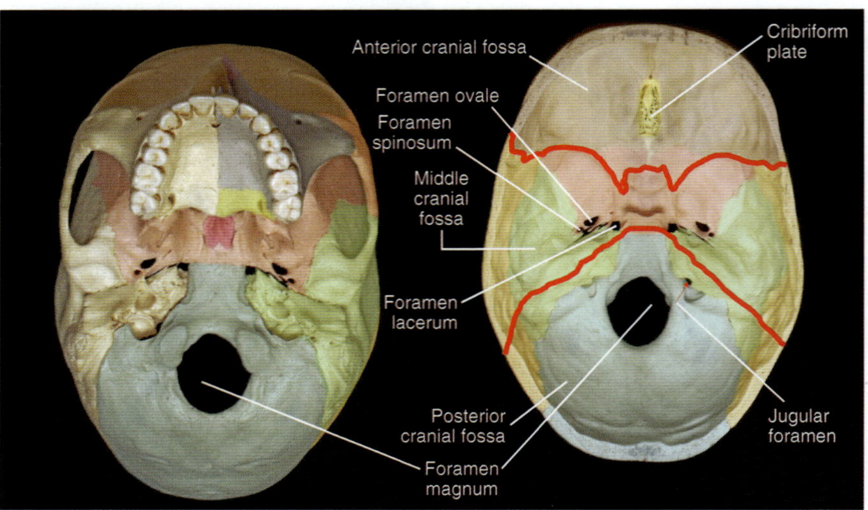

Fig. 5.36 Cranium. Left: Inferior view of the skull (mandible removed). Right: View of the floor of the cranial vault (anterior, middle and posterior cranial fossae).

- Roof of the cranial cavity (calvaria) is formed by the frontal, parietal and occipital bones, and the coronal, sagittal and lambdoid sutures are visible internally, as is the frontal crest (attachment for the falx cerebri)
- There are several foramina and fissures through which major structures enter and leave the cranial cavity, as listed in the table below

TABLE 5.4 ■ **Summary of Foramina and Fissures Through Which Major Structures Enter and Leave the Cranial Cavity**

	Foramen or Opening	**Contents**
Anterior Cranial Fossa	Cribriform plate	Olfactory nerves (CN I)
Middle Cranial Fossa	Optic canal	Optic nerve (CN II) Ophthalmic artery
	Superior orbital fissure	Ophthalmic division of trigeminal nerve (CN V1) Oculomotor nerve (CN III) Trochlear nerve (CN IV) Abducent nerve (CN VI) Superior ophthalmic vein
	Foramen lacerum	(Filled with cartilage during life)
	Foramen rotundum	Maxillary division of trigeminal nerve (CN V2)
	Foramen ovale	Mandibular division of trigeminal nerve (CN V3) Accessory meningeal artery
	Carotid canal	Internal carotid artery
	Foramen spinosum	Middle meningeal artery

TABLE 5.4 ■ **Summary of Foramina and Fissures Through Which Major Structures Enter and Leave the Cranial Cavity** (Continued)

	Foramen or Opening	Contents
Posterior Cranial Fossa	Jugular foramen	Glossopharyngeal nerve (CN IX) Vagus nerve (CN X) Accessory nerve (CN XI) Internal jugular vein
	Internal acoustic meatus	Facial nerve (CN VII) Vestibulocochlear nerve (CN VIII) Labrynnthine artery and vein
	Foramen magnum	Spinal cord Vertebral arteries Roots of accessory nerve pass from the upper region of the spinal cord through the foramen magnum into the cranial cavity and then leave the cranial cavity through the jugular foramen
	Hypoglossal canal	Hypoglossal nerve (CN XII)

CRANIAL MENINGES AND LAYERS

The brain is surrounded by three layers of membranes (the meninges): the dura mater (outer and inner layers), the arachnoid mater and the pia mater.

- **Dura mater**
  - The outer periosteal layer is firmly attached to the skull
  - The inner meningeal layer is in close contact with the arachnoid mater and is continuous with the spinal dura mater through the foramen magnum
  - The two layers of dura separate from each other at numerous locations to form two unique types of structures: intracranial venous structures and dural partitions
- The **arachnoid mater** is a thin, avascular membrane that lines the inner surface of the dura mater. It does not enter the grooves or fissures of the brain, except for the longitudinal fissure between the two cerebral hemispheres
- The **pia mater** is a thin membrane which invests the surface of the brain

BLOOD SUPPLY

Arteries to the dura mater travel in the outer periosteal layer of the dura. These are the anterior meningeal artery, the middle meningeal artery, the accessory meningeal artery and the posterior meningeal artery. All are small arteries except the middle meningeal artery, which supplies the greatest part of the dura. The middle cranial fossa is supplied by the middle meningeal and accessory meningeal arteries. The middle meningeal artery enters the skull through the foramen spinosum and divides into anterior and posterior branches. The anterior branch crosses the pterion (a weak H-shaped junction of sutures about 3 cm above the centre of the zygomatic arch). The accessory meningeal artery enters the middle cranial fossa through the foramen ovale.

NERVE SUPPLY

The dura mater is innervated by cranial nerves V1, V2, V3, X and the first, second and sometimes the third cervical nerves (possible contributions from IX and XII in the posterior cranial fossa have been reported).

VENOUS DRAINAGE OF BRAIN

This begins internally as networks of small venous channels draining to larger veins, and the larger veins drain into dural venous sinuses and eventually to the internal jugular veins. Other veins that also empty into the dural venous sinuses are the diploic veins (these run between the internal and external tables of compact bone) and the emissary veins (these run between the outside of the cranial cavity and the dural venous sinuses).

- The emissary veins are important clinically because they can be a passage for infections to enter the cranial cavity
- Dural venous sinuses include the sigmoid, superior sagittal, inferior sagittal, straight, transverse and occipital sinuses, the confluence of sinuses, and the cavernous, sphenoparietal, inferior and superior petrosal and basilar sinuses

Cavernous Sinus

Cavernous sinuses are part of venous drainage of the brain which receive blood not only from the cerebral veins but also from the ophthalmic vein (from the orbit) and emissary veins (from the pterygoid plexus). These connections provide passways for infection into the skull. Six paired structures, which run in the cavernous sinus or within its lateral wall, are vulnerable to injury due to inflammation; they include the internal carotid artery, the oculomotor nerve (CN III), the trochlear nerve (IV), the ophthalmic division of the trigeminal nerve (CN V1), the maxillary division of the trigeminal nerve (CN V2) and the abducent nerve (CN VI).

DURAL PARTITIONS

The dural partitions formed by the dura mater project inwards and incompletely subdivide the cranial cavity. The dural partitions are named: the falx cerebri, the falx cerebelli, the tentorium cerebelli and the diaphragma sellae.

INTRACRANIAL HAEMORRHAGE

Intracranial haemorrhage can be a result of aneurysm rupture, hypertension, bleeding after cerebral infarction or trauma. Three types of intracranial haemorrage are:

- An **extradural haemorrhage** (epidural haemorrhage), which is arterial in origin, and is classically from a torn branch of the middle meningeal artery in the temporoparietal region. It is almost always associated with a skull fracture. The blood collects between the calvarium and the outer periosteal layer of the dura mater
- A **subdural haemorrhage**, which forms within the layers of the dura mater. Relatively little force is required to expand this space. Damage to cerebral veins that cross this space from the brain to the superior sagittal sinus can cause this bleeding, particularly in individuals with cerebral atrophy or on anticoagulants. Chronic subdural haemorrhage is most common, but an acute bleed may follow high-velocity trauma.
- A **subarachnoid haemorrhage**, which is bleeding into the subarachnoid space. It is usually arterial bleeding from a ruptured cerebral artery aneurysm of the circle of Willis. A subarachnoid haemorrhage may also be associated with an intracerebral bleed. It causes a sudden severe headache, vomiting and frequently loss of consciousness.

Page numbers followed by *f* indicates figures and *t* indicates tables.